Metastases to the Central Nervous System

Editors

EDJAH K. NDUOM
JEFFREY J. OLSON

NEUROSURGERY
CLINICS OF NORTH AMERICA

www.neurosurgery.theclinics.com

Consulting Editors
RUSSELL R. LONSER
DANIEL K. RESNICK

October 2020 • Volume 31 • Number 4

ELSEVIER

1600 John F. Kennedy Boulevard • Suite 1800 • Philadelphia, Pennsylvania, 19103-2899

http://www.theclinics.com

NEUROSURGERY CLINICS OF NORTH AMERICA Volume 31, Number 4
October 2020 ISSN 1042-3680, ISBN-13: 978-0-323-76192-5

Editor: Stacy Eastman
Developmental Editor: Laura Fisher

Neurosurgery Clinics of North America (ISSN 1042-3680) is published quarterly by Elsevier Inc., 360 Park Avenue South, New York, NY 10010-1710. Months of issue are January, April, July, and October. Business and Editorial Offices: 1600 John F. Kennedy Blvd., Suite 1800, Philadelphia, PA 19103-2899. Customer Service Office: 11830 Westline Industrial Drive, St. Louis, MO 63146. Periodicals postage paid at New York, NY, and additional mailing offices. Subscription prices are $434.00 per year (US individuals), $785.00 per year (US institutions), $470.00 per year (Canadian individuals), $974.00 per year (Canadian institutions), $534.00 per year (international individuals), $974.00 per year (international institutions), $100.00 per year (US students), $255.00 per year (international students), and $100.00 per year (Canadian students). International air speed delivery is included in all *Clinics* subscription prices. All prices are subject to change without notice. **POSTMASTER:** Send address changes to *Neurosurgery Clinics of North America*, Elsevier Periodicals Customer Service, 11830 Westline Industrial Drive, St. Louis, MO 63146. **Customer Service: 1-800-654-2452 (US and Canada). From outside the US and Canada, call: 1-314-453-7041. Fax: 1-314-453-5170. E-mail: JournalsCustomerService-usa@elsevier.com (for print support) and journalsonline-support-usa@elsevier.com (for online support).**

Reprints. For copies of 100 or more, of articles in this publication, please contact the Commercial Reprints Department, Elsevier Inc., 360 Park Avenue South, New York, NY 10010-1710. Tel. 212-633-3874; Fax: 212-633-3820; E-mail: reprints@elsevier.com.

Neurosurgery Clinics of North America is covered in *MEDLINE/PubMed (Index Medicus), EMBASE/Excerpta Medica, and Current Contents/Clinical Medicine (CC/CM).*

Printed in the United States of America.

Contributors

CONSULTING EDITORS

DANIEL K. RESNICK, MD, MS
Professor and Vice Chairman, Program
Director, Department of Neurosurgery,
University of Wisconsin-Madison School of
Medicine and Public Health, Madison,
Wisconsin, USA

RUSSELL R. LONSER, MD
Professor and Chair, Department of
Neurological Surgery, The Ohio State
University Wexner Medical Center, Columbus,
Ohio, USA

EDITORS

EDJAH K. NDUOM, MD
Assistant Clinical Investigator, Surgical
Neurology Branch, National Institutes of
Neurological Disorders and Stroke, National
Institutes of Health, Bethesda, Maryland, USA

JEFFREY J. OLSON, MD
Professor, Departments of Hematology,
Medical Oncology, and Neurosurgery,

Director, Neurosurgical Oncology Fellowship,
Emory University School of Medicine, Director,
Clinically Related Neuro-Oncology Laboratory,
Co-Director, Brain Tumor Program, Winship
Cancer Institute of Emory University, Atlanta,
Georgia, USA

AUTHORS

THIAGO ALBONETTE-FELICIO, MD
Fellow, Department of Neurological Surgery,
The Ohio State University Wexner Medical
Center, Columbus, Ohio, USA

CHRISTOPHER ALVAREZ-BRECKENRIDGE
Department of Neurosurgery, Massachusetts
General Hospital, Harvard Medical School,
Boston, Massachusetts, USA

KATHERINE BERRY, MD
Department of Neurosurgery, University of
Miami Miller School of Medicine, Department
of Neurological Surgery, University of Miami/
Jackson Health System, Lois Pope Life Center,
Miami, Florida, USA

HRIDAY P. BHAMBHVANI, BS
Medical Student, Department of Neurosurgery,
Stanford University Medical Center, Stanford,
California, USA

DUKAGJIN M. BLAKAJ, MD, PhD
Department of Radiation Oncology, The Ohio
State University Wexner Medical Center, The
James Cancer Hospital and Solove Research
Institute, Columbus, Ohio, USA

ORIN BLOCH, MD
Associate Professor, Department of
Neurological Surgery, University of
California, Davis School of Medicine,
University of California, Davis, Sacramento,
California, USA

PRISCILLA K. BRASTIANOS
Department of Medical Oncology, Dana-Farber
Cancer Institute, Boston, Massachusetts, USA

RICARDO L. CARRAU, MD
Professor, Departments of Neurological
Surgery and Otolaryngology–Head and Neck
Surgery, The Ohio State University Wexner
Medical Center, Columbus, Ohio, USA

LOLA B. CHAMBLESS, MD
Department of Neurological Surgery, Vanderbilt University Medical Center, Nashville, Tennessee, USA

BRYAN D. CHOI, MD, PhD
Resident, Department of Neurosurgery, Massachusetts General Hospital, Harvard Medical School, Boston, Massachusetts, USA

POOJA DAVE, BS
Medical Student, The GW School of Medicine & Health Sciences, Washington, DC, USA

KHALED DIBS, MD
Department of Radiation Oncology, The Ohio State University Wexner Medical Center, The James Cancer Hospital and Solove Research Institute, Columbus, Ohio, USA

NIKOLAS ECHEVERRY, BS
Florida Atlantic University Charles E. Schmidt College of Medicine, Boca Raton, Florida, USA

DANIEL G. EICHBERG, MD
Department of Neurosurgery, University of Miami Miller School of Medicine, Department of Neurological Surgery, University of Miami/Jackson Health System, Lois Pope Life Center, Miami, Florida, USA

J. BRADLEY ELDER, MD
Department of Neurological Surgery, The Ohio State University Wexner Medical Center, Columbus, Ohio, USA

SHERISE D. FERGUSON, MD
Assistant Professor, Department of Neurosurgery, The University of Texas MD Anderson Cancer Center, Houston, Texas, USA

CHASE H. FOSTER, MD, MS
Resident, Department of Neurological Surgery, George Washington University Hospital, Washington, DC, USA

MELANIE HAYDEN GEPHART, MD, MAS
Associate Professor of Neurosurgery, Department of Neurosurgery, Stanford University Medical Center, Stanford, California, USA; Department of Neurosurgery, Associate Professor of Neurosurgery, Co-Director, Brain Tumor Center, Stanford University School of Medicine, Palo Alto, California, USA

NISHA GIRIDHARAN, MD
Resident, Department of Neurosurgery, The University of Texas MD Anderson Cancer Center, Houston, Texas, USA

ISABELLA C. GLITZA OLIVA, MD, PhD
Assistant Professor, Department of Melanoma Medical Oncology, The University of Texas MD Anderson Cancer Center, Houston, Texas, USA

ADEN HASKELL-MENDOZA, MS
Department of Neurological Surgery, University of California, Davis, Sacramento, California, USA

AMY B. HEIMBERGER, MD
Professor, Department of Neurosurgery, The University of Texas MD Anderson Cancer Center, Houston, Texas, USA

MICHAEL IVAN, MD
Department of Neurosurgery, University of Miami Miller School of Medicine, Department of Neurological Surgery, University of Miami/Jackson Health System, Lois Pope Life Center, Sylvester Comprehensive Cancer Center, University of Miami Health System, Miami, Florida, USA

WILLIAM JIANG, BS
Department of Radiation Oncology, The Ohio State University Wexner Medical Center, The James Cancer Hospital and Solove Research Institute, Columbus, Ohio, USA

PAMELA S. JONES, MD, MS, MPH
Assistant Professor, Department of Neurosurgery, Massachusetts General Hospital, Harvard Medical School, Boston, Massachusetts, USA

MICHAEL KADER, MD
Department of Neurosurgery, University of Miami Miller School of Medicine, Department of Neurological Surgery, University of Miami/Jackson Health System, Lois Pope Life Center, Miami, Florida, USA

PATRICK D. KELLY, MD
Department of Neurological Surgery, Vanderbilt University Medical Center, Nashville, Tennessee, USA

RICARDO KOMOTAR, MD
Department of Neurosurgery, University of Miami Miller School of Medicine, Department of Neurological Surgery, University of Miami/Jackson Health System, Lois Pope Life Center, Sylvester Comprehensive Cancer Center, University of Miami Health System, Miami, Floida, USA

DENNIS LEE, MS
Department of Neurological Surgery, University of California, Davis, Sacramento, California, USA

JAMES K.C. LIU, MD
Neurosurgical Oncology, Department of Neuro-Oncology, H. Lee Moffitt Cancer Center and Research Institute, Tampa, Florida, USA

KEVIN LIU, BS
Department of Radiation Oncology, The Ohio State University Wexner Medical Center, The James Cancer Hospital and Solove Research Institute, Columbus, Ohio, USA

EVAN LUTHER, MD
Department of Neurosurgery, University of Miami Miller School of Medicine, Department of Neurological Surgery, University of Miami/Jackson Health System, Lois Pope Life Center, Miami, Florida, USA

SAMUEL MANSOUR, BS
Florida Atlantic University Charles E. Schmidt College of Medicine, Boca Raton, Florida, USA

MALIA B. McAVOY, BS, MS
Resident, Department of Neurosurgery, University of Washington Medical Center, Seattle, Washington, USA

DAVID McCARTHY, MSc
Department of Neurosurgery, University of Miami Miller School of Medicine, Department of Neurological Surgery, University of Miami/Jackson Health System, Lois Pope Life Center, Miami, Florida, USA

GAUTAM U. MEHTA, MD
Division of Neurosurgery, House Clinic, Los Angeles, California, USA

MEREDITH A. MONSOUR, BS
Vanderbilt University School of Medicine, Nashville, Tennessee, USA

NELSON S. MOSS, MD
Assistant Attending, Department of Neurosurgery and Brain Metastasis Center, Memorial Sloan Kettering Cancer Center, New York, New York, USA

AHMED NADA, MD
Department of Neurosurgery, University of Miami Miller School of Medicine, Department of Neurological Surgery, University of Miami/Jackson Health System, Lois Pope Life Center, Miami, Florida, USA

BRIAN V. NAHED
Departments of Neurosurgery and Neurology, Massachusetts General Hospital, Harvard Medical School, Boston, Massachusetts, USA

BARBARA J. O'BRIEN, MD
Assistant Professor, Department of Neuro-Oncology, The University of Texas MD Anderson Cancer Center, Houston, Texas, USA

KEVIN OH
Department of Radiation Oncology, Massachusetts General Hospital, Boston, Massachusetts, USA

JOSHUA PALMER, MD
Department of Radiation Oncology, The Ohio State University Wexner Medical Center, The James Cancer Hospital and Solove Research Institute, Columbus, Ohio, USA

BRITTANY C. PARKER KERRIGAN, PhD
Scientific Manager, Department of Neurosurgery, The University of Texas MD Anderson Cancer Center, Houston, Texas, USA

ANKUR R. PATEL, MD
Fellow, Department of Neurosurgery and Brain Metastasis Center, Memorial Sloan Kettering Cancer Center, New York, New York, USA

HALEY K. PERLOW, MD
Department of Radiation Oncology, The James Cancer Hospital, The Ohio State University Wexner Medical Center, Columbus, Ohio, USA

DANIEL M. PREVEDELLO, MD
Professor, Departments of Neurological Surgery and Otolaryngology–Head and Neck Surgery, The Ohio State University Wexner Medical Center, Columbus, Ohio, USA

MARYAM RAHMAN, MD, MS, FAANS
Lillian S. Wells Department of Neurosurgery,
University of Florida, Gainesville, Florida, USA

PRAJWAL RAJAPPA, MD, MS
Department of Radiation Oncology, The
James Cancer Hospital, The Ohio State
University Wexner Medical Center,
Departments of Neurologic Surgery and
Pediatrics, Nationwide Children's Hospital,
Columbus, Ohio, USA

RAJU R. RAVAL, MD, DPhil
Department of Radiation Oncology, The Ohio
State University Wexner Medical Center, The
James Cancer Hospital and Solove Research
Institute, Columbus, Ohio, USA

ABHIK RAY-CHAUDHURY, MD, MBBS
Surgical Neurology Branch, National Cancer
Institute, Bethesda, Maryland, USA

SHAAN M. RAZA, MD
Department of Neurosurgery, The University of
Texas M.D. Anderson Cancer Center, Houston,
Texas, USA

ROBERT A. RIESTENBERG, BS
Department of Neurological Surgery, University
of California, Davis, Sacramento, California, USA

ADRIAN J. RODRIGUES, BS
Medical Student, Department of Neurosurgery,
Stanford University Medical Center, Stanford,
California, USA

PATRICIA SACKS, BS
Lillian S. Wells Department of Neurosurgery,
University of Florida, Gainesville, Florida, USA

ASHISH SHAH, MD
Department of Neurosurgery, University of
Miami Miller School of Medicine, Department
of Neurological Surgery, University of Miami/
Jackson Health System, Lois Pope Life Center,
Miami, Florida, USA

MOSTAFA SHAHEIN, MD, MS
Fellow, Department of Neurological Surgery,
The Ohio State University Wexner Medical
Center, Columbus, Ohio, USA; Assistant
Lecturer, Department of Neurological Surgery,
Aswan University, Egypt

**JONATHAN H. SHERMAN, MD, FAANS,
FACS**
Associate Professor of Neurosurgery and
Director of Surgical Neuro-Oncology, West
Virginia University, Eastern Division,
Martinsburg, West Virginia, USA

HELEN SHIH
Department of Radiation Oncology,
Massachusetts General Hospital, Boston,
Massachusetts, USA

CLARA KWON STARKWEATHER
Department of Neurosurgery, Massachusetts
General Hospital, Harvard Medical School,
Boston, Massachusetts, USA

SABER TADROS, MD
Laboratory of Pathology, National Cancer
Institute, Bethesda, Maryland, USA

MAXINE C. UMEH-GARCIA, PhD, MSc
Postdoctoral scholar, Department of
Neurosurgery, Stanford University Medical
Center, Stanford, California, USA

JOSHUA L. WANG, MD
Department of Neurological Surgery, The Ohio
State University Wexner Medical Center,
Columbus, Ohio, USA

NANCY WANG
Department of Radiation Oncology,
Massachusetts General Hospital, Boston,
Massachusetts, USA

KENNY K.H. YU, MBBS, PhD
Fellow, Department of Neurosurgery and Brain
Metastasis Center, Memorial Sloan Kettering
Cancer Center, New York, New York, USA

Contents

Brain metastasis continues to be a devastating complication of systemic malignancy, affecting approximately 20% of all patients suffering from cancer. Despite being a major source of morbidity and mortality for this patient population, a nationwide, systematic mechanism for reporting of brain metastases does not exist. Better understanding the epidemiology of brain metastases will help identify individuals who are at greatest risk of developing them and guide clinicians in selecting patients who are most likely to benefit from brain metastasis surveillance and prophylaxis.

Solitary brain metastasis is defined by a single metastatic brain lesion as the only site of metastasis. The initial approach to this condition consists of radiographical evaluation to establish diagnosis, followed by assessment of functional and prognostic status. Neurologic symptom management consists of using dexamethasone and antiepileptic medications. Treatment consists of a combination of surgical and radiation therapy. Surgical treatment is indicated where there is a need for tissue diagnosis or immediate alleviation of neurologic symptoms and mass effect. Stereotactic radiosurgery has become an effective treatment modality. Whole-brain radiation therapy may have a role as an adjunctive therapy.

Brain metastases are the most common intracranial tumor in adults, with increasing incidence owing to prolonged survival times. Roughly half of patients diagnosed with new brain metastases have greater than 1 brain metastasis at the time of diagnosis, raising the question of how to optimize patient care with multiple brain metastases. The authors review studies relevant to the care of patients with brain metastasis, with emphasis on those relevant to the care of patients with multiple brain metastases. They discuss evolving strategies involving multiple modalities and the benefit of surgical management in patients with a large symptomatic brain metastasis.

Brain metastases (BrM) affect up to 20% of patients with cancer and represent an increasing portion of patients with surgical brain tumors owing to improving prognoses of cancer patients in general and in many cases even of those with brain metastases. With advances in molecular biology and targeted therapy, the indications for neurosurgical sampling and specifically stereotactic biopsy are likely to change in the future. In this review the authors address some of the scientific advances in BrM biology, the clinical rationale and range of techniques currently used to perform stereotactic biopsy, and how the advent of molecular interrogation may potentially alter the way patients with BrM are managed in the future.

Techniques for Open Surgical Resection of Brain Metastases   527

Joshua L. Wang and J. Bradley Elder

Brain metastases are the most common intracranial tumor and a leading cause of morbidity and mortality for patients with systemic cancer. En bloc surgical resection of brain metastases improves survival, local recurrence rates, and functional independence in patients with up to three metastases and controlled extracranial disease. Modern techniques and technologies provide the neurosurgeon with minimally invasive approaches, such as keyhole craniotomies and tubular retractors. Preoperative planning for tumors located in eloquent regions includes mapping with functional MRI and diffusion tensor imaging, and intraoperative mapping and monitoring with electrophysiologic techniques under general or awake anesthesia to preserve normal neurologic function.

Laser Ablation for Cerebral Metastases   537

Evan Luther, Samuel Mansour, Nikolas Echeverry, David McCarthy, Daniel G. Eichberg, Ashish Shah, Ahmed Nada, Katherine Berry, Michael Kader, Michael Ivan, and Ricardo Komotar

Laser interstitial thermal therapy is a minimally invasive surgical alternative to craniotomy that uses laser light through a fiber optic probe placed within a target lesion to create thermal tissue damage, resulting in cellular death. It is used in neuro-oncology to treat inaccessible lesions and obviate morbidity in high-risk patients. Overall complication rates and outcome measures are comparable with those seen in radiation and/or craniotomy. Laser interstitial thermal therapy can be an effective option for recurrent brain metastases. Prospective, randomized trials must be performed to evaluate the efficacy of laser interstitial thermal therapy as a primary treatment for brain metastases.

Pathological Features of Brain Metastases   549

Saber Tadros and Abhik Ray-Chaudhury

Metastases are the most common intracranial tumors in adults. Lung cancer, melanoma, renal cell carcinoma, and breast cancer are the most common primary tumors that metastasize to the brain. Improved detection of small metastases by MRI, and improved systemic therapy for primary tumors, resulted in increased incidence of brain metastasis. Advances in neuroanesthesia and neurosurgery have significantly improved the safety of surgical resection of brain metastases. Surgical approach and active management have become applicable for many patients. Subsequently, brain metastases diagnosis no longer equals palliative treatment. Moreover, the demand for diagnosing brain masses has increased with its associated challenges.

Whole-Brain Radiation Therapy Versus Stereotactic Radiosurgery for Cerebral Metastases   565

Haley K. Perlow, Khaled Dibs, Kevin Liu, William Jiang, Prajwal Rajappa, Dukagjin M. Blakaj, Joshua Palmer, and Raju R. Raval

Whole-brain radiation therapy (WBRT) was frequently used to treat brain metastases in the past. Stereotactic radiosurgery (SRS) is now generally preferred to WBRT for patients with limited brain metastases. SRS can also be used to treat extensive brain metastases (>10–15 metastases), and clinical trials are currently comparing WBRT with SRS for extensive disease. SRS may allow for an increased risk of radiation necrosis or leptomeningeal disease dissemination after treatment. Preoperative SRS and multifraction radiotherapy decrease the risk of these side effects and may soon become standard of care. Combining SRS with immune checkpoint inhibitors may improve patient outcomes.

Radiation necrosis (RN) occurs in 5% to 25% of patients with brain metastases treated with stereotactic radiosurgery. RN must be distinguished from recurrent tumor to determine appropriate treatment. Stereotactic biopsy remains the gold standard for identifying RN. Initial treatment of RN often involves management of edema using corticosteroids, antiangiogenic therapies, and hyperbaric oxygen therapy. For refractory symptoms, surgical resection can be considered. Minimally invasive stereotactic laser ablation has the benefit of providing tissue diagnosis and treating RN or recurrent tumor with similar efficacy. Laser ablation should be considered for lesions in need of intervention where the diagnosis requires tissue confirmation.

Seizures represent a common and debilitating complication of central nervous system metastases. The use of prophylactic antiepileptic drugs (AEDs) in the preoperative period remains controversial, but the preponderance of evidence suggests that it is not helpful in preventing seizure and instead poses a significant risk of adverse events. Studies of postoperative seizure prophylaxis have not shown substantial benefit, but this practice remains widespread. Careful analysis of the risk of seizure based on patient-specific factors, such as tumor location and primary tumor histology, should guide the physician's decision on the initiation and cessation of prophylactic AED therapy.

Chemotherapy has played a minor role as adjuvant therapy in treatment of cerebral metastases from solid cancers. The blood-brain barrier and cerebral metastases' considerable machinery of self-preservation have been significant obstacles to delivery and efficacy of chemotherapy. However, several methods intended to surmount these challenges have arisen alongside advent of technology and with the development of targeted molecular therapies. Focused ultrasound and molecular Trojan horses represent two such novel means of increasing permeability of the blood-brain barrier to effector agents. Published data on efficacy of these targeted therapies remain mostly restricted to retrospective studies and phase II prospective clinical trials.

Leptomeningeal carcinomatosis is a devastating consequence of late-stage cancer, and despite multimodal treatment, remains rapidly fatal. Definitive diagnosis requires identification of malignant cells in the cerebrospinal fluid (CSF), or frank disease on MRI. Therapy is generally palliative and consists primarily of radiotherapy and/or chemotherapy, which is administered intrathecally or systemically. Immunotherapies and novel experimental therapies have emerged as promising options for decreasing patient morbidity and mortality. In this review, the authors discuss a refined view of the molecular pathophysiology of leptomeningeal carcinomatosis, current approaches to disease management, and emerging therapies.

Brain metastases lead to substantial morbidity and mortality among patients with advanced malignancies. Although treatment options have traditionally included largely palliative measures, studies of brain metastasis response to immunotherapy are promising. Immune checkpoint inhibitors have shown efficacy in studies of patients with melanoma, renal cell carcinoma, and lung cancer brain metastases. Patients with brain metastases are more frequently included in clinical trials, ushering in a new era in immunotherapy and management for patients with brain metastases. Gaining an understanding of the molecular determination for response to immunotherapies remains a major challenge and is an active area of future research.

Dynamic interplay between cancer cells and the surrounding microenvironment is a feature of the metastatic process. Successful metastatic brain colonization requires complex mechanisms that ultimately allow tumor cells to adapt to the unique microenvironment of the central nervous system, evade immune destruction, survive, and grow. Accumulating evidence suggests that components of the brain tumor microenvironment (TME) play a vital role in the metastatic cascade. In this review, the authors summarize the contribution of the TME to the development and progression of brain metastasis. They also highlight opportunities for TME-directed targeted therapy.

Sellar metastases account for 0.87% of all intracranial metastases. They are usually asymptomatic and can be the first manifestations of some occult malignancy. The diagnosis is made mainly during the screening of patients with known primary lesions or can present with neurologic or hormonal changes related to compression or invasion of surrounding structures. Differentiating these lesions from other more common lesions such as pituitary adenoma maybe difficult. Management is mainly aimed at the primary lesion and is palliative to improve quality of life or for pathologic confirmation.

Autopsy studies suggest that skull base metastases are likely underrecognized in patients with cancer. Patients frequently present with one or a combination of skull base clinical syndromes that manifest as pain or cranial neuropathy. Once a skull base metastasis is suspected, establishing a histologic diagnosis, dedicated imaging, and restaging (if appropriate) are the first steps in management. A multidisciplinary approach should then be used to identify the optimal histology-based treatment strategy, taking into account the burden of systemic disease. Finally, definitive treatment may include one or a combination of surgical management, radiation therapy, or chemotherapy.

NEUROSURGERY CLINICS OF NORTH AMERICA

SERIES OF RELATED INTEREST

Neurologic Clinics
https://www.neurologic.theclinics.com/
Neuroimaging Clinics
https://www.neuroimaging.theclinics.com/

Preface

Metastases to the Central Nervous System: A Comprehensive Guide on Current Management and Future Directions

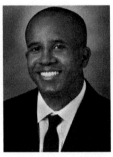   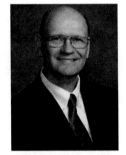

Edjah K. Nduom, MD   Jeffrey J. Olson, MD

Editors

We are pleased to present our issue of *Neurosurgery Clinics of North America* on Metastases to the Central Nervous System. We are particularly thankful to the many colleagues from across the country who have agreed to participate in this undertaking. Cerebral metastases remain the most common malignant lesion of the brain. They cause great morbidity and mortality for cancer patients, even as systemic targeted therapies have become more successful. The approach to treatment of these lesions has evolved over the years. Years ago, whole-brain radiation therapy was widely used for most cerebral metastases, prior to the seminal work of Patchell and colleagues,[1] demonstrating the value of surgical resection. More recently, the development of stereotactic radiosurgery has supplanted surgical resection in many cases. However, even for patients who present with multiple metastases, surgery maintains an important role in the appropriate care of these patients. Whole-brain radiation therapy is also making a comeback with adjunctive treatment to reduce the cognitive impact and hippocampal-sparing therapy, making a case for its continued inclusion in treatment.

Unfortunately, significant ongoing challenges to the treatment of patients suffering from these common brain lesions remain. The efforts to document the prevalence of these lesions are currently lacking. As evidenced in Dr Rahman's article on metastases, many of our primary sources on this topic date back to the 1970s. No US registry is currently mandated to record the incidence of these lesions, making it hard to track their prevalence over time.

Patients with cerebral metastases have historically been excluded from many landmark clinical trials, including those for treatments like checkpoint inhibition. This means that patients with brain metastases are often precluded from benefiting from the most advanced treatments available. This can also lead to their exclusion from the indications of the eventual Food and Drug Administration–approved medication.

Luckily, solutions are coming for many of these challenges, and we have done our best to cover these advances in this collection. Many institutions are developing multidisciplinary tumor boards focused on the care of patients with

Neurosurg Clin N Am 31 (2020) xiii–xiv
https://doi.org/10.1016/j.nec.2020.07.001
1042-3680/20/© 2020 Published by Elsevier Inc.

cerebral metastases. Such multidisciplinary care is evidenced in our articles on the approach to patients with solitary or multiple metastases, which require the consideration of many treatment modalities at once. Ongoing research on the genetic differences between metastases and parent tumors may reveal new targets for therapeutics. Blood-brain opening agents may increase the efficacy of existing systemic therapeutics, and immune therapy has already demonstrated an ability to induce objective responses in the treatment of many brain lesions. Our existing treatment options may improve as we learn more about hippocampal-sparing whole-brain radiotherapy, and surgery for these lesions has never been safer.

Here, our collection provides a review of the landscape of the current treatment of cerebral metastases while exploring some of the topics on the cutting edge. For neurosurgeons, whether subspecialized in neurosurgical oncology or in general practice, a broad understanding of the current approach to these lesions remains an important foundation to effective neurosurgical care.

Edjah K. Nduom, MD
10 Center Drive
10/3D20, MSC 1414
Bethesda, MD 20892, USA

Jeffrey J. Olson, MD
Department of Neurosurgery
Emory University
1365 Clifton Road NE
Suite B6200
Atlanta, GA 30322, USA

E-mail addresses:
edjah.nduom@nih.gov (E.K. Nduom)
jolson@emory.edu (J.J. Olson)

REFERENCE

1. Patchell RA, Tibbs PA, Walsh JW, et al. A randomized trial of surgery in the treatment of single metastases to the brain. N Engl J Med 1990;322(8):494–500.

Epidemiology of Brain Metastases

Patricia Sacks, BS, Maryam Rahman, MD, MS*

KEYWORDS

- Brain metastases • Epidemiology • Incidence • Pathophysiology • Breast cancer • Lung cancer

KEY POINTS

- Brain metastases continue to be a major source of morbidity and mortality for and one-fifth of cancer patients.
- Much of the data that do exist regarding the epidemiology of brain metastases stem from older studies, which carry several methodological limitations and predate important advancements in chemotherapy and neuroimaging.
- Lack of a unified patient registry for reporting of brain metastases limits the ability to estimate their true incidence and prevalence in the United States.
- Brain metastases are most likely to be have spread from breast, lung, renal cell, and melanoma primary cancers.
- Several factors influence the development of brain metastasis. Karnofsky performance scale status and recursive partitioning analysis classification are useful in estimating the prognosis for patients undergoing treatment of brain metastases.

INTRODUCTION

With advancements in screening, imaging, and therapeutics, cancer patients are enjoying improved survival and quality of life. Brain metastases (BMs), however, continue to be a major source of morbidity and mortality for nearly one-fifth of adult cancer patients.[1] BMs are the most common type of intracranial neoplasm in adults[2] and may arise in the brain parenchyma, leptomeninges, dura mater, and calvaria. Historically, BMs have portended a poor prognosis, often resulting in neurologic deficits, such as seizures, paralysis, and cognitive decline, that can devastate patients' quality of life and hinder their eligibility for further treatment or enrollment in clinical trials. Development of BM places an enormous financial, as well as physical, toll on patients. Longer hospital stays, more physician office visits, and higher pharmacy expenditures mean that cancer patients who develop BMs incur more than double the costs compared with those who do not.[3]

Although a precise value for incidence of BM is unknown, more than 100,000 persons are diagnosed annually.[4] The incidence of BM is thought to be climbing due to advancements in neuroimaging and treatment of primary cancers as well as heightened physician and patient awareness of BMs .[5–7] This is thought to have led to earlier diagnosis and prolonged survival among those with primary malignancies,[8] thereby increasing the pool of prevalent cancer patients at risk for metastatic disease.

Despite BMs being 10 times more common than their primary counterparts, there remains a lack of systematic, nationwide reporting of such events, which frustrates efforts to predict the true incidence, prevalence, and prognosis of BMs. Primary central nervous system (CNS) cancers are required to be reported to local and federal cancer registries, such as the Surveillance, Epidemiology,

Lillian S. Wells Department of Neurosurgery, UF Brain Tumor Immunotherapy Program, University of Florida, PO Box 100265, Gainesville, FL 32610, USA
* Corresponding author.
E-mail address: Maryam.Rahman@neurosurgery.ufl.edu

Neurosurg Clin N Am 31 (2020) 481–488
https://doi.org/10.1016/j.nec.2020.06.001
1042-3680/20/© 2020 Elsevier Inc. All rights reserved.

and End Results and the Central Brain Tumor Registry of the United States.[9] BMs, however, are not required to be reported to any particular registry. Due to this lack of a unified reporting mechanism for BMs, accurately estimating the incidence and prevalence of these tumors has proved a difficult task. Much of the current knowledge regarding epidemiology of BMs is based on a limited number of older population-based, hospital-based, and autopsy studies, which carry several methodological shortcomings and predate the era of key advancements in chemotherapy and neuroimaging.

SHORTCOMINGS OF THE EXISTING LITERATURE

Population-based studies have been utilized for the purpose of investigating the epidemiology and time trends of BMs. These studies are scarce, however, with only 4 population-based studies on BMs having been published in fairly recent literature. Among these 4 studies, the findings are widely varied. A study of all cranial neoplasms in Finland revealed 18% of them to be BMs.[10] In Iceland, the incidence of BM was reported to be much lower, with 2.8 per 100,000.[11] Researchers in Minnesota found that 41% of patients with primary malignances had BM.[12] In a national US survey of CNS tumors, 51% were labeled as BMs.[13] Variation in findings among these studies may be due in part to differences in accuracy of data collection, diagnostic practices, referral patterns, access to health care, extent of tissue examination, and selection of subpopulations for study.[14] Some studies include all cranial lesions, which resemble metastases on imaging, whereas other studies include only tumors that have been pathologically verified through tissue biopsy or autopsy. Moreover, completely asymptomatic patients, patients with severely symptomatic primary cancer, and patients with widely metastatic disease may not have been captured by these studies due to lack of recognition and/or inconsistent documentation. Although exact numbers have been difficult to determine, population-based studies conducted over the past 4 decades suggest an incidence rate of at least 10 per 100,000 individuals.[14]

Hospital-based studied have drawn on data from autopsy, radiology, and operative reports as well as reviews of the medical record.[15–19] Like population-based studies, their estimates for BM incidence percentage show great variation, ranging from as low as 3% to as high as 50%. The major limitations of these studies are their age and inherent selection bias. Patients from

large tertiary referral centers 20 years ago are unlikely to be representative of the current population. Findings from more recent hospital-based studies may be more generalizable to the population at large today. Similar to current population-based data, however, these studies are few and far between.

Autopsy studies carry several limitations. Today fewer than 5% of hospital deaths resulted in autopsy (compared with 40-60% before 1970).[20,21] In general, the prevalence of BMs reported by postmortem studies is much higher in comparison to that in antemortem reports. As an example, Posner and Chernick[22] found that a quarter of approximately 2400 cancer patients had BMs at autopsy, with 15% intraparenchymal, 8% leptomeningeal, and 20% dural. This 1978 study was one of few to provide histopathologic confirmation of BM. Studies such as this are unlikely to be repeated because autopsies have become less commonplace and physicians continue to rely heavily on clinical diagnosis and imaging to evaluate for metastases.[22]

MODELS FOR REPORTING OF BRAIN METASTASES

A 2009 study spanning 2 decades conducted by Swedish researchers may be the most accurate, comprehensive study looking at the epidemiology of BMs to date. Researchers found that the incidence of patients hospitalized with BMs in Sweden doubled from 7 to 14 per 100,000 people between 1987 and 2006. This study utilized data from all hospital admissions during this time period, encompassed all primary cancer types, and had virtually complete follow-up.[23] This study was made possible largely due to Sweden's health care system being mainly government-funded and universal for all its citizens.[24] All patients who are admitted to a Swedish hospital are entered into the National Patient Register. For every hospital discharge, up to 8 diagnoses can be recorded according to *International Classification of Diseases* (ICD). Smedby and colleagues[23] were able search the National Patient Register using ICD codes for BMs (C793/*ICD, Tenth Revision*, and 198D/*ICD, Ninth Revision*). Once the cohort of patients who were hospitalized with BMs was identified, further information on the patients' primary cancer sites was obtained by searching the National Cancer Registry by national registration numbers, which are assigned to all Swedish citizens. Because patients who develop BMs are likely to become hospitalized at some point during their disease course, Smedby and colleagues[23] were likely to have captured most, if not all, patients with BMs in Sweden during that 20-year timeframe, making this a landmark epidemiologic study for BMs.

Perhaps the most recent effort to precisely estimate the incidence percentage of BMs within the United States was carried out by researchers in Detroit employing the Metropolitan Detroit Cancer Surveillance System (MDCSS).[8] Similar to the Swedish National Patient Register in Sweden, the MDCSS is a population-based, comprehensive cancer database, which includes information on both primary tumors and their metastases for more than 16,000 patients diagnosed with cancer between 1973 and 2001 in Wayne, Oakland, and Macomb counties. This cancer database organizes information related to incidence, first course of therapy, survival reporting, and cause of death for patients with primary and secondary malignancies in the Detroit area. MDCSS was created through collaboration among approximately 60 local hospitals, pathology laboratories, and private clinics. Active follow-up is maintained for all cases entered into the database, with requests for information sent to treating physicians twice yearly and periodic checks for hospital readmissions for patients in the system. Using information from the MDCSS, Barnholtz-Sloan and colleagues[8] found that the total incidence percentage of BMs was 9.6% for all primary tumors combined. African Americans, women, persons 40 to 49 years old with lung cancer, persons 50 to 59 years old with melanoma, and persons ages 20 to 39 with breast cancer experienced the highest incidence of BMs overall.[8]

Although the precise incidence and prevalence of BMs in the United States is up for debate, it is clear that the weight of problem is considerable, having an impact on nearly as many patients as those affected by the most common primary cancers.[12,13] The need for accurate, unbiased estimates of the incidence and prevalence of BMs is pressing, as BM continues to be an enormous burden on both patients and the health care system across a multitude of medical specialties. Nationwide, organized patient registries that exist in countries with universal health care programs like Sweden may not be feasible in the United States. Nevertheless, increasing the number of smaller-scale population-based registries that implement active and consistent patient follow-up in major cities, such as the MDCSS, may bring the United States closer to addressing this need. This article summarizes the epidemiology of BMs for each of the major primary tumor types in an effort to more accurately identify which patients are at greatest risk and would maximally benefit from BM surveillance and prophylaxis.

NUMBER AND LOCATION OF BRAIN METASTASES

An autopsy study by Pickren and colleagues[25] found solitary metastases without evidence of a systemic malignancy to be relatively rare, discovered in only 0.3% of cancer patients. Single metastases in patients with cancer are found in approximately 39% of patients[25] and comprise 47% of BMs overall.[26] Among patients with BMs, multiple metastases tend to occur in roughly 41% to 47% of cases.[16,25] A particular primary cancer has a proclivity for forming multiple versus single metastases. For example, breast and gastrointestinal cancers are more likely to cause a single metastasis whereas lung cancer and melanoma typically form multiple BMs.[27]

A majority of BMs occur at the gray-white junction due to hematogenous spread of tumor emboli, which become entrapped in the small branches of terminal arteries found at this junction.[28] Accordingly, most metastases are located in the cerebrum whereas only 10% to 15% occur in the cerebellum and 3% in the brainstem[27] Pure hemodynamics cannot account for all metastatic phenomenon to the brain, however. Molecular recognition between tumor cells and healthy cells within the brain parenchyma is also thought to play a vital role.[29]

PRIMARY TUMORS THAT METASTASIZE TO THE BRAIN

The mechanism underlying the spread of primary cancer to the brain is a complex, dynamic process influenced by both the features of the metastasizing cancer cells and the microenvironment of the brain itself. Approximately 15% of cancer cells in a particular tumor are capable of metastasis.[30] Lung cancer, breast cancer, melanoma, and renal cell carcinoma account for a majority of BMs.[16,31,32] These cancers comprise approximately three-quarters of malignancies that result in BM.[33] In 80% of patients, BMs are discovered after a primary cancer already has been diagnosed (metachronous diagnosis). Far less frequently, BMs are diagnosed at the same time as the systemic malignancy (synchronous diagnosis) or, even rarer, BMs are identified before the primary tumor (precocious presentation)[34]; 60% to 80% of patients have synchronous systemic metastases, most commonly to the lungs.[27,35] A retrospective cohort study by She and colleagues[36] revealed that patients with non–small cell lung carcinoma (NSCLC) who had intracranial lesions on initial presentation had an increased risk of death from BM. Although most patients with BM have a known cancer diagnosis, a subset has BM originating from an unknown primary tumor, which is never discovered, even after autopsy[37] (**Table 1**). Most unknown tumors, however, eventually are determined to originate from the lung.

LUNG CANCER

The highest numbers of BMs come from the lung.[38] In a retrospective cohort study by Benna and colleagues,[39] of the 139 individuals found to have BMs from a cohort of 7055 cancer patients, 80% had either a primary lung or breast cancer. Other studies report lung cancer accounting for anywhere between 39% and 72% of BM cases.[40]

Benna and colleagues found that patients with lung cancer primaries and BMs were significantly older compared with those with primary malignancy elsewhere and almost exclusively were male. Just over half of patients had their metastases detected at the same time as their primary lung cancer. Of those who did not, BMs were diagnosed on average 10 months later. Approximately one-third of lung cancer patients who had BMs were asymptomatic.[39]

NSCLC accounted for 80% to 85% of cases of lung cancer with BM, with adenocarcinoma, small cell carcinoma, and small cell lung cancer comprising the minority of cases. Although men are more likely to have NSCLC overall, patients

Table 1
Risk of brain metastasis based on cancer type

Primary Tumor	Nussbaum et al,[29] 1996	Stark et al,[34] 2011	Fabi et al,[28] 2011
	39%	50%	—
	17%	15%	30%
	11%	7%	6%
	5%	—	—

This table shows the percentages of BMs from different primary cancers. According to the investigators, 39% to 50% of BMs develop from lung cancer, 15% to 30% from breast cancer, and 6% to 11% from melanoma.[28,29,34] According to Nussbaum and colleagues,[29] 5% of BMs never have an underlying systemic malignancy identified.

with NSCLC who develop BMs are more likely to be female.[41] Of the cases of synchronous BM at the time of lung cancer diagnosis, one-third were attributable to small cell lung cancer. Patients with NSCLC are estimated to have a 30% to 50% risk of developing BM compared with the 58% risk of those with small cell histology.[42] That is, although NSCLC comprises the majority of cases of BMs, patients with small cell lung cancer are at higher risk of metastasis to the brain. Because of this significant risk, it has become commonplace to include cerebral imaging in the initial diagnostic work-up of suspected NSCLC and small cell lung cancer.[43] Of those with lung cancer who developed BM, 6.7% had received prophylactic cerebral irradiation. Compared with breast cancer patients with BMs who had an average survival of 8 months, lung cancer patients with BMs had a statistically significantly worse average survival of 6 months.[44]

BREAST CANCER

Because the incidence of breast cancer is so high, it represents the second leading cause of BMs; 5% of patients with underlying breast malignancy are found to have BM.[45] Autopsy studies found BMs in 18% to 30% of patients.[39] Typically, BMs develop many months or even years after primary breast cancer is diagnosed. One study found the median time to BM detection to be 48 months after the original breast cancer diagnosis.[16]

Unlike other primary malignancies, young age is a risk factor for breast metastases to the brain, with younger women (less than 35 years old) with larger tumor size (greater than 2 cm), more than 2 metastatic sites, and high-grade tumor histology carrying the greatest risk.[1,46] HER2-positive breast tumors have the highest likelihood of metasta- sizing to the brain.[47] Survival, however, tends to be longer in patients with HER2-positive BMs rela- tive to other subtypes.[48]

MELANOMA

Although lung cancer accounts for the majority of BMs, melanoma has the highest propensity for spread to the brain of all cancers.[49] In a study by Madajewicz and colleagues,[50] as great as 90% of patients who had been diagnosed with mela- noma were found to have BMs at autopsy. Other autopsy studies report incidences of BMs ranging from 10% to 73%.[51] The average time to diagnosis of BMs for patients with melanoma is 22 months to 37 months.[16,52] Risk factors for metastatic mela- noma to the brain include male gender, ulcerated primary lesions, and having nodular or acral

lentiginous subtypes.[53] Melanomas of the head and neck are more likely to metastasize to the brain relative to truncal lesions.[54] Unlike most can- cers, when melanoma spreads to the brain, it is most likely to affect the cortex as opposed to the gray white junction.[31] BMs from an underlying mel- anoma have a tendency to bleed more so than other primary cancers, causing hemorrhage in 40% of patients.[55]

UNKNOWN PRIMARY CANCER

Studies have shown that 2% to 15% of patients develop BMs with unknown underlying systemic cancer.[25] Approximately a third of these patients did not have a systemic malignancy identified even after further extensive diagnostic work-up with neuropathologic examination and imaging and 5% even after autopsy.[56] Fludeoxyglucose-PET/computed tomography has substantially facilitated this process and has been able to iden- tify 20% to 40% of unknown primary cancers.[57,58]

PROGNOSIS AND SURVIVAL OF PATIENTS WITH BRAIN METASTASES

BMs continue to foreshadow a poor prognosis for cancer patients. Benna and colleagues[39] followed patients for 33 months and found average survival to be 4 months. Patients with BM and underlying lung cancer had shorter survival compared with those with primary breast cancer. Those who un- derwent surgery and patients with synchronous BM tended to have better survival, although these findings were not statistically significant. There was no difference in survival between patients with BM alone versus patients with BM and meta- static disease outside of the CNS.[44]

A retrospective cohort study by Pojskic and col- leagues[59] aimed at determining prognostic factors among patients undergoing surgery for BMs. Re- searchers found survival time for patients with a single BM to be 17.6 months and with multiple BMs to be 17.9 months on average.[59] Similar to Benna, Pojskic and colleagues[59] found that pa- tients with metastatic breast cancer had longer mean survival time compared with patients with other primary malignancies. Regarding the best tool to estimate outcomes for cancer patients, re- searchers found that that the recursive partitioning analysis (RPA) classification had superior predic- tive power relative to the Diagnostic-Specific Graded Prognostic Assessment. Favorable fac- tors for enhanced survival in the setting of BMs included Karnofsky performance scale (KPS) score greater than 70%, RPA classification I and

> **Box 1**
> **Favorable prognostic factors in the setting of brain metastasis**
>
> - Synchronous BMs
> - KPS score >70%
> - RPA classification I and II
> - Age <65 years
> - Use of adjuvant therapy

II, female sex, age less than 65 years, and the use of adjuvant therapy (**Box 1**).[60]

SUMMARY

In summary, BMs continue to impart an overwhelming physical and financial toll on approximately one-fifth of patients suffering from systemic cancer. Given the lack of systematic reporting; the small number of studies, which predate advances in imaging and chemotherapeutics; and discrepancies among researchers exploring the topic, it is unclear exactly how the incidence and prevalence of BMs have evolved over time. Patients with a primary cancer and BMs most often also have metastases in other anatomic locations. A single BM without evidence of extracranial disease should raise suspicion for an alternative diagnosis.

The pathophysiology underlying metastasis to the brain is complex and influenced by the particular features of the tumor cells themselves in addition to the microenvironment of the brain, hemodynamics, and molecular recognition between cells. Although most metastases occur at the gray-white junction, certain cancers have a predilection for less commonly affected areas of the CNS. Lung cancer, breast cancer, and melanoma continue to represent a majority of cases of BMs, with melanoma having the greatest proclivity toward dissemination to the brain and breast cancer the least. Renal cell carcinoma, colorectal cancer, and other GI malignancies represent a smaller proportion of primary tumors that metastasize to the brain. A subset of patients, however, develops BMs without ever determining the origin of their primary cancer.

Metastasis to the brain portends a poor prognosis in general, with metastatic breast cancer patients having the longest survival. Older age (except for breast cancer), male sex, and low KPS score predict worse survival outcomes for patients with metastatic disease to the brain. Surgery may help improve survival in some patients, but

further study is needed to gauge whether a significant benefit truly exists. The creation of a national data collection system for BMs, or at least an increase in the number of population-based registries in major metropolitan areas, would help organize important demographical information and risk factors, leading to better identification, surveillance, and prophylactic treatment of cancer patients at greatest risk for this significant morbidity.

DISCLOSURE

The authors have nothing to disclose.

REFERENCES

1. Lin X, DeAngelis L. Treatment of brain metastases. J Clin Oncol 2015;33(30):3475–84.
2. Gavrilovic IT, Posner JB. Brain metastases: epidemiology and pathophysiology. J Neurooncol 2005; 75(1):5–14.
3. Pelletier EM, Shim B, Goodman S, et al. Epidemiology and economic burden of brain metastases among patients with primary breast cancer: results from a US claims data analysis. Breast Cancer Res Treat 2008;108:297–305.
4. Nathoo N, Toms SA, Barnett GH. Metastases to the brain: current management perspectives. Expert Rev Neurother 2004;4:633–40.
5. Brufsky AM, Mayer M, Rugo HS, et al. Central nervous system metastases in patients with HER2-positive metastatic breast cancer: incidence, treatment, and survival in patients from registHER. Clin Cancer Res 2011;17:4834–43.
6. Crivellari D, Pagani O, Veronesi A, et al. High incidence of central nervous system involvement in patients with metastatic or locally advanced breast cancer treated with epirubicin and docetaxel. Ann Oncol 2001;12:353–6.
7. Dawood S, Broglio K, Esteva FJ, et al. Defining prognosis for women with breast cancer and CNS metastases by HER2 status. Ann Oncol 2008;9:1242–8.
8. Barnholtz-Sloan JS, Sloan AE, Davis FG, et al. Incidence proportions of brain metastases in patients diagnosed (1973–2001) in the Metropolitan Detroit Cancer Surveillance System. J Clin Oncol 2004;22: 2865–72.
9. Ostrom Q, Gittleman H, Truitt G, et al. CBTRUS statistical report: primary brain and other central nervous cystem tumors diagnosed in the United States in 2011–2015. Neuro Oncol 2018;20(4): iv1–86.
10. Fogelholm R, Uutela T, Murros K. Epidemiology of central nervous system neoplasms: a regional survey in Central Finland. Acta Neurol Scand 1984; 69:129.

11. Guomundsson KR. A survey of tumors of the central nervous system in Iceland during the 10-year period 1954-1963. Acta Neurol Scand 1970;46(538): 538–52.

12. Percy AK, Elveback LR, Okazaki H, et al. Neoplasms of the central nervous system. Epidemiologic considerations. Neurology 1972;22:40–8.

13. Walker AE, Robins M, Weinfeld FD. Epidemiology of brain tumors: the national survey of intracranial neoplasms. Neurology 1985;35:219–26.

14. Fox BD, Cheung VJ, Patel AJ, et al. Epidemiology of metastatic brain tumors. Neurosurg Clin N Am 2011; 22:1–6.

15. Takakura K, Teramoto A, Nakamura O, et al. Epidemiology of brain tumors [English translation]. No To Shinkei 1982;34:465–72.

16. Delattre JY, Krol G, Thaler HT, et al. Distribution of brain metastases. Arch Neurol 1988;45:741–4.

17. Bartelt S, Lutterbach J. Brain metastases in patients with cancer of unknown primary. J Neurooncol 2003; 64:249–53.

18. Weinberg JS, Lang FF, Sawaya R. Surgical management of brain metastases. Curr Oncol Rep 2001;3: 476–2483.

19. Tremont-Lukats IW, Bobustuc G, Lagos GK, et al. Brain metastasis from prostate carcinoma: The M.D. Anderson Cancer Center experience. Cancer 2003;98:363–2368.

20. Shojana KG, Burton EC. The vanishing nonforensic autopsy. N Engl J Med 2008;358(9):873–5.

21. Hoyert DL. The changing profile of autopsied deaths in the United States, 1972-2007. NCHS Data Brief 2011;67:1–8.

22. Posner JB, Chernik JL. Intracranial metastases from systemic cancer. Adv Neurol 1978;19:579–92.

23. Smedby KE, Brandt L, Backlund ML, et al. Brain metastases admissions in Sweden between 1987 and 2006. Br J Cancer 2009;101(11):1919–24.

24. Anell A, Glenngard AH, Merkur S. Sweden health system review. Health Syst Transit 2012;14(5):1–159.

25. Pickren JW, Lopez G, Tsukada Y, et al. Brain metastases: an autopsy study. Cancer Treat Symp 1983;2: 295–313.

26. Cavallaro U, Christofori G. Cell adhesion in tumor invasion and metastasis: loss of the glue is not enough. Biochim Biophys Acta Rev Cancer 2001; 1552(1):39–45.

27. Fidler IJ, Kripke ML. Metastasis results from preexisting variant cells within a malignant tumor. Science 1977;197(4306):893–5.

28. Fabi A, Felici A, Metro G, et al. Brain metastases from solid tumors: disease outcome according to type of treatment and therapeutic resources of the treating center. J Exp Clin Cancer Res 2011;30:10.

29. Nussbaum ES, Djalilian HR, Cho KH, et al. Brain metastases. Histology, multiplicity, surgery, and survival. Cancer 1996;78:1781–8.

30. Noone AM, Howlader N, Krapcho M, et al, editors. SEER cancer statistics review, 1975-2015. Bethesda (MD): National Cancer Institute. Available at: www. seer.cancer.gov/csr/1975_2015/, based on November 2017 SEER data submission, posted to the SEER website April 2018. Accessed August 25, 2019.

31. Hwang TL, Close TP, Grego JM, et al. Predilection of brain metastasis in gray and white matter junction and vascular border zones. Cancer 1996;77(8): 1551–5.

32. Weiss L. Comments on hematogenous metastatic patterns in humans as revealed by autopsy. Clin Exp Metastasis 1992;10:191–9.

33. DeAngelis LM, Posner JB. Intracranial metastases. In: DeAngelis LM, Posner JB, editors. Neurologic complications of cancer. New York: Oxford University Press; 2009. p. 141–93.

34. Stark AM, Stohring C, Hedderich J, et al. Surgical treatment for brain metastases: prognostic factors and survival in 309 patients with regard to patient age. J Clin Neurosci 2011;18:34–8.

35. Graf AH, Buchberger W, Langmayr H, et al. Site preference of metastatic tumours of the brain. Virchows Arch A Pathol Anat Histopathol 1988;412:492–8.

36. She C, Wang R, Lu C, et al. Prognostic factors and outcome of surgically treated patients with brain metastases of non-small cell lung cancer. Thorac Cancer 2018;10(2):137–42.

37. Vuong DA, Rades D, Vo SQ. Extracranial metastatic patterns on occurrence of brain metastases. J Neurooncol 2011;105(1):83–90.

38. Sawaya R, Bindal RK, Lang FF, et al. Metastatic brain tumors. In: Kaye EL, editor. Brain tumors 2nd edition: an encyclopedic approach. London: Churchill Livingstone; 2001. p. 999–1026.

39. Benna M, Mejri N, Mabrouk M, et al. Brain metastases epidemiology in a Tunisian population: trends and outcome. CNS Oncol 2018;7(1):35–9.

40. Hutter A, Schwetye KE, Bierhals AJ, et al. Brain neoplasms: epidemiology, diagnosis, and prospects for cost-effective imaging. Neuroimaging Clin N Am 2003;13(2):237–42.

41. Ruda R, Borgognone M, Benech F, et al. Brain metastases from unknown primary tumour: a prospective study. J Neurol 2001;248:394–8.

42. Nieder C, Hintz M, Grosu AL. Predicted survival in patients with brain metastases from colorectal cancer: is a current nomogram helpful? Clin Neurol Neurosurg 2016;143:107–10.

43. Goncalves PH, Peterson SL, Vigneau FD, et al. Risk of brain metastases in patients with nonmetastatic lung cancer: analysis of the Metropolitan Detroit Surveillance, Epidemiology, and End Results (SEER) data. Cancer 2016;122:1921–7.

44. Taillibert S, Le Rhun É. Epidemiology of brain metastases. Cancer Radiother 2015;19(1):3–9 [in French].

45. Kawabe T, Phi JH, Yamamoto M, et al. Treatment of brain metastasis from lung cancer. Prog Neurol Surg 2012;25:148–55.

46. Weil RJ, Palmieri DC, Bronder JL, et al. Breast cancer metastasis to the central nervous system. Am J Pathol 2005;167:913–20.

47. Schouten LJ, Rutten J, Huveneers HA, et al. Incidence of brain metastases in a cohort of patients with carcinoma of the breast, colon, kidney, and lung and melanoma. Cancer 2002;94:2698–705.

48. Tsukada Y, Fouad A, Pickren JW, et al. Central nervous system metastasis from breast carcinoma. Autopsy study. Cancer 1983;52:2349–54.

49. Musolino A, Ciccolallo L, Panebianco M, et al. Multifactorial central nervous system recurrence susceptibility in patients with HER2-positive breast cancer: epidemiological and clinical data from a population-based cancer registry study. Cancer 2011;117:1837–46.

50. Madajewicz S, Karakousis C, West CR, et al. Malignant melanoma brain metastases. Review of Roswell Park Memorial Institute experience. Cancer 1984; 53(11):2550–2.

51. Sul J, Posner JB. Brain metastases: epidemiology and pathophysiology. Cancer Treat Res 2007;136: 1–21.

52. Dasgupta T, Brasfield R. Metastatic melanoma. A clinicopathological study. Cancer 1964;17:1323–39.

53. Patel JK, Didolkar MS, Pickren JW, et al. Metastatic pattern of malignant melanoma. A study of 216 autopsy cases. Am J Surg 1978;135:807–10.

54. Fife KM, Colman MH, Stevens GN, et al. Determinants of outcome in melanoma patients with cerebral metastases. J Clin Oncol 2004;22:1293–300.

55. Sampson JH, Carter JH Jr, Friedman AH, et al. Demographgics, prognosis, and therapy in 702 patients with brain metastases from malignant melanoma. J Neurosurg 1988;88:11–20.

56. Sperduto PW, Kased N, Roberge D, et al. Summary report on the graded prognostic assessment: an accurate and facile diagnosis-specific tool to estimate survival for patients with brain metastases. J Clin Oncol 2012;30:419–25.

57. Vosoughi E, Lee JM, Miller JR, et al. Survival and clinical outcomes of patients with melanoma brain metastasis in the era of checkpoint inhibitors and targeted therapies. BMC Cancer 2018;18(1):490.

58. Giordana MT, Cordera S, Boghi A. Cerebral metastases as first symptom of cancer: a clinicopathologic study. J Neurooncol 2000;50:265–73.

59. Pojskic M, Bopp MH, Schymalla M, et al. Retrospective study of 229 surgically treated patients with brain metastases: prognostic factors, outcome and comparison of recursive partitioning analysis and diagnosis-specific graded prognostic assessment. Surg Neurol Int 2017;8:259.

60. Pavlidis N, Briasoulis E, Hainsworth J, et al. Diagnostic and therapeutic management of cancer of an unknown primary. Eur J Cancer 2003;39: 1990–2005.

Initial Approach to Patients with a Newly Diagnosed Solitary Brain Metastasis

James K.C. Liu, MD

KEYWORDS

- Solitary brain metastasis • Surgical resection • Stereotactic radiosurgery
- Whole-brain radiation therapy

KEY POINTS

- Solitary brain metastasis is defined by a single metastatic brain tumor as the only site of metastasis.
- The initial approach to patients with newly diagnosed solitary brain metastases consists of radiographical diagnosis, identification of a primary malignancy, prognostic and molecular assessment, symptom management, and treatment planning.
- The indications for surgical resection of a solitary brain metastasis includes obtaining tissue diagnosis, relief of mass effect, reversal of neurologic symptoms, oncologic control not amendable to radiation, and supplementation of systemic therapy.
- Stereotactic radiosurgery (SRS), alone or as an adjunct to surgery, is an effective treatment of metastatic tumors less than 3 cm.
- With strategies that provide cognitive protection, whole-brain radiation therapy may have a role as an adjunct to surgery or SRS for distant tumor control.

INTRODUCTION

Brain metastases (BMs) occur in up to 30% of all solid tumors. The most common originating sites of BMs are lung cancer, breast cancer, and melanoma, followed by gastrointestinal and renal cancers. Although a singular metastatic brain tumor denotes 1 lesion in the brain with the presence of extracranial metastasis sites, a solitary BM indicates the cranial lesion is the only site of metastasis.[1] Treatment of a solitary metastatic brain tumor provides a unique situation in treating a singular lesion of the brain in a patient that is likely to present with a favorable performance status given the lack of extracranial sites of disease. This situation allows an aggressive treatment plan that combines advances in surgery, radiation, and targeted chemotherapies to achieve the overall goal of local and distant tumor control. The initial approach to a patient with a newly diagnosed solitary BM consists of diagnosis through intracranial and systemic imaging, followed by symptom management, and application of an optimal treatment combination of surgery and/or radiation, taking into the account the lesion itself as well as the overall condition of the patient (**Fig. 1**).

CLINICAL PRESENTATION

Diagnosis of a solitary BM typically occurs as a result of clinical imaging performed because of acute onset of neurologic symptoms. The most common presentation is headaches, which accounts for approximately 20% of presenting symptoms for newly diagnosed BM.[1] This symptom is followed by seizures, which account for

Department of Neuro-Oncology, Moffitt Cancer Center, 12902 USF Magnolia Drive, CSB 6141, Tampa, FL 33612, USA
E-mail address: James.liu@moffitt.org

Neurosurg Clin N Am 31 (2020) 489–503
https://doi.org/10.1016/j.nec.2020.05.001
1042-3680/20/© 2020 Elsevier Inc. All rights reserved.

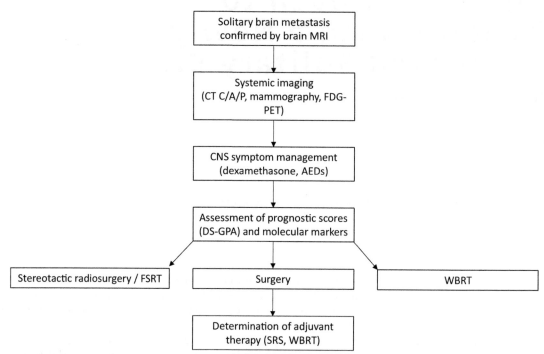

Fig. 1. Algorithm for initial approach to the patient with a newly diagnosed solitary BM. AED, anti-epileptic drug; CNS, central nervous system; CT, computed tomography; CT C/A/P, CT chest/abdomen/pelvis; DS-GPA, disease-specific graded prognostic assessment; FDG, 18F-fluoro-2-deoxy-ᴅ-glucose; SRS, stereotactic radiosurgery; WBRT, whole-brain radiation therapy.

approximately 10% to 15% of new diagnoses. Other presenting symptoms include motor weakness, sensory related apraxia, visual field deficits, and speech disturbances. Localizing the neurologic deficits may help to isolate the location of the offending lesion within the intracranial cavity before obtaining imaging studies. The temporal distribution of onset of symptoms may also help to determine the disorder in question. A history of gradual onset of motor weakness, which may have been preceded by occult symptoms such as dyscoordination or imbalance, or a history of progressive headaches may indicate a slow-growing mass lesion. This presentation may be in contrast with sudden hemibody weakness, which is more indicative of an acute process such as an intracranial hemorrhage or acute infarct.

IMAGING

The initial imaging work-up for a patient who presents with acute headaches, neurologic deficits, or changes in alertness or mentation is typically a noncontrast computed tomography (CT) scan. Noncontrast CT is the imaging modality of choice for initial screening modality because of its fast acquisition time, ease of access, and ability to identify acute neurologic injuries that require

immediate attention, such as cerebral hemorrhages, acute infarcts, or hydrocephalus. CT imaging can detect brain tumors but does not provide the sensitivity in detecting small tumors or precise characterization of visualized tumors.[2] Noncontrast CT scan may be able to note increased areas of edema but does not allow for fine delineation of mass lesions to determine the type of tumor. Contrast-enhanced CT can provide improved delineation of tumors but is still inferior to MRI for detection of smaller lesions.[2] Contrast CT may serve as a substitute for patients who are unable to obtain MRI because of implanted devices. CT imaging does have an advantage over MRI for visualization of bony detail and assessment of osseous metastasis.

MRI is the gold standard for detection and monitoring disease progression in brain tumors (**Table 1**). A typical MRI protocol that allows for full assessment and diagnosis of BM consists of a standard set of sequences, including precontrast and postcontrast T1-weighted imaging (T1WI), T2-weighted imaging (T2WI), fluid-attenuated inversion recovery (FLAIR), diffusion-weighted imaging (DWI), and apparent diffusion coefficient (ADC) sequences. BMs can be located anywhere in the intracranial cavity, most commonly as intra-axial lesions but also as extra-axial, dural, or

Table 1
MRI characteristics of brain metastases and similar-appearing lesions

Lesion	Location	T1WI	CE T1WI	T2WI	FLAIR	DWI	ADC
Brain metastasis	Gray-white junction	Isointense to hypointense	Peripheral enhancing or solidly enhancing	Hyperintense	Hyperintense surrounding area	Low signal	High signal
GBM	Supratentorial >>infratentorial	Isointense to hypointense	Peripheral enhancing,	Hyperintense	Hyperintense surrounding area	Low signal	High signal
Cerebral abscess	Variable	Hypointense	Peripheral enhancing	Central hyperintensity	Hyperintense	High signal centrally	Low signal
Lymphoma	Periventricular May cross corpus callosum	Hypointense	Solidly enhancing, rare peripheral enhancing	Variable	Hyperintense	High signal	Low signal
Demyelinating disease	Variable	Isointense to hypointense	Open ring enhancement	Hyperintense	Hyperintense	Variable	Variable

Abbreviations: ADC, apparent diffusion coefficient; DWI, diffusion-weighted imaging; FLAIR, fluid-attenuated inversion recovery; GBM, glioblastoma multiforme; T1WI, T1-weighted imaging, T2WI, T2-weighted imaging.

osseous-based lesions.[3] Intra-axial lesions are often located in gray-white junction as a result of the vascular architecture of the brain.[4] Contrast-enhanced T1WI is the most essential sequence to the evaluation and diagnosis of metastatic brain tumors. Contrast enhancement of a lesion is a hallmark of a high-grade intracranial neoplasm secondary to blood-brain barrier breakdown. Confirmation of contrast enhancement must be confirmed by comparing with the precontrast T1WI sequence in order to rule out acute hemorrhage, fat, or proteinaceous fluid. These lesions also appear hyperintense on T1WI without contrast and may be mistaken for enhancement if the contrast-enhanced T1WI is evaluated alone. The T1WI enhancement of the lesion may be solid or isolated to the periphery (ring enhancement).[5] Lesions are typically solidly enhancing at a smaller size, and later develop peripheral enhancement as a result of tumor growth surpassing its blood supply, leading to central necrosis. Hemorrhage within the lesions can be noted as hyperintensity on T1WI depending on the age of the blood products, or as decreased signal on susceptibility-weighted index (SWI) (**Fig. 2**).

On T2WI, BMs can have a variable appearance but typically appear as hyperintense lesions. Among the imaging hallmarks for metastatic brain tumor is the significant vasogenic edema around the tumor secondary to increased capillary permeability.[6] Vasogenic edema is best noted as hyperintensity surrounding the tumor on T2WI or FLAIR sequences because of its greater sensitivity to water content (**Fig. 3**). Vasogenic edema associated with BMs can often be disproportionate to the size of the tumor. Edema patterns typically are confined to the white matter, and involvement of the cortical gray matter should question an alternative diagnosis, such as cerebral infarct. FLAIR sequences suppress cerebrospinal fluid (CSF) signal for greater accuracy in showing edema, and can also be used to detect smaller metastatic brain tumors that are difficult to detect on contrast-enhanced T1WI alone.[7]

DWI sequences show the diffusion of water molecules, which can be affected by the disease processes and the cytoarchitecture of the brain parenchyma. Restricted diffusion is seen as high signal intensity on DWI sequences and low signal on the corresponding ADC maps. Diffusion imaging can be helpful in differentiating BMs from other brain lesions that have otherwise similar findings on MRI. Vasogenic edema (seen with BMs and high-grade brain tumors) does not restrict diffusion, whereas cytotoxic edema (seen with acute infarcts) does restrict diffusion.

Malignancies such as breast, colon, renal cell, and thyroid cancer often develop singular metastases in the brain, whereas lung and melanoma tend to present as multiple metastases.[8] In the

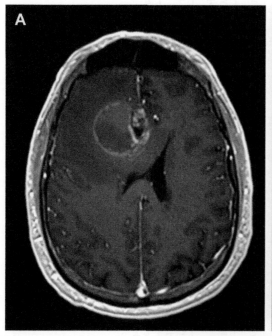
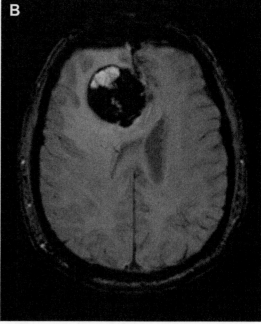

Fig. 2. Right frontal metastatic melanoma tumor. (*A*) Contrast-enhanced T1WI, (*B*) SWI indicating hemorrhagic products within the tumor.

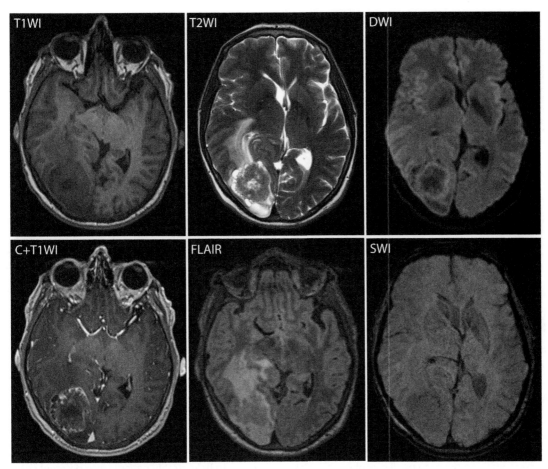

Fig. 3. Right occipital metastatic colon tumor.

case of a solitary lesion with a peripherally enhancing appearance on contrast-enhanced T1WI, it can be challenging to distinguish between BMs and other intracranial lesions with similar MRI characteristics, such as primary gliomas, lymphoma, cerebral abscess, and demyelinating disease. For a solitary metastasis, the most challenging diagnostic distinction may be from glioblastoma (GBM). Metastatic lesions are often well circumscribed, compared to primary brain tumors, which often possess a more irregular shape, although variations exist. BMs can show very different edema patterns compared with GBMs because of the lack of neurovascular unit components within BMs, resulting in significant surrounding vasogenic edema, compared with GBMs, which contain irregular neurovascular units.[3]

Analysis of the peritumoral edema using diffusion imaging may also help to differentiate GBMs from BMs. Peritumoral edema surrounding BM represents areas of vasogenic edema, unlike in GBMs, which represents edema as well as infiltrative tumor cells. Infiltration of tumor cells

results in restricted diffusion and therefore decreased ADC values in GBMs compared with BMs.[5] DWI can also be used to differentiate BM from cerebral abscess. Significant restricted diffusion is a hallmark of brain abscess and is seldom seen in primary or metastatic brain tumors (**Fig. 4**). Although most brain tumors do not restrict diffusion, lymphoma typically does show moderate restricted diffusion, but can usually be easily distinguished from abscess because untreated lymphoma typically presents as a solid homogeneously enhancing mass rather than a peripheral enhancing lesion with central area of necrosis. Central nervous system lymphoma is typically located in periventricular locations and shows increased signal on DWI.[5] These lesions often show marked radiographic response with steroids or high-dose methotrexate[9] (**Fig. 5**). Active demyelinating lesions such as multiple sclerosis can be distinguished from BM because of an open ring peripheral enhancement pattern as well as restricted diffusion on DWI.[10,11]

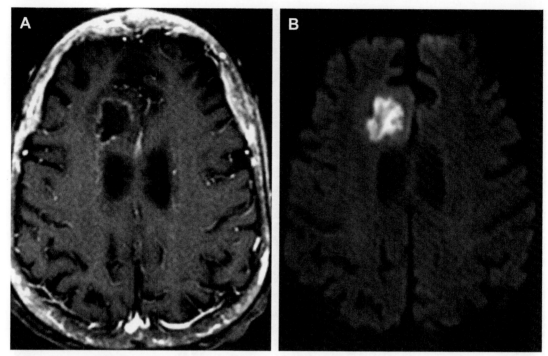

Fig. 4. MRI of right frontal cerebral abscess. (*A*) Contrast-enhanced T1WI. (*B*) DWI indicating diffusion restriction.

ADDITIONAL WORK-UP

As an adjunct to radiographical diagnosis of BM, there have been sparse reports of certain serum tumor markers that have an association with BM.[12,13] Markers such as neuron-specific enolase, S100B, lactate dehydrogenase, albumin, and proapolipoprotein A1 have shown various association in lung cancer, but overall the associations are not strong enough to provide a predictive value or are too inconsistent to be of clinical value.[13–15]

In the presence of a primary malignancy with a known predilection for metastasizing to the brain, an intracranial lesion consistent with classic features on MRI is presumed to be metastatic disease. In approximately 20% of cases, BMs are the first site detected of advanced cancer.[16] In these instances, work-up for a primary malignancy is required and starts with contrast CT of the chest, abdomen, and pelvis, followed by tissue diagnosis of the primary lesion if possible. Lack of detection on body CT imaging may necessitate PET with 18F-fluoro-2-deoxy-ᴅ-glucose (FDG) PET scanning. FDG-PET has shown greater sensitivity in detecting primary malignancies not visualized using conventional imaging techniques.[16] Despite this work-up, approximately 18% to 26% of intracranial lesions consistent with metastasis on histologic evaluation can be without a site of primary malignancy within the first 3 months of initial diagnosis of a BM.[16,17]

PROGNOSTIC AND MOLECULAR CLASSIFICATIONS

Understanding the patients' clinical status plays an important role in treatment decision making. In order to help stratify patients into different categories, the recursive partitioning analysis (RPA) was established based on retrospective analysis of multiple Radiation Therapy Oncology Group (RTOG) clinical trial data to take into account patient age, Karnofsky Performance Status (KPS), primary tumor control, and extracranial metastases (ECMs), to offer survival estimates of patients stratified into 3 classes[18] (**Table 2**). Because of evidence in subsequent studies that showed the importance of the role that the number of BMs plays in prognosis, the graded prognostic assessment (GPA) was established, which takes into account number of intracranial metastases in addition to age, KPS, and ECM[19,20] (**Table 3**). Further evaluation of the GPA noted that different prognostic factors played a larger role in different primary malignancies. Therefore, a disease-specific GPA (DS-GPA) scoring system was created and later further refined to consider disease-specific prognostic factors[21,22] (**Table 4**). For non–small cell and small cell lung cancer, the prognostic factors that were found to play a role in determining patient outcome were KPS, age, ECM, and number of BMs. For melanoma and renal cell cancer, prognostic factors were primarily

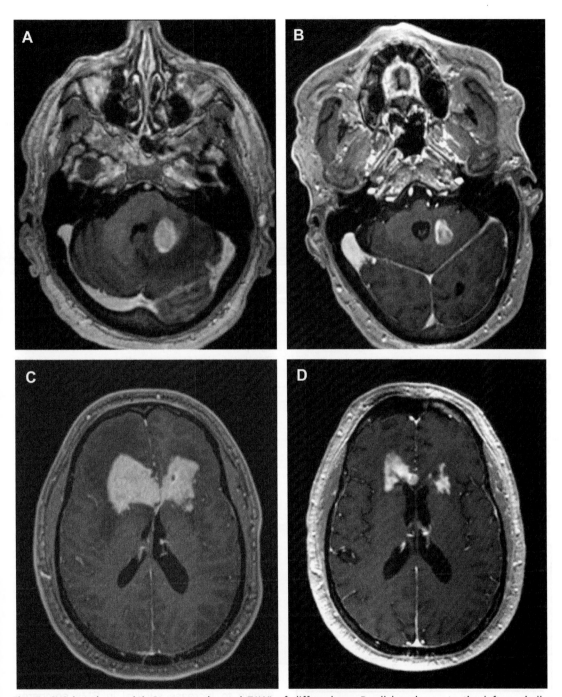

Fig. 5. CNS lymphoma. (*A*) Contrast-enhanced T1WI of diffuse large B-cell lymphoma to the left cerebellar peduncle. (*B*) Contrast-enhanced T1WI after 9 days of dexamethasone. (*C*) Contrast-enhanced T1WI of diffuse large B-cell lymphoma in the bifrontal lobe. (*D*) Contrast-enhanced T1WI after 1 month of high-dose methotrexate.

KPS and number of BMs. For breast cancer, the prognostic factors were tumor, KPS, and age. For gastrointestinal cancers, the only prognostic factor was KPS.

In addition to the prognostic values identified by the DS-GPA, molecular alterations present within both the primary site of malignancy as well as within the metastatic brain tumor must also be considered when considering treatment options for BMs. For example, in breast cancer, patients treated concurrently with radiosurgery and HER2/epidermal growth factor receptor

Table 2
Recursive partitioning analysis

	RPA Class	
I	II	III
Age<65 y	—	—
KPS>70	Not class I or III	KPS<70
Controlled primary tumor	—	—
(−) ECM	—	—
Score	Median Survival (mo)	
0	2.6	
1.5–2.5	3.8	
3	6.9	
3.5–4.0	11.0	

Data from Gaspar L, Scott C, Rotman M, et al. Recursive partitioning analysis (RPA) of prognostic factors in three Radiation Therapy Oncology Group (RTOG) brain metastases trials. Int J Radiat Oncol Biol Phys. 1997;37(4):745–51.

tyrosine kinase inhibitors showed improved local control and survival.[23] Patients with lung adenocarcinoma with epidermal growth factor receptor (EGFR) or anaplastic lymphoma kinase (ALK) gene alterations showed delayed development of initial BMs, and EGFR-positive patients treated with tyrosine kinase inhibitor showed improvement in median survival.[24] In addition to the identified genetic alterations within the parental tumor, consideration of novel actionable mutations within the brain tumor must also be taken

Table 3
Graded prognostic assessment

	GPA Score		
	0	0.5	1.0
Age (y)	>60	50–59	<50
KPS	<70	70–80	90–100
No. of BMs	>3	2–3	1
ECM	Present	—	None
Score	Median Survival (mo)		
0–1	2.6		
1.5–2.5	3.8		
3	6.9		
3.5–4.0	11.0		

Data from Sperduto PW, Berkey B, Gaspar LE, Mehta M, Curran W. A new prognostic index and comparison to three other indices for patients with brain metastases: an analysis of 1,960 patients in the RTOG database. Int J Radiat Oncol Biol Phys. 2008;70(2):510–4.

into account when pathology is available. Whole-exome sequencing analysis of matched metastatic brain and primary tumor samples has shown actionable mutations present in the metastatic brain tumors that were not present in the parental tumor.[25] Understanding the presence of these genetic alterations may help guide the use of targeted systemic therapies with improved central nervous system penetration for distant tumor control, and may ultimately result in overall survival benefits.

SYMPTOM MANAGEMENT

Before initiation of definitive therapy, management of the presenting neurologic symptoms needs to be addressed. Headaches, motor weakness, and visual field deficits are often secondary to edema and mass effect. This condition can be treated in the acute period with dexamethasone. Dexamethasone has been proved to reduce peritumoral edema on imaging as well as reverse neurologic symptoms secondary to intracranial metastases.[26] Typical dosing for dexamethasone ranges from 6 to 16 mg/d, with mixed evidence of dose-dependent improvement.[27] Dosing regimen for dexamethasone must be weighed against increased risk of side effects, which can include peptic ulcer disease, hyperglycemia, and steroid myopathy.[28] An attempt to wean steroids to the lowest possible dosage or after definitive management of the intracranial lesion should be attempted to reduce adverse side effects.

The second most common presenting symptom of newly diagnosed BM is seizures. Acute-onset seizures are typically self-limiting, but, once they occur, require initiating treatment with an antiepileptic medication. At present there is no evidence to support prophylactic antiepileptic therapy for newly diagnosed BMs without a history of seizures.[29,30]

TREATMENT
Surgery

Surgical resection of a solitary BM has been shown to increase survival in BMs compared with whole-brain radiotherapy alone.[31,32] Despite the advancements of radiation therapy, surgical treatment of solitary metastatic brain tumors continues to occupy definitive roles depending on the clinical scenario and treatment goals. Among the indications that necessitate surgical intervention is the need for tissue diagnosis, either for an unknown primary disease or to provide further molecular characterization of the intracranial lesion.[25]

Table 4
Diagnosis-specific graded prognostic assessment

DS-GPA Scoring Criteria					
NSCLC/SCLC	Score	0	0.5	1.0	—	—
	Age (y)	>60	50–60	<50	—	—
	KPS	<70	70–80	90–100	—	—
	ECM	Present	—	Absent	—	—
	No. of BMs	>3	2–3	1	—	—
Melanoma/Renal	Score	0	1.0	2.0	—	—
	KPS	<70	70–80	90–100	—	—
	No. of BMs	>3	2–3	1	—	—
Breast	Score	0	0.5	1.0	1.5	2.0
	KPS	≤50	60	70-80	90-100	—
	Subtype	Basal	NA	LumA	HER2	LumB
	Age (y)	≥60	<60	—	—	—
GI	Score	0	1	2	3	4
	KPS	<70	70	80	90	100

Median Survival (mo)					
Score	Lung	Melanoma	Breast	Renal	GI
0–1.0	3.0	3.4	3.4	3.3	3.1
1.5–2.0	5.5	4.7	7.7	7.3	4.4
2.5–3.0	9.4	8.8	15.1	11.3	6.9
3.5–4.0	14.8	13.2	25.3	14.8	13.5

Abbreviations: GI, gastrointestinal; NA, not applicable; NSCLC, non–small cell lung cancer; SCLC, small cell lung cancer.
Data from Sperduto PW, Kased N, Roberge D, et al. Summary report on the graded prognostic assessment: an accurate and facile diagnosis-specific tool to estimate survival for patients with brain metastases. J Clin Oncol. 2012;30(4):419–25.

The most common indications for surgical intervention are often palliation or oncologic control. Surgical resection is required for tumors that require immediate decompression of neural structures to reduce mass effect, or for reversal of neurologic symptoms (**Fig. 6**). These situations include compression of the motor and speech cortices; posterior fossa lesions causing, or at risk of causing, obstructive hydrocephalus; as well as large tumors causing significant mass effect with risk of supratentorial herniation. Surgery is also indicated for expectant palliation for lesions that may result in future neurologic deterioration without immediate treatment or secondary to inflammatory response from radiation treatments, as may be seen with posterior fossa or hemorrhagic lesions.[33]

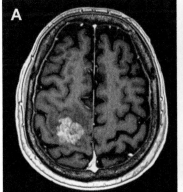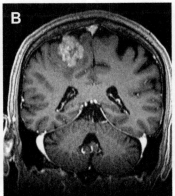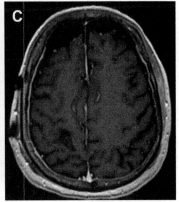

Fig. 6. Right motor cortex metastatic non–small cell lung cancer tumor. (*A*, *B*) Contrast-enhanced T1WI showing right perimotor cortex metastasis causing left upper extremity weakness. (*C*) Postsurgical contrast-enhanced T1WI.

Surgery may also be indicated for oncologic control, when alternative therapies such as stereotactic radiosurgery (SRS) or whole-brain radiation therapy (WBRT) alone have proved to be less effective. The effectiveness of SRS has been shown to decrease for lesions greater than 3 cm.[34] Therefore, lesions that exceed this size limit may be indicated for surgical resection. Oncologic control as an indication for surgical resection of solitary metastases must take into account the patient's performance and prognostic status, which may affect overall life expectancy.

The final indication for surgery is that it may serve as an adjunct to systemic treatment management. With the emergence of immune therapy, surgical resection of symptomatic lesions that may be otherwise amenable to radiation therapy may allow more rapid reduction of dexamethasone usage to avoid conflict with immune therapy.[35]

Contraindications for surgical resection may include deep-seated locations such as the thalamus or brainstem. Surgical resection has also shown a potential risk of seeding that leads to leptomeningeal disease. Some studies have shown an increased risk of leptomeningeal disease following piecemeal resection or tumor with proximity to the CSF space.[36,37] These studies indicate

a role in radiation as an adjunct to surgical resection.

Stereotactic Radiosurgery

SRS delivers a single dose of highly conformed ionizing radiation to a defined target using image guidance, which allows minimal toxicity to surrounding structures (**Fig. 7**).[38] Its effectiveness in the treatment of BMs has allowed it to become a dominant treatment option for solitary BMs that do not require surgical resection for relief of mass effect, or that are in locations not amenable to surgical resection. Multiple studies have compared the effectiveness of SRS with surgery in the treatment of single or solitary BMs, and none have shown a significant difference in overall survival, making SRS comparable with surgery for lesions less than 3 to 3.5 cm.[39–42] SRS has also been proved in some studies to show equivalent survival benefit to WBRT without evidence of neurocognitive decline.[43,44]

In addition to stand-alone treatment of solitary metastases, SRS also serves as an adjunct surgical resection. Studies have shown that SRS to the surgical resection site with a 2-mm margin around the edge of the cavity results in improvement in local recurrence.[45,46] SRS has primarily replaced WBRT as the adjuvant treatment modality of

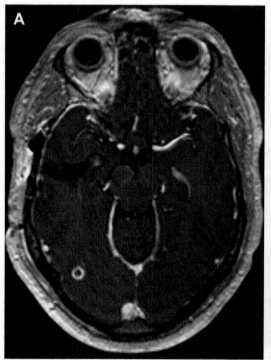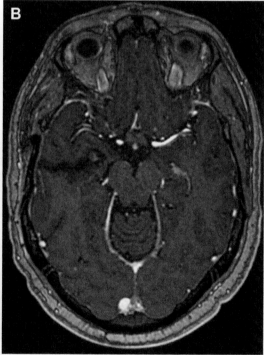

Fig. 7. Right occipital metastatic melanoma tumor treated with SRS. (*A*) Contrast-enhanced T1WI showing right occipital metastasis. (*B*) Contrast-enhanced T1WI 2 months after SRS (24 Gy).

choice because of concerns of cognitive decline from WBRT.[47] Because of challenges in treatment planning around surgical resection cavities, and the risk of leptomeningeal disease secondary to tumor spillage, the use of neoadjuvant SRS has been applied.[48–50] Initial studies on neoadjuvant SRS have shown a potential for decrease in leptomeningeal disease, but further evidence is needed to definitively define its effectiveness.[50]

For lesions larger than 3 cm, SRS has been shown to be less effective.[34] Hypofractionated radiotherapy has been used to treat large BMs with a reduced risk of radiation necrosis, which can be higher following SRS to larger tumors.[51] An alternative to hypofractionated radiotherapy is the use of 2-stage SRS for treatment of large (≥2 cm) metastatic lesions.[52]

Whole-Brain Radiation Therapy

WBRT consists of irradiating the entire brain and was once a mainstay of therapy for the treatment of BMs. The standard WBRT dose fractionation schedule for optimal treatment consists of 30 Gy in 10 fractions.[53] In patients with poor performance status or shortened predictive survival, the fractionation may be shortened to consist of 20 Gy in 5 fractions. The advantages of whole-brain therapy include ease of administration and the potential ability to target micrometastases that are not detectable on clinical imaging, allowing improvement in distant recurrence.[54]

The role of WBRT as the primary treatment of BM has been supplanted since the introduction of studies that have shown that surgical resection in addition to WBRT provides advantages in both local control and overall survival.[31,32] Since then, WBRT therapy has been relegated to adjunctive therapy following surgical resection or SRS. Early studies of WBRT in addition to SRS showed overall survival advantage and benefits in local recurrence rates, particularly in the treatment of singular BM and patients with good prognostic factors as defined by RPA class I.[19,55] Despite these data, concerns for the cognitive toxicities of WBRT, as well as an apparent lack of overall survival benefit from subsequent studies, have prevented its widespread use as an adjunctive

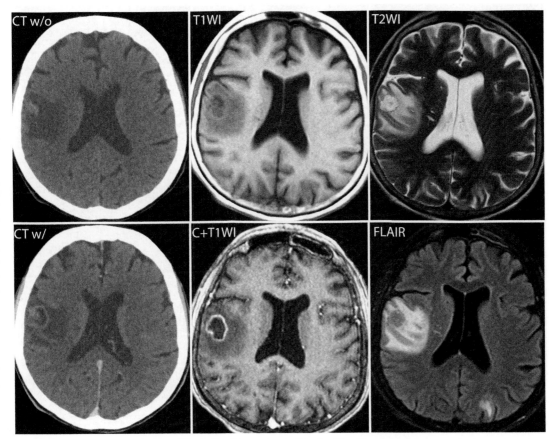

Fig. 8. Right motor cortex lesion. CT w/, CT with contrast; CT w/o, CT without contrast.

therapy.[47,56,57] Cognitive decline has been addressed through the use of memantine, an *N*-methyl-D-aspartate agonist, as well as hippocampal-sparing WBRT techniques.[58,59] A recent phase III clinical trial showed the effectiveness of memantine with hippocampal-avoidance WBRT to reduce the risk of cognitive failure. Reevaluation of previous studies using WBRT have indicated that there may be a survival benefit associated with distant tumor control in patients with favorable prognostic factors.[60]

Despite strategies for cognitive protection and reevaluation of possible survival advantages as a result of WBRT, there does not seem to be a definitive role for WBRT in the treatment of solitary BMs. Further focused studies may be able to define whether it provides an overall survival benefit in a select patient population.

CASE EXAMPLES
Case 1

A 69-year-old woman with a diagnosis of non–small cell lung cancer following a left lower lobe segmental resection 1 year prior presented with a short history of intermittent headaches. CT of the head detected a possible lesion in the right frontal lobe (**Fig. 8**). Follow-up MRI was performed and showed a single peripherally enhancing lesion in the lateral frontal lobe. The patient was placed on dexamethasone at a dosage of 4 mg twice a day, with relief of her headaches and improvement in her left arm strength. Treatment options, including surgery and SRS, were discussed with the patient and her oncology team. Although the lesion was amenable to SRS, the patient's lung cancer was positive for programmed death-ligand 1 (PD-L1) and she was a candidate for immune therapy. Therefore, the patient was offered surgical resection of the lesion to allow for an immediate taper of steroids to prevent interference with immune therapy. She underwent successful surgical resection of her lesion with adjuvant SRS and was placed on immune therapy.

Case 2

A 73-year-old man with a history of prostate cancer resected 9 years prior presented with left leg weakness, dizziness, and diplopia. He has noticed

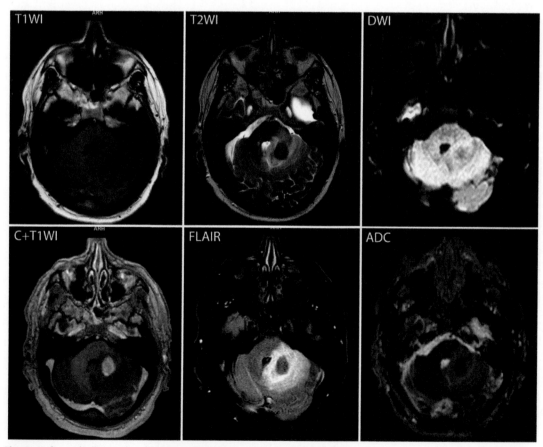

Fig. 9. Left cerebellar peduncle lesion. C+T1WI, contrast enhance T1WI.

an increase of imbalance and falls. The symptoms began 2 weeks before his presentation and have progressively worsened. MRI was performed and showed an irregularly shaped solidly enhancing mass in the deep left cerebellum near the peduncle (**Fig. 9**). The patient was placed on dexamethasone at 4 mg 4 times daily, with relief of headaches and significant improvement in left leg strength. Given the distant history of prostate cancer and the low likelihood of prostate cancer metastasizing to the brain, CT of the chest, abdomen, and pelvis was performed to survey for another malignancy source. A right thyroid nodule was found, and an ultrasonography-guided fine-needle aspiration was performed, which showed follicular neoplasm. Given the low likelihood of thyroid metastasis to the brain, a stereotactic biopsy was planned. Repeat MRI before the biopsy showed decrease in size of the lesion from the initial MRI. A biopsy was performed and pathology confirmed large B-cell lymphoma. The patient was treated with methotrexate.

SUMMARY

The initial approach to patients with newly diagnosed solitary BMs involves definitive radiographic diagnosis, management of neurologic symptoms, assessing the patient's clinical and molecular status, and application of the treatment modality best suited to the goals of the treatment. The ultimate objective is to achieve local and distant intracranial tumor control that results in a benefit to overall survival. Advances in surgery and radiation therapies, along with ongoing studies, are providing more information regarding the best combination of therapy to achieve long-term overall survival, whereas advances in molecular medicine contribute to defining treatment plans that are tailored specifically to each patient's tumor.

DISCLOSURE

Novocure, advisory board. BMS, scientific grant funding.

REFERENCES

1. Westphal M, Heese O, de Wit M. Intracranial metastases: therapeutic options. Ann Oncol 2003; 14(Suppl 3):iii4–10.
2. Schellinger PD, Meinck HM, Thron A. Diagnostic accuracy of MRI compared to CCT in patients with brain metastases. J Neurooncol 1999;44(3):275–81.
3. Barajas RF Jr, Cha S. Metastasis in adult brain tumors. Neuroimaging Clin N Am 2016;26(4):601–20.
4. Delattre JY, Krol G, Thaler HT, et al. Distribution of brain metastases. Arch Neurol 1988;45(7):741–4.
5. Pope WB. Brain metastases: neuroimaging. Handb Clin Neurol 2018;149:89–112.
6. Strugar J, Rothbart D, Harrington W, et al. Vascular permeability factor in brain metastases: correlation with vasogenic brain edema and tumor angiogenesis. J Neurosurg 1994;81(4):560–6.
7. Okubo T, Hayashi N, Shirouzu I, et al. Detection of brain metastasis: comparison of Turbo-FLAIR imaging, T2-weighted imaging and double-dose gadolinium-enhanced MR imaging. Radiat Med 1998;16(4): 273–81.
8. Barajas RF Jr, Cha S. Imaging diagnosis of brain metastasis. Prog Neurol Surg 2012;25:55–73.
9. Bromberg JE, Siemers MD, Taphoorn MJ. Is a "vanishing tumor" always a lymphoma? Neurology 2002; 59(5):762–4.
10. Abdoli M, Chakraborty S, MacLean HJ, et al. The evaluation of MRI diffusion values of active demyelinating lesions in multiple sclerosis. Mult Scler Relat Disord 2016;10:97–102.
11. Masdeu JC, Quinto C, Olivera C, et al. Open-ring imaging sign: highly specific for atypical brain demyelination. Neurology 2000;54(7):1427–33.
12. Ishibashi N, Maebayashi T, Aizawa T, et al. Serum tumor marker levels at the development of intracranial metastasis in patients with lung or breast cancer. J Thorac Dis 2019;11(5):1765–71.
13. Jacot W, Quantin X, Boher JM, et al. Brain metastases at the time of presentation of non-small cell lung cancer: a multi-centric AERIO analysis of prognostic factors. Br J Cancer 2001;84(7):903–9.
14. Li BT, Lou E, Hsu M, et al. Serum biomarkers associated with clinical outcomes fail to predict brain metastases in patients with stage IV non-small cell lung cancers. PLoS One 2016;11(1):e0146063.
15. Marchi N, Mazzone P, Fazio V, et al. ProApolipoprotein A1: a serum marker of brain metastases in lung cancer patients. Cancer 2008;112(6):1313–24.
16. Wolpert F, Weller M, Berghoff AS, et al. Diagnostic value of (18)F-fluordesoxyglucose positron emission tomography for patients with brain metastasis from unknown primary site. Eur J Cancer 2018;96: 64–72.
17. Giordana MT, Cordera S, Boghi A. Cerebral metastases as first symptom of cancer: a clinico-pathologic study. J Neurooncol 2000;50(3):265–73.
18. Gaspar L, Scott C, Rotman M, et al. Recursive partitioning analysis (RPA) of prognostic factors in three Radiation Therapy Oncology Group (RTOG) brain metastases trials. Int J Radiat Oncol Biol Phys 1997;37(4):745–51.
19. Andrews DW, Scott CB, Sperduto PW, et al. Whole brain radiation therapy with or without stereotactic radiosurgery boost for patients with one to three brain metastases: phase III results of the RTOG

9508 randomised trial. Lancet 2004;363(9422): 1665–72.

20. Sperduto PW, Berkey B, Gaspar LE, et al. A new prognostic index and comparison to three other indices for patients with brain metastases: an analysis of 1,960 patients in the RTOG database. Int J Radiat Oncol Biol Phys 2008;70(2):510–4.

21. Sperduto PW, Chao ST, Sneed PK, et al. Diagnosis-specific prognostic factors, indexes, and treatment outcomes for patients with newly diagnosed brain metastases: a multi-institutional analysis of 4,259 patients. Int J Radiat Oncol Biol Phys 2010;77(3):655–61.

22. Sperduto PW, Kased N, Roberge D, et al. Summary report on the graded prognostic assessment: an accurate and facile diagnosis-specific tool to estimate survival for patients with brain metastases. J Clin Oncol 2012;30(4):419–25.

23. Miller JA, Kotecha R, Ahluwalia MS, et al. Overall survival and the response to radiotherapy among molecular subtypes of breast cancer brain metastases treated with targeted therapies. Cancer 2017; 123(12):2283–93.

24. Sperduto PW, Yang TJ, Beal K, et al. The effect of gene alterations and tyrosine kinase inhibition on survival and cause of death in patients with adenocarcinoma of the lung and brain metastases. Int J Radiat Oncol Biol Phys 2016;96(2):406–13.

25. Brastianos PK, Carter SL, Santagata S, et al. Genomic characterization of brain metastases reveals branched evolution and potential therapeutic targets. Cancer Discov 2015;5(11):1164–77.

26. Jessurun CAC, Hulsbergen AFC, Cho LD, et al. Evidence-based dexamethasone dosing in malignant brain tumors: what do we really know? J Neurooncol 2019;144(2):249–64.

27. Vecht CJ, Hovestadt A, Verbiest HB, et al. Dose-effect relationship of dexamethasone on Karnofsky performance in metastatic brain tumors: a randomized study of doses of 4, 8, and 16 mg per day. Neurology 1994;44(4):675–80.

28. Pezner RD, Lipsett JA. Peptic ulcer disease and other complications in patients receiving dexamethasone palliation for brain metastasis. West J Med 1982;137(5):375–8.

29. Mikkelsen T, Paleologos NA, Robinson PD, et al. The role of prophylactic anticonvulsants in the management of brain metastases: a systematic review and evidence-based clinical practice guideline. J Neurooncol 2010;96(1):97–102.

30. Tremont-Lukats IW, Ratilal BO, Armstrong T, et al. Antiepileptic drugs for preventing seizures in people with brain tumors. Cochrane Database Syst Rev 2008;(2):CD004424.

31. Patchell RA, Tibbs PA, Walsh JW, et al. A randomized trial of surgery in the treatment of single metastases to the brain. N Engl J Med 1990; 322(8):494–500.

32. Vecht CJ, Haaxma-Reiche H, Noordijk EM, et al. Treatment of single brain metastasis: radiotherapy alone or combined with neurosurgery? Ann Neurol 1993;33(6):583–90.

33. Leeman JE, Clump DA, Flickinger JC, et al. Extent of perilesional edema differentiates radionecrosis from tumor recurrence following stereotactic radiosurgery for brain metastases. Neuro Oncol 2013;15(12): 1732–8.

34. Vogelbaum MA, Angelov L, Lee SY, et al. Local control of brain metastases by stereotactic radiosurgery in relation to dose to the tumor margin. J Neurosurg 2006;104(6):907–12.

35. Tawbi HA, Forsyth PA, Algazi A, et al. Combined nivolumab and ipilimumab in melanoma metastatic to the brain. N Engl J Med 2018;379(8):722–30.

36. Suki D, Hatiboglu MA, Patel AJ, et al. Comparative risk of leptomeningeal dissemination of cancer after surgery or stereotactic radiosurgery for a single supratentorial solid tumor metastasis. Neurosurgery 2009;64(4):664–74 [discussion: 674–6].

37. Ahn JH, Lee SH, Kim S, et al. Risk for leptomeningeal seeding after resection for brain metastases: implication of tumor location with mode of resection. J Neurosurg 2012;116(5):984–93.

38. Aoyama H, Shirato H, Onimaru R, et al. Hypofractionated stereotactic radiotherapy alone without whole-brain irradiation for patients with solitary and oligo brain metastasis using noninvasive fixation of the skull. Int J Radiat Oncol Biol Phys 2003;56(3): 793–800.

39. Auchter RM, Lamond JP, Alexander E, et al. A multiinstitutional outcome and prognostic factor analysis of radiosurgery for resectable single brain metastasis. Int J Radiat Oncol Biol Phys 1996; 35(1):27–35.

40. Muacevic A, Kreth FW, Horstmann GA, et al. Surgery and radiotherapy compared with gamma knife radiosurgery in the treatment of solitary cerebral metastases of small diameter. J Neurosurg 1999; 91(1):35–43.

41. Schoggl A, Kitz K, Reddy M, et al. Defining the role of stereotactic radiosurgery versus microsurgery in the treatment of single brain metastasis. Acta Neurochir (Wien) 2000;142(6):621–6.

42. O'Neill BP, Iturria NJ, Link MJ, et al. A comparison of surgical resection and stereotactic radiosurgery in the treatment of solitary brain metastases. Int J Radiat Oncol Biol Phys 2003;55(5):1169–76.

43. Chang EL, Wefel JS, Hess KR, et al. Neurocognition in patients with brain metastases treated with radiosurgery or radiosurgery plus whole-brain irradiation: a randomised controlled trial. Lancet Oncol 2009; 10(11):1037–44.

44. Aoyama H, Shirato H, Tago M, et al. Stereotactic radiosurgery plus whole-brain radiation therapy vs stereotactic radiosurgery alone for treatment of brain

metastases: a randomized controlled trial. JAMA 2006;295(21):2483–91.

45. Mahajan A, Ahmed S, McAleer MF, et al. Post-operative stereotactic radiosurgery versus observation for completely resected brain metastases: a single-centre, randomised, controlled, phase 3 trial. Lancet Oncol 2017;18(8):1040–8.

46. Choi CY, Chang SD, Gibbs IC, et al. Stereotactic radiosurgery of the postoperative resection cavity for brain metastases: prospective evaluation of target margin on tumor control. Int J Radiat Oncol Biol Phys 2012;84(2):336–42.

47. Brown PD, Ballman KV, Cerhan JH, et al. Postoperative stereotactic radiosurgery compared with whole brain radiotherapy for resected metastatic brain disease (NCCTG N107C/CEC.3): a multicentre, randomised, controlled, phase 3 trial. Lancet Oncol 2017; 18(8):1049–60.

48. Suki D, Abouassi H, Patel AJ, et al. Comparative risk of leptomeningeal disease after resection or stereotactic radiosurgery for solid tumor metastasis to the posterior fossa. J Neurosurg 2008;108(2):248–57.

49. Siomin VE, Vogelbaum MA, Kanner AA, et al. Posterior fossa metastases: risk of leptomeningeal disease when treated with stereotactic radiosurgery compared to surgery. J Neurooncol 2004;67(1–2): 115–21.

50. Asher AL, Burri SH, Wiggins WF, et al. A new treatment paradigm: neoadjuvant radiosurgery before surgical resection of brain metastases with analysis of local tumor recurrence. Int J Radiat Oncol Biol Phys 2014;88(4):899–906.

51. Minniti G, D'Angelillo RM, Scaringi C, et al. Fractionated stereotactic radiosurgery for patients with brain metastases. J Neurooncol 2014;117(2):295–301.

52. Angelov L, Mohammadi AM, Bennett EE, et al. Impact of 2-staged stereotactic radiosurgery for treatment of brain metastases >/= 2 cm. J Neurosurg 2018;129(2):366–82.

53. Gaspar LE, Prabhu RS, Hdeib A, et al. Congress of neurological surgeons systematic review and evidence-based guidelines on the role of whole brain radiation therapy in adults with newly diagnosed metastatic brain tumors. Neurosurgery 2019;84(3):E159–62.

54. Kocher M, Soffietti R, Abacioglu U, et al. Adjuvant whole-brain radiotherapy versus observation after radiosurgery or surgical resection of one to three cerebral metastases: results of the EORTC 22952-26001 study. J Clin Oncol 2011;29(2):134–41.

55. Sanghavi SN, Miranpuri SS, Chappell R, et al. Radiosurgery for patients with brain metastases: a multi-institutional analysis, stratified by the RTOG recursive partitioning analysis method. Int J Radiat Oncol Biol Phys 2001;51(2):426–34.

56. Patil CG, Pricola K, Sarmiento JM, et al. Whole brain radiation therapy (WBRT) alone versus WBRT and radiosurgery for the treatment of brain metastases. Cochrane Database Syst Rev 2017;(9):CD006121.

57. Sahgal A, Aoyama H, Kocher M, et al. Phase 3 trials of stereotactic radiosurgery with or without whole-brain radiation therapy for 1 to 4 brain metastases: individual patient data meta-analysis. Int J Radiat Oncol Biol Phys 2015;91(4):710–7.

58. Brown PD, Pugh S, Laack NN, et al. Memantine for the prevention of cognitive dysfunction in patients receiving whole-brain radiotherapy: a randomized, double-blind, placebo-controlled trial. Neuro Oncol 2013;15(10):1429–37.

59. Gondi V, Pugh SL, Tome WA, et al. Preservation of memory with conformal avoidance of the hippocampal neural stem-cell compartment during whole-brain radiotherapy for brain metastases (RTOG 0933): a phase II multi-institutional trial. J Clin Oncol 2014;32(34):3810–6.

60. Mehta MP. The controversy surrounding the use of whole-brain radiotherapy in brain metastases patients. Neuro Oncol 2015;17(7):919–23.

Initial Approach to the Patient with Multiple Newly Diagnosed Brain Metastases

Clara Kwon Starkweather[a], Bryan D. Choi[a],
Christopher Alvarez-Breckenridge[a], Priscilla K. Brastianos[b], Kevin Oh[c],
Nancy Wang[c], Helen Shih[c], Brian V. Nahed[a,d],*

KEYWORDS

- Brain metastasis • Stereotactic radiosurgery • Neurosurgical oncology • Multiple metastases

KEY POINTS

- The management of brain metastases involves multiple modalities, including surgery, radiation, and targeted therapy.
- There is an increasing need for therapies that preserve cognitive function and quality of life.
- The management of patients with 2 to 3 brain metastases has evolved toward a multidisciplinary approach.
- Patients with a large brain metastasis benefit from surgical resection followed by radiation or targeted therapy.

INTRODUCTION

Brain metastases are the most common intracranial tumor in adults.[1] Historically, metastatic brain cancer signaled a dismal prognosis with median survival times of 3 to 4 months with treatment; however, modern therapies have led to a more promising picture.[2] For example, patients with 1 to 2 intracranial metastases from breast cancer, with controlled extracranial disease and no functional deficits, have median survival times of 29 months.[3] Increased survival is multifactorial, owing to advancements in radiation therapy, improved systemic therapy, and earlier identification of metastatic cancer in patients with preserved functional status. Systemic therapies have led to longer survival, which in turn extends the time window for cancer to disseminate to the brain; as a result, the incidence of brain metastases is expected to increase.[1] The number of operations for brain metastases has increased by 79% from 1998 to 2010.[4] This increase reflects the increased incidence of brain metastases as well as a demonstrated survival benefit of surgery in certain patients, particularly when combined with radiation therapy. Given the longer survival of patients with intracranial metastases, therapeutic strategies addressing brain metastases must preserve neurocognitive function and quality of life.

Patients with multiple metastases require multidisciplinary approaches. Among all patients with newly diagnosed brain metastases, 47% to 51% will have multiple metastases (≥2 metastases),[5,6] and 41% will have ≥3 brain metastases.[7] Some

[a] Department of Neurosurgery, Massachusetts General Hospital, Harvard Medical School, 55 Fruit Street, Boston, MA 02114, USA; [b] Department of Medical Oncology, Dana-Farber Cancer Institute, Boston, MA, USA; [c] Department of Radiation Oncology, Massachusetts General Hospital, Boston, MA, USA; [d] Department of Neurology, Massachusetts General Hospital, Boston, MA, USA
* Corresponding author.
E-mail address: bnahed@partners.org

Neurosurg Clin N Am 31 (2020) 505–513
https://doi.org/10.1016/j.nec.2020.05.002
1042-3680/20/© 2020 Elsevier Inc. All rights reserved.

patient classification schemes relegate patients with higher intracranial metastatic burden to poorer prognostic tiers, yet this may ultimately be less relevant to surgical candidacy.[2] Because of poor prognosis, some landmark clinical trials for surgical and systemic therapies have excluded patients with multiple metastases. Nonetheless, surgery is often recommended for patients with multiple brain metastases, especially those who have a large, dominant lesion or one causing significant edema or symptoms. Herein, the authors discuss therapeutic strategies for patients with brain metastasis, with an emphasis on studies relevant to patients with multiple metastases.

TISSUE DIAGNOSTICS

In any patient with newly discovered brain metastases, tissue diagnosis is often required for confirmation of histology or genotyping. In patients without a diagnosis of cancer (2%–14%), brain metastases can be the first manifestation of cancer.[1,8] Surgical resection or biopsy of these lesions is often used to histologically confirm metastasis, because other causes, including primary intracranial malignancy, infection, and vascular malformations, may mimic metastasis on imaging.[9]

More recent advances in systemic therapy for specific mutations place a spotlight on tissue diagnosis for molecular diagnostics. A 2015 study of whole-exome sequencing of metastatic brain tumor tissue showed that 53% of tumors had clinically informative genetic alterations that were not present in the primary tumor.[10] For instance, mutations that predicted sensitivity to HER2/EGFR inhibitors were found in brain metastases, but not in the primary tumor of 10 out of 86 patients. Brain metastases in the same patient are genetically homogeneous, despite often differing substantially from extracranial sites or primary site.[10] Therefore, resection of a brain metastasis provides valuable diagnostic information in patients with heavy metastatic burden and will likely become increasingly important as molecular diagnostics continue to expand in areas such as epigenetic profiling.[11]

In addition to tissue diagnosis, additional workup should be performed. In patients with unknown primary tumor, this workup should include a thorough physical examination (particularly breasts, testes, and skin), abdominal computed tomography (CT), chest CT, and mammography, if applicable.[12] If this additional workup is negative, whole-body fluorodeoxyglucose PET should be considered. In patients with a known primary, further workup for systemic staging should be performed as appropriate for the specific tumor type.[12]

WHOLE-BRAIN RADIATION THERAPY

Radiation therapy has been a mainstay in the treatment of brain metastases for many decades. However, given recent advances in targeted therapy and increasing evidence supporting the use of stereotactic radiosurgery (SRS), whole-brain radiation therapy (WBRT) is often reserved for very diffuse disease or leptomeningeal disease for which there is no reliable systemic agent. WBRT first became available in the1960s and involves irradiation of the entire brain (total dose: 25–40 Gy).[13,14] WBRT was thought to treat radiologically occult lesions, or "micrometastases," reducing the propensity of developing new intracranial metastases. Indeed, WBRT reduces the rate of intracranial progression (ie, both at the initial metastatic sites and at new sites).[15–17] In 1 study by Kocher and colleagues,[17] studying patients with 1 to 3 brain metastases, the 2-year intracranial relapse rate was 48% in patients treated exclusively with SRS and 33% in patients treated with SRS followed by WBRT. However, reduced rates of intracranial relapse do not translate into significant prolongation of overall survival or functionally independent survival in patients treated with WBRT in addition to SRS, versus SRS alone.[15–18] Furthermore, WBRT is associated with significant neurocognitive decline.[19] Post-WBRT patients show decreased performance on a battery of cognitive tests, such as delayed recall,[20] with greater than 90% of patients showing cognitive decline in the 3 months following WBRT + SRS versus 63.5% who underwent SRS alone.[16] The deleterious effects of WBRT persisted over time in those surviving 12 months, which is particularly troublesome given the increasing life expectancy of patients with brain metastases.[1] Accordingly, in their 2014 "Choosing Wisely" initiative, the American Society of Radiation Oncology advised that WBRT not be routinely added to SRS for patients with a limited number of brain metastases.

Upfront WBRT is reserved for patients with very high metastatic tumor burden, with palliation being the main goal of therapy.[21] However, there is a dearth of studies comparing WBRT with supportive therapy. In 1 randomized trial, Mulvenna and colleagues[22] assessed the use of WBRT in patients with non–small-cell lung cancer (NSCLC) with brain metastases. Patients were randomized to WBRT or supportive therapy alone. The study included patients with Karnofsky performance status (KPS) <70, most of whom had greater than 1 intracranial metastasis, in whom surgery and radiosurgery were not options, and in whom the clinical benefit of WBRT was thought to be equivocal. This study found no difference in overall survival or quality-of-life measures between the 2 groups, calling into question whether WBRT should always be deployed invariant of primary diagnosis. For other primary tumor types, studies investigating whether WBRT yields a benefit over SRS for $\geq$4 metastases are currently underway, such as a phase 3 trial at MD Anderson (ClinicalTrials.gov identifier: NCT01592968) and a phase 3 trial in The Netherlands (ClinicalTrials.gov identifier: NCT02353000), with primary endpoints including cognitive function and quality-of-life measures, respectively. Currently, when WBRT is the only option, hippocampal-avoidant WBRT (HA-WBRT) is used to mitigate the neurocognitive side effects. A recent study demonstrated a 7% mean decline in the Hopkins Verbal Learning Test-Revised Delayed Recall (HVLT-RDR) at 4 months, versus a 30% decline in a historical control that underwent WBRT.[23] A randomized phase 2/3 trial (ClinicalTrials.gov identifier: NCT02635009) recently showed that HA-WBRT results in a lower risk of deterioration on various cognitive tests (including HVLT-RDR) in patients undergoing WBRT for metastatic small-cell lung cancer.[24] With regard to pharmacologic mitigation, 1 study, although underpowered, showed a significantly longer time to cognitive decline if patients received memantine within 3 days of initiating WBRT,[20] and memantine is now considered standard of care if WBRT is performed. In conclusion, WBRT is reserved for patients for whom SRS and other localized radiation therapies, targeted therapy, and immunotherapy are not options. Given the significant side effects of WBRT, active investigation aims to determine the limited role of WBRT in patients with higher metastatic burden.

STEREOTACTIC RADIOSURGERY

SRS has become more widely used as monotherapy in recent years given the lack of survival benefit provided by SRS + WBRT with 1 to 3 intracranial metastases, and the minimal neurocognitive side-effect profile.[15–18] Although SRS was traditionally deployed in patients with less than 4 brain metastases,[25,26] more recent studies suggest a broader range of patients may be amenable to SRS. One retrospective cohort study showed no difference in survival between patients with greater than 10, versus 2 to 9 brain metastases, all of whom underwent SRS monotherapy targeting all lesions.[27] A more recent retrospective cohort study showed that total tumor volume greater than 10 cc corresponded to decreased survival in patients receiving SRS, whereas the

number of metastases had no effect on survival (4–5 vs $\geq$6 metastases).[28] For larger tumors, greater than 3 cm, the risk for substantial neurotoxicity scales with tumor diameter.[29] Hypofractionation, in which the dose of radiation delivered is divided between 2 and 5 sessions,[30,31] may reduce radiation necrosis (incidence of SRS-induced radiation necrosis estimated to be 25% by 1 study[32]) and allow larger tumors to be effectively targeted. An ongoing trial at Stanford (ClinicalTrials.gov identifier: NCT00928226) aims to determine the maximum tolerated dose of hypofractionated radiation in brain metastases greater than 4.2 cc in volume. Although SRS alone produces fewer neurocognitive side effects than SRS + WBRT, further studies are needed to characterize the neurocognitive effects of SRS as it becomes more widely used for treatment of multiple brain metastases.[16] Current efforts include an ongoing prospective trial in The Netherlands, which will evaluate cognitive functioning in patients with 1 to 10 brain metastases undergoing SRS (ClinicalTrials.gov identifier: NCT02953756).

In summary, radiation therapy has been a cornerstone of the treatment of brain metastases, which now largely involves SRS. As molecular and immunotherapy improve in efficacy, the timing and use of SRS will continue to evolve as a treatment modality for patients with multiple brain metastases.

SURGERY

As aforementioned, surgical resection provides a diagnosis, while removing mass effect, particularly for larger masses greater than 3 cm in diameter (because smaller lesions are often deemed more appropriate for SRS[33]) and lesions with edema. A classic randomized study by Patchell and colleagues[34] showed that surgical resection improves survival when combined with WBRT, compared with WBRT alone, in patients with KPS $\geq$70 and nonradiosensitive primary tumor with only 1 intracranial metastasis. Importantly, patients in the "surgery + WBRT" group maintained an average of 38 weeks of functionally independent survival (KPS $\geq$70) versus 8 weeks in the "WBRT-only" group. A similar randomized study by Vecht and colleagues[35] showed both a survival benefit and functionally independent survival benefit in patients who underwent surgery + WBRT, versus those who underwent WBRT alone. One study failed to show survival benefit of surgery + WBRT versus WBRT alone,[36] but was noted to have unequal distribution of primary pathologic conditions between patient groups.[37] Surgery is typically combined with radiation therapy in order to prevent local recurrence, with the exception of lung cancers with targetable mutations and melanoma treated with immunotherapy.[38] One randomized study showed that surgery alone results in a 57% chance of local recurrence at 12 months, compared with surgery + postoperative SRS, which results in a 28% chance of local recurrence.[39] However, this study found no difference in survival or functionally independent survival between the 2 groups. Similarly, 2 other randomized studies found that "surgery only" is associated with higher rates of local recurrence compared with "surgery + WBRT,"[17,40] yet neither study showed a difference in overall survival between the 2 groups. This lack of survival benefit of WBRT has led to it being considered "salvage therapy" or in cases not amenable to SRS.[41] Patients who undergo complete resection of a solitary brain metastasis may currently undergo SRS, whereas the role of immunotherapy in place of SRS has led to active investigation on timing and efficacy of SRS.

To summarize, the benefit of surgery in addition to radiation is well established for patients with metastasis. In general, postoperative radiotherapy following surgical resection continues to be used to prevent intracranial recurrence. It is important to reconsider the above historic studies,[34,35] which use "WBRT only" as a comparison, in light of SRS being increasingly favored as the postoperative radiation therapy of choice (see "Radiation therapy" discussion above).[42] Although SRS has emerged as an attractive option for postoperative radiotherapy, the role of SRS in patients with multiple brain metastases and in patients undergoing targeted therapy or immunotherapy is under active investigation.

Some retrospective cohort studies specifically examine the role of surgical resection in patients with multiple metastases. Most of these studies are at least 15 years old, in the setting of postoperative WBRT,[43–46] making the results difficult to interpret in light of current trends toward postoperative SRS. Nonetheless, 1 study showed that patients with 2 to 3 brain metastases, who underwent surgical resection of all metastases, experienced postoperative survival rates similar to those with single metastases who underwent resection.[43] Of note, patients who underwent multiple craniotomies during a single operation did not experience higher complication rates than those who underwent single craniotomies. A 2018 study,[46] which included only patients with KPS greater than 60, produced similar results, with no difference in survival between patients who underwent resection of a single brain metastasis and those who underwent resection of 2 to 3 brain metastasis. In another study, Paek and colleagues[44] showed no difference in mean survival time (MST) between patients with single (8-month MST) or 2 to 3 metastases (11-month MST) who underwent surgical resection (**Table 1**). Furthermore, there was no difference in MST between patients with multiple metastases who underwent resection of all intracerebral metastases, versus those who underwent resection of just 1 metastasis. Importantly, recursive partitioning analysis[a] (RPA) class I patients with multiple metastases had MST of 16.1 months, versus RPA class II or III patients, with MST of 7 months, suggesting that the dogma that those with higher functional status show increased postsurgical survival holds true, even in the presence of multiple metastases. Most postsurgical patients in the study by Paek and colleagues underwent WBRT and could be compared favorably with SRS cases in the RTOG 9508 trial, which included a WBRT + SRS group. RTOG 9508-eligible patients with multiple metastases in the Paek and colleagues[25] study had an MST of 11 months, versus 5.8 months for patients with multiple metastases in the RTOG 9508 trial. However, given that the study by Paek and colleagues represents data from a retrospective cohort study, it remains difficult to ascertain whether surgery truly holds a survival benefit for multiple metastases over SRS. Nonetheless, these studies suggest that surgical resection of 2 to 3 metastases is safe and possibly prolongs survival, particularly in patients with higher functional status.

Posterior fossa metastases account for approximately 20% of all intracranial metastases.[47] In patients with brain metastases (single or multiple), the presence of a posterior fossa metastasis is associated with poorer survival, compared with those with supratentorial metastases alone.[48–50] Posterior fossa metastases must be evaluated for their size, perilesional edema, and associated mass effect to determine the role of surgical resection. Lesions with compression of the cerebellum fourth ventricle, or brainstem, may warrant

[a]Recursive partitioning analysis (RPA) is a prognostic classification system derived from a database of 3 trials conducted by the Radiation Therapy Oncology Group[72]: RPA class 1: patients with KPS 70+, age ≤65, and controlled primary tumor with no extracranial metastases; RPA class 3: patients with KPS less than 70; RPA class 2: all others.

Table 1
Retrospective studies capturing overall survival following surgical resection of multiple brain metastases

	Study Type	Performance	Patients (No.)	Groups	Overall Survival (mo)
Bindal et al,[43] 1993	Retrospective	92% with KPS >70	208	A: Single lesion B: Multiple (2–3 lesions)	A: 8 B: 11
Paek et al,[44] 2005	Retrospective	KPS >60	62	A: Single lesion B: Multiple (2–3 lesions)	A: 17.4 B: 14.6
Salvati et al,[46] 2018	Retrospective	KPS 70 (mean)	82	A: Multiple lesions, >1 lesion left unresected B: Multiple lesions, all resected C: Single lesion, resected	A: 6 B: 14 C: 14

Trials may be able to include more w disseminated disease.

surgical resection based on the tumor size or the tumor's edema regardless of size.[51] Given the concern of acute neurologic decline from compression of the fourth ventricle resulting in hydrocephalus, surgery often is essential to relieve mass effect through mechanical cytoreduction.[52] Multiple retrospective cohort studies have shown that surgery combined with SRS or WBRT confers a survival benefit over SRS alone[53,54] or surgery alone.[51,53] One study in patients, most of whom had multiple intracranial metastases, with at least 1 metastasis in the posterior fossa, showed that aggressive treatment combining WBRT, SRS, and resection of the posterior fossa metastasis provided the best survival benefit in RPA class II patients,[55] compared with SRS, WBRT, or surgery alone. Thus, although the above studies are retrospective, and are therefore confounded by the determination of suitability for patients who underwent postoperative radiation therapy, the existing data support the use of multimodal therapy, including both surgery and postoperative radiotherapy in patients with posterior fossa metastases. With regard to surgical morbidity, 1 study of 44 operated patients reported 9 postoperative complications, 8 of which were cerebellar hematomas requiring surgical evacuation,[56] whereas another study of 50 operated patients reported just 2 complications.[52] This second study also demonstrated that 76% of patients avoided undergoing subsequent procedures for cerebrospinal fluid diversion despite more than half of patients having hydrocephalus on initial imaging.[52] In summary, evaluation and treatment of patients with posterior fossa metastasis, by a neurosurgeon experienced in treating brain metastases,

may confer immediate symptom relief and likely survival benefit, in addition to sparing patients further cerebrospinal fluid diversion procedures.

TARGETED THERAPY

Systemic therapies are emerging as promising options for some patients with brain metastasis. Although traditional chemotherapies showed limited efficacy in patients because of their inability to cross the blood-brain barrier, small-molecule tyrosine kinase inhibitors have shown activity in the central nervous system.[57,58] Specific targets thus far include ALK and EGFR in NCSLC, the MAPK pathway in melanoma, and HER2 in breast cancer. In a prospective study of patients with NSCLC harboring EGFR mutations, 83% of patients had a partial response (>30% decrease in diameter of all intracranial metastases) to gefitinib or erlotinib, both EGFR inhibitors.[59] Osimertinib, a third-generation irreversible EGFR inhibitor, has shown progression-free survival benefit in EGFR-mutant NSCLC over gefitinib and erlotinib, even in patients with brain metastases.[60] In a phase 2 study that deployed WBRT in addition to EGFR inhibitor erlotinib, patients with EGFR mutations had a survival benefit (median survival 19.1 months) when compared with historical controls with EGFR mutations (12.4 months by 1 account[61]).[62] More than 70% of patients included in this study had 4 or more brain metastases, although subgroup analyses quantifying the effect of number of metastases on survival benefit are not reported.[62] Overall, data addressing whether addition of an EGFR inhibitor to radiation therapy is beneficial in patients with EGFR mutation are limited. Therefore, although there are promising initial results for intracranial effect of new systemic therapies in NSCLC, how they will fit into prevailing treatments such as radiotherapy and surgery is an area of active investigation.

Targeted therapy has also made inroads in metastatic melanoma, particularly in tumors harboring BRAF mutations. One prospective trial showed that the BRAF inhibitor vemurafenib reduced the diameter of intracranial metastasis by 30% or more, in 7 out of 19 patients with intracranial metastases.[63] More than half of the patients included in this study had 3 or more brain lesions, although the small number of enrolled patients may have prevented meaningful subgroup analysis. Another prospective study of vemurafenib in patients with BRAF-mutant tumors, all of whom had brain metastases and 55% of whom had multiple brain metastases, showed an 18% best overall response for intracranial metastases.[64] Subgroup analysis showed that patients with higher numbers of intracranial lesions tended to have poorer response rates, although the data are somewhat limited by small sample size. Interestingly, however, the rate of response was not significantly different for patients who had previously undergone WBRT, SRS, and/or surgery, suggesting that local treatments did not select for brain metastases resistant to vemurafenib. A similar finding was reported for dabrafenib, which was found to have similar efficacy in both a treatment-naïve group and a previously treated (surgery, WBRT, or SRS) group.[65] More recently, dabrafenib combined with trametinib, an MEK inhibitor, produced an intracranial response rate of 58% in patients with BRAF V600E-mutated tumors,[66] showing that the MAPK pathway can be targeted combinatorially.[66,67] At least half of the patients enrolled in all of these dabrafenib studies had 2 or more brain lesions[65–67]; however, subgroup analyses are not available to address response rates in those with more metastases. Finally, whether combinatorial targeted therapy may be safely and effectively used in conjunction with SRS is currently being investigated by a phase 2 clinical trial (ClinicalTrials.gov identifier: NCT02974803).

IMMUNOTHERAPY

Immunotherapy has made significant inroads in brain metastasis, with several phase 2 clinical trials being completed in the past decade. A 2012 study showed that ipilimumab, which targets CTLA-4, showed activity in melanoma patients with brain metastases, particularly in those with stable, asymptomatic metastases who were not on corticosteroids.[68] A more recent study showed that ipilimumab combined with PD-1 inhibitor nivolumab halted intracranial progression at 6 months in 64% of metastatic melanoma patients and also provided an increased intracranial benefit compared with ipilimumab alone.[69] Patients with more than 1 lesion were included in these ipilimumab studies. In fact, half of the patients included in the ipilimumab + nivolumab study had more than 1 brain lesion, with a subgroup analysis showing that patients with 1 to 2 brain lesions had intracranial response rates slightly (but not significantly) higher than those with 3+ brain lesions.[69] Finally, immunotherapy shows efficacy outside of metastatic melanoma. PD-1 inhibitor pembrolizumab produced a brain metastasis response rate (assessed by radiographic response[70]) of 33% in patients with NSCLC.[71] Importantly, patients with multiple brain metastases (mean = 6 lesions) were included, and patients with brain metastasis diameters of up to 2 cm were enrolled. Of the 6 out of 18 patients who showed clinical benefit in NSCLC, 5 had more than 2 brain lesions. Ongoing clinical trials, such as one that includes an SRS + pembrolizumab arm for melanoma patients with brain metastases (ClinicalTrials.gov identifier: NCT02886585), will further clarify how immunotherapy can be used alongside localized treatment modalities. Furthermore, as the survival of patients with brain metastasis increases, trials will be able to include patients with higher intracranial disease burden.

SUMMARY

The management of brain metastases is multifaceted and multidisciplinary and includes surgery, radiation, and systemic therapy. Patients with multiple metastases (particularly those with 2–3 metastases) lend to a multidisciplinary discussion to determine the best strategy for therapy. Patients with a large lesion, or one with significant edema, patients with mass effect, or patients suffering symptoms from their lesion, benefit from surgical resection followed by radiation and/or molecular or targeted therapy. As new therapies are developed, investigation is needed to compare the efficacy, timing, and combination of therapies to help guide the future of management of patients with brain metastases.

ACKNOWLEDGMENTS

The project described was supported by award Number T32GM007753 from the National Institute of General Medical Sciences (C.K.S.). The content is solely the responsibility of the authors and does not necessarily represent the official views of the

National Institute of General Medical Sciences or the National Institutes of Health.

DISCLOSURE

Dr Nahed BV is a consultant for Genentech-Roche, Tesaro, Angiochem, Lilly, Elevate-Bio. He received speaker's Honoraria from Merck and Genentech-Roche. He received research funds from Lilly, Merck, and BMS.

REFERENCES

1. Nayak L, Lee EQ, Wen PY. Epidemiology of brain metastases. Curr Oncol Rep 2012;14(1):48–54.
2. Stelzer K. Epidemiology and prognosis of brain metastases. Surg Neurol Int 2013;4(Suppl4). https://doi.org/10.4103/2152-7806.111296.
3. Niwińska A, Murawska M. New breast cancer recursive partitioning analysis prognostic index in patients with newly diagnosed brain metastases. Int J Radiat Oncol Biol Phys 2012;82(5):2065–71.
4. Barker FG. Craniotomy for the resection of metastatic brain tumors in the U.S., 1988-2000: decreasing mortality and the effect of provider caseload. Cancer 2004;100(5):999–1007.
5. Delattre JY, Krol G, Thaler HT, et al. Distribution of brain metastases. Arch Neurol 1988;45(7):741–4.
6. Nussbaum ES, Djalilian HR, Cho KH, et al. Brain metastases: histology, multiplicity, surgery, and survival. Cancer 1996;78(8):1781–8.
7. Fabi A, Felici A, Metro G, et al. Brain metastases from solid tumors: disease outcome according to type of treatment and therapeutic resources of the treating center. J Exp Clin Cancer Res 2011;30(1):10.
8. Giordana MT, Cordera S, Boghi A. Cerebral metastases as first symptom of cancer: a clinico-pathologic study. J Neurooncol 2000;50(3):265–73.
9. Pope WB. Brain metastases: neuroimaging. vol. 149. 2018. https://doi.org/10.1016/B978-0-12-811161-1.00007-4.
10. Brastianos PK, Carter SL, Santagata S, et al. Genomic characterization of brain metastases reveals branched evolution and potential therapeutic targets. Cancer Discov 2015;5(11):1164–77.
11. Orozco JIJ, Knijnenburg TA, Manughian-Peter AO, et al. Epigenetic profiling for the molecular classification of metastatic brain tumors. Nat Commun 2018;9(1). https://doi.org/10.1038/s41467-018-06715-y.
12. Soffietti R, Abacioglu U, Baumert B, et al. Diagnosis and treatment of brain metastases from solid tumors: guidelines from the European Association of Neuro-Oncology (EANO). Neuro Oncol 2017;19(2):162–74.
13. Chu FCH, Hilaris BB. Value of radiation therapy in the management of intracranial metastases. Cancer 1961;14(3):577–81.
14. Lokich JJ. Management of cerebral metastasis. JAMA 1975;234(7):748–51.
15. Chang EL, Wefel JS, Hess KR, et al. Neurocognition in patients with brain metastases treated with radiosurgery or radiosurgery plus whole-brain irradiation: a randomised controlled trial. Lancet Oncol 2009;10(11):1037–44.
16. Brown PD, Jaeckle K, Ballman KV, et al. Effect of radiosurgery alone vs radiosurgery with whole brain radiation therapy on cognitive function in patients with 1 to 3 brain metastases a randomized clinical trial. JAMA 2016;316(4):401–9.
17. Kocher M, Soffietti R, Abacioglu U, et al. Adjuvant whole-brain radiotherapy versus observation after radiosurgery or surgical resection of one to three cerebral metastases: results of the EORTC 22952-26001 study. J Clin Oncol 2011;29(2):134–41.
18. Aoyama H, Shirato H, Tago M, et al. Stereotactic radiosurgery plus whole-brain radiation therapy vs stereotactic radiosurgery alone for treatment of brain metastases: a randomized controlled trial. J Am Med Assoc 2006;295(21):2483–91.
19. Wefel JS, Parsons MW, Gondi V, et al. 1st edition. Neurocognitive aspects of brain metastasis, vol. 149. Elsevier B.V.; 2018. https://doi.org/10.1016/B978-0-12-811161-1.00012-8.
20. Brown PD, Pugh S, Laack NN, et al. Memantine for the prevention of cognitive dysfunction in patients receiving whole-brain radiotherapy: a randomized, double-blind, placebo-controlled trial. Neuro Oncol 2013;15(10):1429–37.
21. Brown PD, Ahluwalia MS, Khan OH, et al. Whole-brain radiotherapy for brain metastases: evolution or revolution? J Clin Oncol 2018;36(5):483–91
22. Mulvenna P, Nankivell M, Barton R, et al. Dexamethasone and supportive care with or without whole brain radiotherapy in treating patients with non-small cell lung cancer with brain metastases unsuitable for resection or stereotactic radiotherapy (QUARTZ): results from a phase 3, non-inferiority. Lancet 2016;388(10055):2004–14.
23. Gondi V, Pugh SL, Tome WA, et al. Preservation of memory with conformal avoidance of the hippocampal neural stem-cell compartment during whole-brain radiotherapy for brain metastases (RTOG 0933): a phase II multi-institutional trial. J Clin Oncol 2014;32(34):3810–6.
24. Gondi V, Deshmukh S, Brown PD, et al. NRG oncology CC001: a phase III trial of hippocampal avoidance (HA) in addition to whole-brain radiotherapy (WBRT) plus memantine to preserve neurocognitive function (NCF) in patients with brain metastases (BM). J Clin Oncol 2019;37(15_suppl):2009.

25. Andrews DW, Scott CB, Sperduto PW, et al. Whole brain radiation therapy with or without stereotactic radiosurgery boost for patients with one to three brain metastases: phase III results of the RTOG 9508 randomised trial. Lancet 2004;363:1665–72.

26. Kondziolka D, Patel A, Lunsford LD, et al. Stereotactic radiosurgery plus whole brain radiotherapy versus radiotherapy alone for patients with multiple brain metastases. Int J Radiat Oncol Biol Phys 1999;45(2):427–34.

27. Yamamoto M, Kawabe T, Sato Y, et al. Stereotactic radiosurgery for patients with multiple brain metastases: a case-matched study comparing treatment results for patients with 2-9 versus 10 or more tumors. J Neurosurg 2014;121(December):16–25.

28. Limon D, McSherry F, Herndon J, et al. Single fraction stereotactic radiosurgery for multiple brain metastases. Adv Radiat Oncol 2017;2(4):555–63.

29. Shaw E, Scott C, Souhami L, et al. Single dose radiosurgical treatment of recurrent previously irradiated primary brain tumors and brain metastases: final report of RTOG protocol 90-05. Int J Radiat Oncol Biol Phys 2000;47(2):291–8.

30. Minniti G, D'Angelillo RM, Scaringi C, et al. Fractionated stereotactic radiosurgery for patients with brain metastases. J Neurooncol 2014;117(2):295–301.

31. Kirkpatrick JP, Soltys SG, Lo SS, et al. The radiosurgery fractionation quandary: single fraction or hypofractionation? Neuro Oncol 2017;19(2):ii38–49.

32. Kohutek ZA, Yamada Y, Chan TA, et al. Long-term risk of radionecrosis and imaging changes after stereotactic radiosurgery for brain metastases. J Neurooncol 2015;125(1):149–56.

33. Schöggl A, Kitz K, Reddy M, et al. Defining the role of stereotactic radiosurgery versus microsurgery in the treatment of single brain metastases. Acta Neurochir (Wien) 2000;142(6):621–6.

34. Patchell RA, Tibbs PA, Walsh JW, et al. A randomized trial of surgery in the treatment of single metastases to the brain. N Engl J Med 1990; 322(8):494–500.

35. Vecht CJ, Haaxma-Reiche H, Noordijk EM, et al. Treatment of single brain metastasis: radiotherapy alone or combined with neurosurgery. Ann Neurol 1993;33(6):583–90.

36. Mintz AH, Kestle J, Rathbone MP, et al. A randomized trial to assess the efficacy of surgery in addition to radiotherapy in patients with a single cerebral metastasis. Cancer 1996;78(7):1470–6.

37. Vogelbaum MA, Suh JH. Resectable brain metastases. J Clin Oncol 2006;24(8):1289–94.

38. Fecci PE, Champion CD, Hoj J, et al. The evolving modern management of brain metastasis. Clin Cancer Res 2019;1–11.

39. Mahajan A, Ahmed S, McAleer MF, et al. Post-operative stereotactic radiosurgery versus observation for completely resected brain metastases: a single-centre, randomised, controlled, phase 3 trial. Lancet Oncol 2017;18(8):1040–8.

40. Patchell RA, Tibbs PA, Regine WF, et al. Postoperative radiotherapy in the treatment of single metastases to the brain: a randomized trial. J Am Med Assoc 1998;280(17):1485–9.

41. Kalkanis SN, Kondziolka D, Gaspar LE, et al. The role of surgical resection in the management of newly diagnosed brain metastases: a systematic review and evidence-based clinical practice guideline. J Neurooncol 2010;96(1):33–43.

42. Brown PD, Ballman KV, Cerhan JH, et al. Postoperative stereotactic radiosurgery compared with whole brain radiotherapy for resected metastatic brain disease (NCCTG N107C/CEC·3): a multicentre, randomised, controlled, phase 3 trial. Lancet Oncol 2017; 18(8):1049–60.

43. Bindal RK, Sawaya R, Leavens ME, et al. Surgical treatment of multiple brain metastases. J Neurosurg 1993;79(2):210–6.

44. Paek SH, Audu PB, Sperling MR, et al. Reevaluation of surgery for the treatment of brain metastases: review of 208 patients with single or multiple brain metastases treated at one institution with modern neurosurgical techniques. Neurosurgery 2005; 56(5):1021–33.

45. Pollock BE, Brown PD, Foote RL, et al. Properly selected patients with multiple brain metastases may benefit from aggressive treatment of their intracranial disease. J Neurooncol 2003;61(1):73–80.

46. Salvati M, Tropeano MP, Maiola V, et al. Multiple brain metastases: a surgical series and neurosurgical perspective. Neurol Sci 2018;39(4):671–7.

47. Ghia A, Tomé WA, Thomas S, et al. Distribution of brain metastases in relation to the hippocampus: implications for neurocognitive functional preservation. Int J Radiat Oncol Biol Phys 2007;68(4):971–7.

48. Wroński M, Arbit E. Resection of brain metastases from colorectal carcinoma in 73 patients. Cancer 1999;85(8):1677–85.

49. Wronski M, Arbit E, Burt M, et al. Survival after surgical treatment of brain metastases from lung cancer: a follow-up study of 231 patients treated between 1976 and 1991. J Neurosurg 1995;83(4):605–16.

50. Chaichana KL, Rao K, Gadkaree S, et al. Factors associated with survival and recurrence for patients undergoing surgery of cerebellar metastases. Neurol Res 2014;36(1):13–25.

51. Sunderland GJ, Jenkinson MD, Zakaria R. Surgical management of posterior fossa metastases. J Neurooncol 2016;130(3):535–42.

52. Ghods A, Byrne R, Munoz L. Surgical treatment of cerebellar metastases. Surg Neurol Int 2011;2(1):159.

53. Yoshida S, Takahashi H. Cerebellar metastases in patients with cancer. Surg Neurol 2009;71(2):184–7.

54. Ampil FL, Nanda A, Willis BK, et al. Metastatic disease in the cerebellum: the LSU experience in 1981-1993. Am J Clin Oncol 1996;19(5). Available at: https://journals.lww.com/amjclinicaloncology/Fulltext/1996/10000/Metastatic_Disease_in_the_Cerebellum__The_LSU.16.aspx.

55. Kanner AA, Suh JH, Siomin VE, et al. Posterior fossa metastases: aggressive treatment improves survival. Stereotact Funct Neurosurg 2003;81(1–4): 18–23.

56. Pompili A, Carapella CM, Cattani F, et al. Metastases to the cerebellum. Results and prognostic factors in a consecutive series of 44 operated patients. J Neurooncol 2008;88(3):331–7.

57. Venur VA, Karivedu V, Ahluwalia MS. 1st edition. Systemic therapy for brain metastases, vol. 149. Elsevier B.V.; 2018. https://doi.org/10.1016/B978-0-12-811161-1.00011-6.

58. Rick JW, Shahin M, Chandra A, et al. Systemic therapy for brain metastases. Crit Rev Oncol Hematol 2019;142:44–50.

59. Park SJ, Kim HT, Lee DH, et al. Efficacy of epidermal growth factor receptor tyrosine kinase inhibitors for brain metastasis in non-small cell lung cancer patients harboring either exon 19 or 21 mutation. Lung Cancer 2012;77(3):556–60.

60. Soria JC, Ohe Y, Vansteenkiste J, et al. Osimertinib in untreated EGFR-mutated advanced non-small-cell lung cancer. N Engl J Med 2018;378(2):113–25.

61. Hsu F, De Caluwe A, Anderson D, et al. EGFR mutation status on brain metastases from non-small cell lung cancer. Lung Cancer 2016;96:101–7.

62. Welsh JW, Komaki R, Amini A, et al. Phase II trial of erlotinib plus concurrent whole-brain radiation therapy for patients with brain metastases from non-small-cell lung cancer. J Clin Oncol 2013;31(7): 895–902.

63. Dummer R, Goldinger SM, Turtschi CP, et al. Vemurafenib in patients with BRAFV600 mutation-positive melanoma with symptomatic brain metastases: final results of an open-label pilot study. Eur J Cancer 2014;50(3):611–21.

64. McArthur GA, Maio M, Arance A, et al. Vemurafenib in metastatic melanoma patients with brain metastases: an open-label, single-arm, phase 2, multicentre study. Ann Oncol 2017;28(3):634–41.

65. Long GV, Trefzer U, Davies MA, et al. Dabrafenib in patients with Val600Glu or Val600Lys BRAF-mutant melanoma metastatic to the brain (BREAK-MB): a multicentre, open-label, phase 2 trial. Lancet Oncol 2012;13(11):1087–95.

66. Davies MA, Saiag P, Robert C, et al. Dabrafenib plus trametinib in patients with BRAFV600-mutant melanoma brain metastases (COMBI-MB): a multicentre, multicohort, open-label, phase 2 trial. Lancet Oncol 2017;18(7):863–73.

67. Holbrook K, Lutzky J, Davies MA, et al. Intracranial antitumor activity with encorafenib plus binimetinib in patients with melanoma brain metastases: a case series. Cancer 2019;1–8. https://doi.org/10.1002/cncr.32547.

68. Margolin K, Ernstoff MS, Hamid O, et al. Ipilimumab in patients with melanoma and brain metastases : an open-label, phase 2 trial. Lancet Oncol 2020;13(5): 459–65.

69. Tawbi HA, Forsyth PA, Algazi A, et al. Combined nivolumab and ipilimumab in melanoma metastatic to the brain. N Engl J Med 2018;379(8):722–30.

70. Eisenhauer EA, Therasse P, Bogaerts J, et al. New response evaluation criteria in solid tumours: revised RECIST guideline (version 1.1). Eur J Cancer 2009; 45(2):228–47.

71. Goldberg SB, Gettinger SN, Mahajan A, et al. Pembrolizumab for patients with melanoma or non-small-cell lung cancer and untreated brain metastases: early analysis of a non-randomised, open-label, phase 2 trial. Lancet Oncol 2016;17(7): 976–83.

72. Gaspar L, Scott C, Rotman M, et al. Recursive partitioning analysis (RPA) of prognostic factors in three Radiation Therapy Oncology Group (RTOG) brain metastases trials. Int J Radiat Oncol Biol Phys 1997;37(4):745–51.

The Role of Stereotactic Biopsy in Brain Metastases

Kenny K.H. Yu, MBBS, PhD, Ankur R. Patel, MD, Nelson S. Moss, MD*

KEYWORDS

- Stereotactic techniques • Image-guided biopsy • Brain metastasis

KEY POINTS

- Stereotactic biopsy plays an important role in the management of brain metastases, and knowledge of underlying pathobiology of brain metastases can influence treatment decisions.
- Neurosurgical oncology surgeons should be aware of the techniques available to perform stereotactic biopsies and the current and potential future indications of stereotactic biopsies. Recent scientific research has uncovered differences in the underlying pathbiology of brain metastases compared to their primary counterparts.
- The utility of a stereotactic biopsy must be evaluated on a case by case basis and is influenced by a patient's history and radiographic findings.

INTRODUCTION

Brain metastases (BrM) are the most common brain tumor in adults, affecting some 8 to 14 people per 100,000 population, and up to 20% of patients with cancer will develop clinically- or radiographically-apparent BrM.[1–5] Some autopsy studies estimate the true incidence as higher still, up to some 30% of patients with cancer,[6] and this represents a growing concern for oncologists and neurosurgeons. The most common primary brain-metastatic malignancies are lung and breast carcinomas and melanoma, largely reflecting their extra-central nervous system (CNS) incidence, and colorectal and renal cell carcinomas are also seen in increasing numbers.[3] Although improvements in CNS and extracranial systemic control have resulted in steady gains in both survival and morbidity, the prognosis for BrM remains poor with a median survival of between 4 and 8 months depending on cancer type[3,7,8] and a 5-year survival rate of 2.4%.[9]

Prognosis and thus decision support for treatment remains partially defined with considerable variation among cancer types and molecular features, systemic manifestations, and treatment tolerance.[8,10] Prognostic factors include age, performance status, extra-cranial metastases, treatment history, and most importantly the extent of primary disease control.[1,9,11,12] The degree of heterogeneity in primary cancer types and the patterns of BrM spread and presentations presents formidable challenges in terms of patient stratification and management. To this end, data-driven prognostic models have been used to better understand key risk factors. These models include Recursive Partition Analysis (RPA)[11,13] and Graded Prognostic Assessment,[14–16] which takes into account histologic grade, and now also integrates molecular subtype.[17] However, the clinical value of these scoring systems has historically been limited due to the overall poor prognosis of BrM.[1,9]

Symptomatic patients are often referred to neurosurgical care for signs and symptoms of raised intracranial pressure such as headache and papilledema, focal neurologic deficits such as weakness or paresthesias, obstruction of cerebrospinal fluid (CSF) flow, acute lesional hemorrhage (more frequently seen in renal cell carcinoma and melanoma), and for seizure. BrM should always be suspected in patients with previous known primary cancers, and diagnosis can be made on neuroimaging modalities such as computed tomography (CT) and MRI. The gold

Department of Neurosurgery and Brain Metastasis Center, Memorial Sloan Kettering Cancer Center, 1275 York Avenue, New York City, NY 10065, USA
* Corresponding author.
E-mail address: mossn@mskcc.org

Neurosurg Clin N Am 31 (2020) 515–526
https://doi.org/10.1016/j.nec.2020.06.002
1042-3680/20/© 2020 Elsevier Inc. All rights reserved.

standard for diagnosis remains histologic diagnosis, which can be obtained either through surgical resection or stereotactic biopsy.

From a neurosurgical standpoint, resective surgery is offered for palliation, for example, where significant mass effect is present, for local control of large or growing previously irradiated tumors, and where cerebrospinal fluid obstruction is present or imminent. Retrospective studies support the contention that RPA class I patients benefit the most from surgical resection of solitary BrM.[18–21] This, along with the opportunity to concurrently obtain tissue diagnosis, has made surgical resection a primary treatment option in solitary and oligometastatic BrM, with several studies showing no differences in surgical outcome for patients with solitary versus with up to 4 lesions.[22–26] Neurosurgical considerations include patient fitness; extent of extracranial disease; and lesion site, number, and proximity to eloquent brain circuitry.

In contrast, stereotactic biopsy for BrM is reserved for patients where there is diagnostic uncertainty, such as suspected BrM of unknown primary or ring-enhancing lesions in immunocompromised patients that could represent either infectious or neoplastic lesions or in patients with conditions with lesions that can mimic BrM, such as tumefactive multiple sclerosis or primary central nervous system lymphoma. Additional indications may also include patients with multiple primary cancers or those individuals who have undergone stereotactic radiosurgery (SRS) in order to differentiate between radiation necrosis and viable tumor growth. Recent advances in our understanding of the pathobiology of brain tumors, however, may further expand the role of stereotactic biopsy.

PATHOBIOLOGY OF BRAIN METASTASES

The formation of BrM requires successful adaptation to the CNS host environment through a process of intravasation of tumor cells into the circulation, followed by adhesive arrest in the circulation, extravasation, and migration across the blood brain barrier and successful growth within the brain. A growing literature is defining tumor-specific biological adaptations that allow for CNS-specific colonization. For example, expression of specific adhesion molecules including the membrane glycosyltransferase ST6GALNAC5 in breast cancer tumor cells has been shown to facilitate circulating tumor cell adhesion to brain endothelial cells.[1,27] Tumor and stromal angiogenic factors such as vascular endothelial growth factor and matrix metalloproteinases, permeability

factors, and integrins all aid in the successful extravasation and establishment of a metastatic foothold in the CNS.[1]

Significantly, recent studies have highlighted clonal divergence between primary lesions and their BrM counterparts. BrM seem to harbor, with some frequency, targetable mutations that are not identifiable in the primary tumor or in other sampled extracranial metastases. Examples include epidermal growth factor receptor (EGFR) and anaplastic large-cell lymphoma kinase (ALK) gene rearrangements in lung cancer BrM formation, which are increasingly targetable CNS-penetrant tyrosine kinase inhibitors.[28–30] In addition, breast cancer subtype switching in the CNS has been established.[31,32]

Data gleaned from comparative analyses of paired BrM and primary cancer tissue from individual patients may inform mechanisms of CNS-specific metastasis. Mutations, not yet targetable, which have been implicated in the development of BrM in lung adenocarcinomas include upregulation of Wnt signaling pathways via LEF1, HOXB mutation, and mutations in the serpin family. The Wnt/TCF signaling pathways have been shown to mediate chemotactic invasion in lung adenocarcinoma models,[33] and tumor-derived serpins suppress of stromal antitumor effects through inhibition of plasminogen activators.[34] Breast cancer BrM display differential patterns of BrM propensity depending on subtype, with human epidermal growth factor receptor 2 (HER-2) positive and triple-negative subtypes most likely to metastasize to the brain; however, the extent to which this may be related to relative CNS inefficacy of established systemic treatment options remains to be determined. Genetic driver mutations commonly found in breast BrM include the tumor suppressors TP53 and PTEN, as well as ERBB2, CCDN1, CDKN2A, and CDKN2B, reflecting common alterations particularly in triple-negative and HER-2 positive subtypes. Activation of the PI3K-AKT pathway is correlated with poor prognosis in patients with breast BrM, and the presence of membranous HER-3 may provide an escape mechanism for PI3K pathway inhibitors.[35] In melanoma BrM, mutations in BRAF, CTNNB1, and RAS-family genes have been implicated[36,37] with BrM response seen in patients treated with BRAF inhibitors such as dabrafenib.[38] The PI3K-Akt pathway was again associated with poorer overall survival.[39] There has also been interest in studying the immune cell infiltrate of melanoma and other cancer BrM due to the efficacy of immune checkpoint inhibitors in systemic melanoma,[40,41] and further understanding in the immune composition of BrM, including how microglia/macrophages modulate the adaptive immune response,[42,43] may help guide immunotherapeutic options for BrM going forward. Mutations in PTEN, CDKN2A, and PIK3CA are also found in RCC BrM but not in the primary tumor,[2,44] and PIK3CA, KRAS, and NRAS have been described in high frequency in CRC BrM.[45]

The most mature studies in this domain have identified nonconcordance between primary and BrM in both breast cancer and lung cancers.[46,47] Specifically, patients with squamous lung cancer harboring aberrations in the PI3K pathway had a much higher incidence of BrM. In addition, whole exome sequencing of 2 patients with paired primary and BrM samples suggested a high degree of clonal divergence.[48] This view was reinforced in 86 paired primary-BrM samples from patients across a range of cancers.[2] Consistent clonal divergence between primary and BrM mutations was again noted; however, BrM retained similarities between distinctly sampled BrM within the same patient, suggesting although clonally divergent from their primary lesion, BrM are relatively homogenous within the CNS. Overall, 53% of patients in their cohort had clinically actionable mutations exclusive to the BrM, which were not detected in the primary tumor. The relative homogeneity of intracranial lesions suggests that biopsy of even a single CNS BrM may yield significant information regarding the mutational profile of the BrM population as a whole within a given patient.

This information provides a paradigm shift in the way BrM are viewed. Instead of considering BrM as simply part of a monolithic primary disease that has spread beyond the confines of systemic treatment and control, these data suggest that BrM harbor subclones that have specifically adapted to the brain host environment, which may harbor unique fitness attributes that cannot be identified by simply sampling their parent tumor.

Information regarding unique BrM specific–mutations is of high clinical value, as it implies potential differential susceptibility to drug targeting and radiation treatment. The availability and rapid fall in the cost of genetic sequencing has led to many institutions, including our own, to offer targeted gene panel sequencing to patients in order to find actionable mutations. For example, the Memorial Sloan Kettering—Integrated Mutational Profiling of Actionable Cancer Targets (MSK-IMPACT) uses next-generation sequencing to target several hundred genes at depth.[49,50] The increasing availability of such assays can provide BrM-specific mutation information with the potential to change neurosurgical management of BrM in the future.

THE ROLE OF STEREOTACTIC BIOPSY IN BRAIN METASTASES

Historically, BrM were treated with whole brain radiation therapy (WBRT) alone. However, despite good local and distant CNS control[51] and in the setting of improved cancer survival overall making long-term considerations increasingly relevant, WBRT has fallen into disfavor for patients with few metastases owing to its associated significant long-term neurocognitive dysfunction.[52] In recent decades, the effectiveness of systemic therapies for cancers that commonly metastasize to the brain such as lung, breast, and melanoma has significantly improved from the historical figure of less than 6 months frequently cited, with the advent of targeted therapies and checkpoint inhibitors.[51,53–55]

The management of BrM can be divided into patient factors and disease factors—patient factors include age/performance status, concomitant disease, and tolerance for a procedure under general anesthesia and disease factors include the status of extracranial disease, number and location of lesions, and suitability for resective surgery. Neurosurgery is offered to patients who are able to tolerate an operation with stable extracranial disease and have a suspected primary cancer that is not considered highly radiosensitive, such as small cell lung cancer, germ cell tumors, or leukemia.[26,56,57]

Currently the predominant indication for BrM biopsy is diagnostic uncertainty, typically where concurrent patient features such as lack of other metastatic disease, immunosuppression/associated infections, or autoimmune disease can give rise to plausible differentials. Surgery in these instances would provide definitive tissue diagnosis that could substantially alter the treatment goals.

The possibility of identifying targetable molecular lesions, exclusive to a given BrM, may increase the role of BrM sampling. Although this is not currently common practice, advances in oncology drug design and recent studies informing the evolution of BrM may alter this, should drugs ultimately prove more effective/less toxic than current paradigms including whole-brain and targeted irradiation, which are very effective at controlling individual BrM. Specifically, identification of alterations that are effectively treated with CNS-penetrant agents, or those that are associated with treatment resistance, has the potential to abrogate the need for potentially more toxic therapy, for example, WBRT with its concomitant neurotoxicity, or to point to a change in targeted therapeutic strategy. Key examples include EGFR mutations and ALK rearrangement in non-small cell lung cancer, with targeted and CNS-penetrant tyrosine kinase inhibitors available.[58,59] Specific EGFR mutations such as T790M are effectively targeted by third-generation TKIs including osimertinib, which have the added advantage of traversing the blood brain barrier and demonstrate clinical activity against BrM.[29,60] Knowledge of specific resistance mutations such as C797S[61] and EGFR L858R could potentially guide treatment decisions.[61,62] Similarly, ALK-positive (EML4-ALK fusion) BrM have seen responses to ALK inhibitors such as crizotinib, and newer drugs in the same family, such as alectinib, ceritinib, brigatinib, and loratinib, have defined CNS penetration profiles.[63] In breast cancer, HER-2 lesions constitute some half of all patients with BrM, in part owing to the success of antibody-based (and non–CNS-penetrant) therapy including trastuzumab and its derivative antibody-drug conjugate ado-trastuzumab emtansine.[64,65] In this setting, CNS-penetrant small molecule TKIs including tucatinib and neratinib have been developed with promising early data.[66,67] Cell cycle inhibitors targeting CDK4/6 such as abemaciclib have been used in estrogen or progesterone receptor positive breast BrM.[68,69] In BRAF-mutated melanoma BrM, BRAF inhibitors such as dabrafenib and vemurafenib have shown efficacy, both alone and in combination with MAPK inhibitors such as trametinib; however response durability is unclear.[70] Melanoma has also seen significant extracranial and CNS efficacy with immunotherapy. Immune checkpoint inhibitors such as drugs against PD-L1 (pembrolizumab and nivolumab) and CTLA-4 (ipilimumab) have conferred response rates of up to 60% when given in combination (ipilimumab and nivolumab).[70,71] An increased understanding of the underlying immunomodulatory mechanisms will help better identify biomarkers to help response prediction. Finally, as more BrM are treated with focused stereotactic irradiation modalities and immunotherapy, radiation necrosis and pseudoprogression are inflammatory entities that are increasingly encountered as radiographic differentials that can mimic disease progression and raise more situations of diagnostic uncertainty that would require definitive surgical biopsy.

One of the key findings from BrM genome sequencing studies is the presence of private, discordant clinically actionable mutations in BrM, which were found to be prevalent in 53% of lesions by Brastianos and colleagues.[2] It should be noted, however, that the term "clinically actionable" was based on genes identified on the TARGET computational platform by Van Allen and colleagues,[72] which are not fully clinically validated. The decision

to operate must therefore necessarily be multifactorial, taking into account the tumor's location and ease with which a sample can be taken, the performance status of the patient, extent of disease and known features of the primary cancer, and likelihood of identifying a treatment-altering paradigm, against the risk of surgery and nondiagnostic yield, with the current mainstay indication remaining radiologically inconclusive lesions.

SURGICAL CONSIDERATIONS

Although a detailed description of the different technical methods of brain biopsy is beyond the scope of this review, there are many different techniques for brain biopsy currently in use. In general, BrM biopsy follows the same principles as other forms of brain biopsy with the overall goal of providing a safe, consistent, and reliable method of sampling lesional tissue. The principles of stereotaxy apply whether frame-based or frameless methods are used, with consideration given to the depth and location of the lesion, relevant neurovascular anatomy, and the constraints of stereotaxy based on preoperative imaging. Recent series have reported diagnostic yields of 84% to 100% with frame-based techniques and 86.6% to 100% with frameless procedures.[73,74] Future diagnostic yields may improve with the increased utilization of sequencing for pathognomonic genomic alterations, which may prove more sensitive than histologic diagnosis alone. Overall morbidity from stereotactic biopsy has been reported in 3.8% to 27.8% of frame-based procedures and 1.3% to 24.5% of frameless procedures.[73,74] Postbiopsy radiographic hemorrhage rates ranged from 5.1% to 14.2% and 2.4% to 17.8% in frame-based and frameless methods and lower for clinical neurologic deficits at 2.8% to 13.9% and 1.3% to 15.4% for frame-based and frameless biopsies, respectively.[73] A more recent meta-analysis has described the morbidity associated with frame-based biopsy to be between 0.7% and 13% and mortality between 0% and 4%. Asymptomatic hemorrhages can be up to 59%; however, symptomatic hemorrhages have been reported in about 0% to 8.6% of cases. Neurologic deficits are most frequently the result of larger hemorrhages.[73,74] Freehand biopsy no longer has a role in the modern neurosurgical setting.

Biopsy has 4 important procedural steps: (1) identification of a safe trajectory, (2) burr hole placement, (3) maintenance of trajectory alignment, and (4) fixation at target point. Complications related to stereotactic biopsy are invariably caused by an issue with one or more of these factors.

Frame-based methods have advantages of being more accurate but require rigid fixation of the patient while the patient undergoes cross-sectional imaging, typically CT and in some cases MRI. Frames used include the Leksell frame or Cosman-Roberts-Wallis frame. Burr hole placement, maintenance of trajectory, and fixation at target is facilitated by attachment of a targeting frame. The slightly higher accuracy for frame-based techniques has led to some surgeons preferring this approach for deep cranial lesions.

Frameless techniques use alignment tools such as the Stealth Navigus (Medtronic, USA) or Brainlab VarioGuide (Brainlab AG, Germany), and navigation systems based on surface facial landmarks cross-referenced to an array fixed to the operating table allow matching of preoperative imaging to the patient. Burr hole placement is planned using neuronavigation. The biopsy itself is typically performed through a linear scalp incision. Either a twist drill or a high-speed drill is then used to make a burr hole. Some systems use burr hole anchors secured to the calvarium to help maintain the trajectory of the biopsy catheter (**Fig. 1**) (Navigus, Medtronic, USA). Alternatively, manufacturers such as Brainlab have engineered a multiarticulated arm (VarioGuide) connected to a fixed array to help neuronavigate and maintain the trajectory (Brainlab AG, Germany). Use of intraoperative CT or MRI can be used to both improve registration and confirm biopsy location. These modalities can also be used following completion of the biopsy to evaluate for intracranial hemorrhage. For suspected metastases, which are typically encapsulated, there is the additional possibility that a tumor could be deflected by a blunt needle end, a yielding nondiagnostic biopsy despite correct alignment. For this reason, our center advocates intraoperative pathologic assessment and in some cases intraoperative imaging. Intraoperative modalities such as simulated

Raman scattering microscopy may increase the rapidity of pathologic evaluation.[75]

The one significant drawback for both frame-based and frameless technologies is the reliance on historical images to plan trajectories. Brain compliance and its lack of rigid fixation to the dura allows for some deformation during surgery. In atrophic brains or those not harboring large/edema-inducing tumors, significant deviations can exist between the preoperative image and the actual trajectory in a phenomenon known as brain shift.[76,77] In principle it is therefore advisable when performing biopsies to minimize the dural opening to prevent CSF egress as much as possible when passing the needle. Alternatively, repeat imaging can be performed intraoperatively to verify neuronavigational registration and landmarks before cannula insertion.

Novel technologies such as interventional MRI (MRI Interventions, USA) use MR compatible, non-ferromagnetic instruments to perform biopsies while the patient is within the bore of the MRI scanner. Planning is first performed by scanning the patient with a series of fiducials to select the optimum entry point, then with the patient anesthetized and in the MR scanner, a linear incision is made and bone-anchored burr hole needle holder is placed, the trajectory is calculated, and the needle is sequentially advanced and adjusted through serial imaging as it traverses the parenchyma to its target. This technique allows near real-time visualization of the target and trajectory and can warn the clinician of any adverse complication during the procedure. An alternative but slightly more cost-effective method of providing real time guidance is to use ultrasound-guided biopsy. This method, which has been successfully used in other neurosurgical conditions,[78–80] uses a combination of a burr hole ultrasound probe along with a needle attachment to the probe to provide real-time image guidance to the target of interest; this

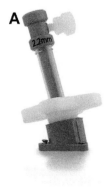 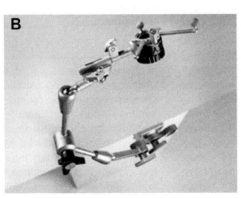

Fig. 1. (*A*) Navigus brain biopsy bone anchor. (*B*) VarioGuide biopsy arm. ([*A*] Reprinted with the permission of Medtronic, Inc. ©; and [*B*] *Courtesy of* Brainlab AG.)

can be used in after standard neuronavigation is used to plan the entry burr hole to achieve real-time image-guided sampling. The drawback of this technique is its poor resolution, particularly at depth and making it not suitable for some small lesions; however, this technique when fused with intraoperative CT/MRI can help improve accuracy even further.

Robotic-assisted surgery is an area that has been gradually gaining acceptance in stereotaxy procedures. Although the procedure differs slightly between manufacturers, all currently available systems rely on preoperative registration and calibration of the robot arm, with robotic assistance in maintaining trajectory and target guidance. Robotic-assisted stereotactic biopsy has been described in multiple case series combining to a total of more than 290 procedures in a variety of different robotic systems. The quoted in vivo target error rate ranged from 0.81 ± 0.39 (ROSA, Zimmer Biomet) to 3.3 to 4.5 mm (Zeiss MKM). The nondiagnostic rate (NDR), hemorrhage rate (HmR), and mortality rate (MR) compares favorably with manual methods, with robotic series having an NDR of 2.2% to 4.3%, HmR of 8% to 10%, and MR of 0% to 0.5% compared with NDR of 0.3% to 4.2%, HmR of 3.7% to 8.8%, and MR of 0% to 2% in frameless manual case series and NDR of 9%, HmR of 3.5% to 8.0%, and MR of 0.7% to 1% in frame-based series.[81] The drawbacks, however, for these newer methods include the need for dedicated or adapted suites for equipment, and the time and resources required to perform these procedures may limit their use in the wider neurosurgical setting at least in the short term.

Other related surgical treatment options include laser interstitial thermal therapy (LITT). Available at several specialized centers, this technique relies on the guided insertion of catheters to the target lesions, which provides target ablation through directed thermal energy (NeuroBlate, Monteris Medical Inc, USA). A 1024 nm laser probe (which can be robotically advanced) in combination with real-time MRI thermometry predicts lesioning area. This approach has recently been used to treat patients who have undergone SRS for BrM with evidence of progression and/or radionecrosis.[82,83] With adequate planning for suspected LITT-responsive diseases (tumors, radionecrosis), stereotactic biopsy can be performed either within the bore of an MRI scanner just before LITT or in an operating room immediately before transfer to a diagnostic MRI with the requisite LITT setup. Should sampling volume be a concern, another option is to use tubular-based stereotactic biopsy

methods, which permits sampling of greater volumes down the same trajectory path.[84]

In rare cases where intraoperative pathology is not available or conclusive, intraoperative or immediate postoperative MRI can be useful to confirm that the correct location has been biopsied; in the absence of easily accessible MRI facilities, some surgeons have described gently introducing a small amount of air after biopsy in order to highlight the biopsy location on postoperative CT.

Finally, the capacity to obtain rapid histologic diagnosis has the potential to increase diagnostic yield through immediate resampling in cases where the tissue obtained is nondiagnostic and to reduce the risk of morbidity from oversampling once a diagnosis has been made. Traditionally this has been performed through intraoperative frozen section analysis; however, the practicalities and speed of obtaining an expert neuropathological opinion intraoperatively varies among institutions. Alternative intraoperative methods have been developed, including optical spectroscopy, such as Raman spectroscopy, which differentiates tissue types based on their light scattering properties. This modality provides the intraoperative pathologist with images within minutes, and a recent study has described its use in combination with machine learning classifier algorithms to identify malignant tissue types in the intraoperative setting to obtain near real-time tissue diagnosis.[75,82] Other technologies currently in development include optical coherence tomography, multiphoton microscopy, video-rate structured illumination microscopy, ex vivo fluorescence confocal microscopy, and ambient mass spectrometry, all aiming to improve the speed, accuracy, and yield of stereotactic biopsies.[85,86]

CLINICAL CASE STUDIES

The following illustrative cases discuss clinical scenarios where the results of a stereotactic biopsy helped to guide therapy in patients with brain metastases.

Case 1

A 60-year-old man with a history of metastatic melanoma presented subacutely with right hemiparesis. He had been receiving treatment with ipilimumab and nivolumab, but therapy was discontinued due to the development of hypophysitis. Brain MRI revealed a 2.5-cm ring-enhancing cystic mass in the left internal capsule without associated restricted diffusion (**Fig. 2**A, B). There were no other intracranial lesions. Given the cystic appearance in the setting of an existing immune-

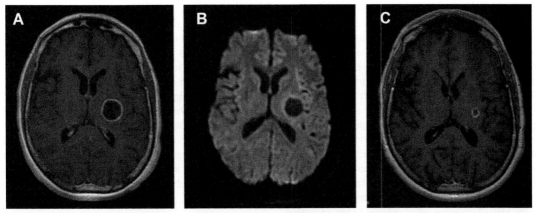

Fig. 2. Axial T1-weighted postcontrast (*A*) and diffusion-weighted images (DWI) (*B*). MRIs of the brain demonstrating a ring-enhancing mass in the left internal capsule without restricted diffusion. Two-month posttreatment axial T1-weighted postcontrast MRI of the brain (*C*) reveals a resolving cystic lesion.

related adverse event from checkpoint inhibitor therapy, the differential diagnosis included a metastatic lesion as well as an inflammatory or infectious process. Given that surgical resection would carry significant risk of neurologic morbidity, consideration was given to stereotactic biopsy and cyst decompression, which would permit simultaneous histologic diagnosis and lesion size reduction, which, if the lesion was confirmed to be metastatic, would also provide an attractive radiosurgical target. The decision was therefore made to perform a stereotactic biopsy of the cyst wall with aspiration of its intrinsic fluid. The biopsy and aspiration were performed through a single burr hole using a frameless technique. The pathology returned as metastatic melanoma, and the patient underwent postoperative stereotactic radiosurgery to a significantly reduced clinical treatment volume for definitive treatment of the metastasis. Two-month posttreatment brain MRI revealed a resolving lesion (**Fig. 2**C). The patient went on to develop progression of disease 10 months later confirmed on brain MRI with perfusion. He was retreated with proton beam radiotherapy at that time and continues to undergo regular radiographic surveillance.

Case 2

A 73-year-old woman with a history of recently treated small cell lung cancer, previously treated stage I triple-negative breast cancer, and anal cancer presented with headaches and double vision. MRI of the brain revealed a 1.5-cm right occipital mass centered around the calcarine sulcus (**Fig. 3**A). The patient was advised to undergo stereotactic biopsy for diagnosis given the history of multiple primary cancers, with possible differential

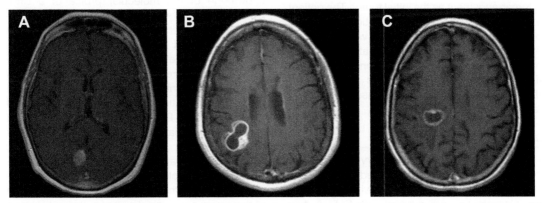

Fig. 3. (*A*) Axial T1-weighted postcontrast MRI of the brain displaying a right medial occipital enhancing mass. (*B*) Axial T1-weighted postcontrast MRI of the brain demonstrates a multicystic peripherally enhancing mass in the right parietal lobe. (*C*) Axial T1-weighted postcontrast MRI of the brain demonstrates a ring-enhancing mass in the right posterior frontal lobe.

diagnoses including glioblastoma in the setting of a potential underlying germline cancer syndrome. In addition, the patient was hesitant to undergo resective surgery in part due to the risk of worsened postoperative vision and the possibility that this tumor represented progression of small cell disease, which is known to be both radiosensitive and likely to progress throughout the CNS. The biopsy was performed through a single burr hole using a frameless technique. The pathology returned as metastatic small cell lung cancer, and given this diagnosis, the patient received whole brain radiation therapy as opposed to stereotactic radiosurgery. Germline genetic testing was unrevealing. Brain MRI 2 months after whole brain radiation therapy revealed complete resolution of the metastatic lesion with no new areas of disease.

Case 3

An 83-year-old woman with a history of ALK-rearranged lung cancer and without active disease for over 10 years presented with left-sided tremulousness, bradykinesia, and micrographia. Her symptoms responded to treatment with carbidopa-levodopa consistent with a diagnosis of Parkinson disease, but MRI of the brain performed in workup for this revealed a multicystic peripherally enhancing mass in the right parietal lobe (**Fig. 3**B). Systemic restaging was negative for extracranial metastatic disease, and the differential diagnosis included BrM versus high-grade glioma. Given the patient's advanced age, relative morbidity of open craniotomy and resection, and potential responsiveness of the lesion to ALK inhibition via CNS-penetrant agents, the decision was made to proceed with stereotactic biopsy. The biopsy was performed through a single burr hole using a frameless technique. The pathology returned as metastatic lung adenocarcinoma with the same ALK rearrangement as the initial tumor. The patient subsequently underwent stereotactic radiosurgery for treatment of the lesion that was stable on repeat MRI 1 month following treatment. Confirmation of ALK rearrangement opened the option of treatment of her CNS-centric process with ALK-directed therapy should her disease progress despite radiosurgery.

Case 4

A 54-year-old woman with a history of metastatic small cell lung carcinoma developed a right frontal lobe metastasis that was treated with single fraction stereotactic radiosurgery (18 Gy). A few months later, she developed left-sided weakness. Brain MRI revealed an increase in the size of the treated lesion (**Fig. 3**C). The time course and

imaging characteristics were ambiguous, with the concurrent possibilities of either disease progression or radiation necrosis, which are managed differently. As a result, a stereotactic biopsy was recommended for diagnosis. The biopsy was performed through a single burr hole using a frameless technique. Pathology revealed predominantly radiation necrosis with a very small amount of viable tumor. As a result, the patient was advised to undergo laser interstitial thermal therapy for treatment that was performed as a separate operation 2 weeks later, and this achieved durable local control at 31-month follow-up.

DISCUSSION

Stereotactic biopsy is a safe and reliable procedure that has been a core part of neurosurgical practice. Its accuracy and yield have steadily improved with the advent of frame-based and frameless techniques, and associated morbidity and mortality are low.[73] Clinically, stereotactic biopsy of BrM has traditionally been seldom performed except for specific indications such as lesions that are inconclusive on radiology and not amenable to open resection or suspected BrM with unknown primary source. This core diagnostic indication is unlikely to change in the near future.

However, the increasingly prominent role of surgical resection for oligometastatic BrM will provide molecular profiling data that will further increase our understanding of the pathobiology of BrM. The finding that BrM harbor targetable mutations, in some cases divergent from the patients' primary tumor site, suggests that in the future a lower clinical threshold may be applied for biopsying lesions in easily accessible locations in order to gain knowledge of the molecular profile of a BrM. Currently the overall proportion of clinically actionable genetic alterations detected exclusively in BrM via targeted genetic sequencing panels remains small. Whether such management strategies become more commonplace will depend on the establishment of clinically validated and actionable mutations for BrM. Knowledge of disease-specific BrM mutational profiles, along with an ever-expanding menu of CNS-penetrant agents targeting specific molecular pathways, will influence treatment decisions, and it is expected that the role of stereotactic biopsy will assume a more prominent role in the armamentarium of the neuro-oncological surgeon. It is anticipated that molecular profiling of both primary and BrM will become *de rigeur*, and our experience with routine tumor panel sequencing at our institution has highlighted situations where biopsy may be particularly helpful. Currently, however, the primary indication remains diagnosis for unresectable or ambiguous but otherwise treatable lesions.

From a surgical perspective, safety and good technique remain critical regardless of modality, and technological improvements in this domain including image guidance, robotic-assisted surgery, and simultaneous therapeutic strategies such as LITT are, together with improving survival of patients with cancer in general, likely to usher an increase in the biopsy of BrM. Therefore, a good understanding of principles of stereotaxy, its utility and risk profile, and familiarity with a variety of techniques that obtain safe, reliable, and accurate results are essential skills in modern neurosurgical practice.

ACKNOWLEDGMENTS

This research was funded in part through the National Institutes of Health/National Cancer Institute (NIH/NCI) Cancer Center Support Grant P30 CA008748.

DISCLOSURE

NM has consulted for AstraZeneca. KY has consulted for BrainLab AG.

REFERENCES

1. Achrol AS, Rennert RC, Anders C, et al. Brain metastases. Nat Rev Dis Primers 2019;5(1):5.
2. Brastianos PK, Carter SL, Santagata S, et al. Genomic Characterization of Brain Metastases Reveals Branched Evolution and Potential Therapeutic Targets. Cancer Discov 2015;5(11):1164–77.
3. Nayak L, Lee EQ, Wen PY. Epidemiology of brain metastases. Curr Oncol Rep 2012;14(1):48–54.
4. Barnholtz-Sloan JS, Sloan AE, Davis FG, et al. Incidence proportions of brain metastases in patients diagnosed (1973 to 2001) in the Metropolitan Detroit Cancer Surveillance System. J Clin Oncol 2004; 22(14):2865–72.
5. Tabouret E, Chinot O, Metellus P, et al. Recent trends in epidemiology of brain metastases: an overview. Anticancer Res 2012;32(11):4655–62.
6. Tsukada Y, Fouad A, Pickren JW, et al. Central nervous system metastasis from breast carcinoma. Autopsy study. Cancer 1983;52(12):2349–54.
7. Berghoff Anna S, Schur S, Füreder Lisa M, et al. Descriptive statistical analysis of a real life cohort of 2419 patients with brain metastases of solid cancers. ESMO Open 2016;1(2):e000024.
8. Nieder C, Spanne O, Mehta MP, et al. Presentation, patterns of care, and survival in patients with brain metastases: what has changed in the last 20 years? Cancer 2011;117(11):2505–12.
9. Hall WA, Djalilian HR, Nussbaum ES, et al. Long-term survival with metastatic cancer to the brain. Med Oncol 2000;17(4):279–86.
10. Jung J, Tailor J, Dalton E, et al. Management evaluation of metastasis in the brain (MEMBRAIN)—a United Kingdom and Ireland prospective, multicenter observational study. Neuro Oncol Pract 2019. https://doi.org/10.1093/nop/npz063.
11. Gaspar L, Scott C, Rotman M, et al. Recursive partitioning analysis (RPA) of prognostic factors in three Radiation Therapy Oncology Group (RTOG) brain metastases trials. Int J Radiat Oncol Biol Phys 1997;37(4):745–51.
12. Nieder C, Grosu Anca L, Gaspar Laurie E. Stereotactic radiosurgery (SRS) for brain metastases: a systematic review. Radiat Oncol 2014;9:155.
13. Gaspar LE, Scott C, Murray K, et al. Validation of the RTOG recursive partitioning analysis (RPA) classification for brain metastases. Int J Radiat Oncol Biol Phys 2000;47(4):1001–6.
14. Sperduto PW, Berkey B, Gaspar LE, et al. A new prognostic index and comparison to three other indices for patients with brain metastases: an analysis of 1,960 patients in the RTOG database. Int J Radiat Oncol Biol Phys 2008;70(2):510–4.
15. Sperduto PW, Kased N, Roberge D, et al. Summary report on the graded prognostic assessment: an accurate and facile diagnosis-specific tool to estimate survival for patients with brain metastases. J Clin Oncol 2012;30(4):419–25.
16. Sperduto PW, Kased N, Roberge D, et al. Effect of tumor subtype on survival and the graded prognostic assessment for patients with breast cancer and brain metastases. Int J Radiat Oncol Biol Phys 2012;82(5):2111–7.
17. Sperduto PW, Yang TJ, Beal K, et al. Estimating Survival in Patients With Lung Cancer and Brain Metastases: An Update of the Graded Prognostic Assessment for Lung Cancer Using Molecular Markers (Lung-molGPA). JAMA Oncol 2017;3(6):827–31.
18. Tendulkar Rahul D, Liu Stephanie W, Barnett Gene H, et al. RPA classification has prognostic significance for surgically resected single brain metastasis. Int J Radiat Oncol Biol Phys 2006;66(3):810–7.
19. Patchell RA, Tibbs PA, Walsh JW, et al. A randomized trial of surgery in the treatment of single metastases to the brain. N Engl J Med 1990; 322(8):494–500.
20. Vecht CJ, Haaxma-Reiche H, Noordijk EM, et al. Treatment of single brain metastasis: radiotherapy alone or combined with neurosurgery? Ann Neurol 1993;33(6):583–90.

21. Mintz AH, Kestle J, Rathbone MP, et al. A randomized trial to assess the efficacy of surgery in addition to radiotherapy in patients with a single cerebral metastasis. Cancer 1996; 78(7):1470–6.

22. Salvati M, Tropeano MP, Maiola V, et al. Multiple brain metastases: a surgical series and neurosurgical perspective. Neurol Sci 2018;39(4):671–7.

23. Bindal Rajesh K, Sawaya R, Leavens Milam E, et al. Surgical treatment of multiple brain metastases. J Neurosurg 1993;210–6. https://doi.org/10.3171/jns.1993.79.2.0210.

24. Hatiboglu MA, Wildrick DM, Sawaya R. The role of surgical resection in patients with brain metastases. Ecancermedicalscience 2013;7:308.

25. Melike M. Surgical treatment of brain metastasis: A review. Clin Neurol Neurosurg 2012;1–8. https://doi.org/10.1016/j.clineuro.2011.10.013.

26. Ranasinghe Moksha G, Sheehan Jonas M. Surgical management of brain metastases. Neurosurg Focus 2007;1–7. https://doi.org/10.3171/foc.2007.22.3.3.

27. Bos Paula D, Zhang Xiang H-F, Nadal C, et al. Genes that mediate breast cancer metastasis to the brain. Nature 2009;459(7249):1005–9.

28. Peters S, Camidge DR, Shaw AT, et al. Alectinib versus Crizotinib in Untreated ALK-Positive Non–Small-Cell Lung Cancer. N Engl J Med 2017; 829–38. https://doi.org/10.1056/nejmoa1704795.

29. Mok TS, Wu Y-L, Ahn M-J, et al. Osimertinib or Platinum-Pemetrexed in EGFR T790M-Positive Lung Cancer. N Engl J Med 2017;376(7):629–40.

30. Ko R, Kenmotsu H, Serizawa M, et al. Frequency of EGFR T790M mutation and multimutational profiles of rebiopsy samples from non-small cell lung cancer developing acquired resistance to EGFR tyrosine kinase inhibitors in Japanese patients. BMC Cancer 2016;16(1):864.

31. Priedigkeit N, Hartmaier RJ, Chen Y, et al. Intrinsic Subtype Switching and Acquired ERBB2/HER2 Amplifications and Mutations in Breast Cancer Brain Metastases. JAMA Oncol 2017;3(5):666–71.

32. Hulsbergen AFC, Claes A, Kavouridis VK, et al. Subtype switching in breast cancer brain metastases: a multicenter analysis. Neuro Oncol 2020. https://doi.org/10.1093/neuonc/noaa013.

33. Nguyen DX, Chiang AC, Zhang Xiang H-F, et al. WNT/TCF signaling through LEF1 and HOXB9 mediates lung adenocarcinoma metastasis. Cell 2009; 138(1):51–62.

34. Valiente M, Obenauf AC, Jin X, et al. Serpins promote cancer cell survival and vascular co-option in brain metastasis. Cell 2014;156(5):1002–16.

35. Kodack DP, Askoxylakis V, Ferraro GB, et al. The brain microenvironment mediates resistance in luminal breast cancer to PI3K inhibition through HER3 activation. Sci Transl Med 2017;eaal4682. https://doi.org/10.1126/scitranslmed.aal4682.

36. Chen G, Chakravarti N, Aardalen K, et al. Molecular profiling of patient-matched brain and extracranial melanoma metastases implicates the PI3K pathway as a therapeutic target. Clin Cancer Res 2014; 20(21):5537–46.

37. Jakob John A, Bassett Roland L, Ng Chaan S, et al. NRAS mutation status is an independent prognostic factor in metastatic melanoma. Cancer 2012; 4014–23. https://doi.org/10.1002/cncr.26724.

38. Long Georgina V, Trefzer U, Davies MA, et al. Dabrafenib in patients with Val600Glu or Val600Lys BRAF-mutant melanoma metastatic to the brain (BREAK-MB): a multicentre, open-label, phase 2 trial. Lancet Oncol 2012;13(11): 1087–95.

39. Bucheit AD, Chen G, Siroy A, et al. Complete Loss of PTEN Protein Expression Correlates with Shorter Time to Brain Metastasis and Survival in Stage IIIB/C Melanoma Patients with BRAFV600 Mutations. Clin Cancer Res 2014;5527–36. https://doi.org/10.1158/1078-0432.ccr-14-1027.

40. Kluger HM, Zito CR, Barr ML, et al. Characterization of PD-L1 Expression and Associated T-cell Infiltrates in Metastatic Melanoma Samples from Variable Anatomic Sites. Clin Cancer Res 2015;3052–60. https://doi.org/10.1158/1078-0432.ccr-14-3073.

41. Strik HM, Stoll M, Meyermann R. Immune cell infiltration of intrinsic and metastatic intracranial tumours. Anticancer Res 2004;24(1):37–42.

42. He BP, Wang JJ, Zhang X, et al. Differential reactions of microglia to brain metastasis of lung cancer. Mol Med 2006;12(7-8):161–70.

43. Lorger M, Felding-Habermann B. Capturing changes in the brain microenvironment during initial steps of breast cancer brain metastasis. Am J Pathol 2010;176(6):2958–71.

44. Han Catherine H, Brastianos Priscilla K. Genetic Characterization of Brain Metastases in the Era of Targeted Therapy. Front Oncol 2017;7:230.

45. Yaeger R, Cowell E, Chou Joanne F, et al. RAS mutations affect pattern of metastatic spread and increase propensity for brain metastasis in colorectal cancer. Cancer 2015;121(8):1195–203.

46. Koo JS, Jung W, Jeong J. Metastatic breast cancer shows different immunohistochemical phenotype according to metastatic site. Tumori 2010;96(3): 424–32.

47. Adamo B, Deal AM, Burrows E, et al. Phosphatidylinositol 3-kinase pathway activation in breast cancer brain metastases. Breast Cancer Res 2011;13(6): R125.

48. Paik Paul K, Johnson Melissa L, D'Angelo Sandra P, et al. Driver mutations determine survival in smokers and never-smokers with stage IIIB/IV lung adenocarcinomas. Cancer 2012;118(23):5840–7.

49. Zehir A, Benayed R, Shah RH, et al. Mutational landscape of metastatic cancer revealed from

prospective clinical sequencing of 10,000 patients. Nat Med 2017;23(6):703–13.

50. Cheng DT, Mitchell TN, Zehir A, et al. Memorial Sloan Kettering-Integrated Mutation Profiling of Actionable Cancer Targets (MSK-IMPACT): A Hybridization Capture-Based Next-Generation Sequencing Clinical Assay for Solid Tumor Molecular Oncology. J Mol Diagn 2015;251–64. https://doi.org/10.1016/j.jmoldx.2014.12.006.

51. Patchell RA, Tibbs PA, Regine WF, et al. Postoperative radiotherapy in the treatment of single metastases to the brain: a randomized trial. JAMA 1998; 280(17):1485–9.

52. Gaspar LE, Prabhu RS, Hdeib A, et al. Congress of Neurological Surgeons Systematic Review and Evidence-Based Guidelines on the Role of Whole Brain Radiation Therapy in Adults With Newly Diagnosed Metastatic Brain Tumors. Neurosurgery 2019; 84(3):E159–62.

53. Brahmer J, Reckamp KL, Baas P, et al. Nivolumab versus Docetaxel in Advanced Squamous-Cell Non-Small-Cell Lung Cancer. N Engl J Med 2015; 373(2):123–35.

54. Brahmer JR, Tykodi SS, Chow LQM, et al. Safety and Activity of Anti–PD-L1 Antibody in Patients with Advanced Cancer. N Engl J Med 2012;2455–65. https://doi.org/10.1056/nejmoa1200694.

55. Larkin J, Chiarion-Sileni V, Gonzalez R, et al. Combined Nivolumab and Ipilimumab or Monotherapy in Untreated Melanoma. N Engl J Med 2015; 373(1):23–34.

56. Kalkanis SN, Kondziolka D, Gaspar LE, et al. The role of surgical resection in the management of newly diagnosed brain metastases: a systematic review and evidence-based clinical practice guideline. J Neuro-Oncology 2010;33–43. https://doi.org/10.1007/s11060-009-0061-8.

57. Moravan MJ, Fecci PE, Anders CK, et al. Current multidisciplinary management of brain metastases. Cancer 2020. https://doi.org/10.1002/cncr.32714.

58. Welsh JW, Komaki R, Amini A, et al. Phase II Trial of Erlotinib Plus Concurrent Whole-Brain Radiation Therapy for Patients With Brain Metastases From Non–Small-Cell Lung Cancer. J Clin Oncol 2013;895–902. https://doi.org/10.1200/jco.2011.40.1174.

59. Ceresoli GL, Cappuzzo F, Gregorc V, et al. Gefitinib in patients with brain metastases from non-small-cell lung cancer: a prospective trial. Ann Oncol 2004; 1042–7. https://doi.org/10.1093/annonc/mdh276.

60. Ahn M-J, Kim D-W, Cho BC, et al. Phase I study (BLOOM) of AZD3759, a BBB penetrable EGFR inhibitor, in patients with TKI-naïve, EGFRm NSCLC with CNS metastases. J Clin Oncol 2017. https://doi.org/10.1200/jco.2017.35.15_suppl.2006.

61. Thress KS, Paweletz CP, Felip E, et al. Acquired EGFR C797S mutation mediates resistance to AZD9291 in non-small cell lung cancer harboring EGFR T790M. Nat Med 2015;21(6):560–2.

62. Ercan D, Choi HG, Yun CH, et al. EGFR Mutations and Resistance to Irreversible Pyrimidine-Based EGFR Inhibitors. Clin Cancer Res 2015; 3913–23. https://doi.org/10.1158/1078-0432.ccr-14-2789.

63. Lin NU, Freedman RA, Miller K, et al. Determination of the maximum tolerated dose (MTD) of the CNS penetrant tyrosine kinase inhibitor (TKI) tesevatinib administered in combination with trastuzumab in HER2 patients with metastatic breast cancer (BC). J Clin Oncol 2016;514. https://doi.org/10.1200/jco.2016.34.15_suppl.514.

64. Kabraji S, Ni J, Lin NU, et al. Drug Resistance in HER2-Positive Breast Cancer Brain Metastases: Blame the Barrier or the Brain? Clin Cancer Res 2018;24(8):1795–804.

65. Askoxylakis V, Kodack DP, Ferraro GB, et al. Antibody-based therapies for the treatment of brain metastases from HER2-positive breast cancer: time to rethink the importance of the BBB? Breast Cancer Res Treat 2017;467–8. https://doi.org/10.1007/s10549-017-4351-0.

66. Murthy RK, Loi S, Okines A, et al. Tucatinib, Trastuzumab, and Capecitabine for HER2-Positive Metastatic Breast Cancer. N Engl J Med 2020;382(7): 597–609.

67. Freedman RA, Gelman RS, Anders CK, et al. TBCRC 022: A Phase II Trial of Neratinib and Capecitabine for Patients With Human Epidermal Growth Factor Receptor 2-Positive Breast Cancer and Brain Metastases. J Clin Oncol 2019;37(13): 1081–9.

68. Venur V, Leone J. Targeted Therapies for Brain Metastases from Breast Cancer. Int J Mol Sci 2016; 1543. https://doi.org/10.3390/ijms17091543.

69. Sahebjam S, Le RE, Kulanthaivel P, et al. Assessment of concentrations of abemaciclib and its major active metabolites in plasma, CSF, and brain tumor tissue in patients with brain metastases secondary to hormone receptor positive (HR) breast cancer. J Clin Oncol 2016;526. https://doi.org/10.1200/jco.2016.34.15_suppl.526.

70. Davies MA, Saiag P, Robert C, et al. Dabrafenib plus trametinib in patients with BRAFV600-mutant melanoma brain metastases (COMBI-MB): a multicentre, multicohort, open-label, phase 2 trial. Lancet Oncol 2017;863–73. https://doi.org/10.1016/s1470-2045(17)30429-1.

71. Tawbi HA, Forsyth PA, Algazi A, et al. Combined Nivolumab and Ipilimumab in Melanoma Metastatic to the Brain. N Engl J Med 2018;722–30. https://doi.org/10.1056/nejmoa1805453.

72. Van Allen EM, Wagle N, Stojanov P, et al. Whole-exome sequencing and clinical interpretation of formalin-fixed, paraffin-embedded tumor samples

to guide precision cancer medicine. Nat Med 2014; 682–8. https://doi.org/10.1038/nm.3559.

73. Dhawan S, He Y, Bartek J, et al. Comparison of Frame-Based Versus Frameless Intracranial Stereotactic Biopsy: Systematic Review and Meta-Analysis. World Neurosurg 2019;607–16.e4. https://doi.org/10.1016/j.wneu.2019.04.016.

74. Riche M, Amelot A, Peyre M, et al. Complications after frame-based stereotactic brain biopsy: a systematic review. Neurosurg Rev 2020. https://doi.org/10.1007/s10143-019-01234-w.

75. Orringer DA, Pandian B, Niknafs YS, et al. Rapid intraoperative histology of unprocessed surgical specimens via fibre-laser-based stimulated Raman scattering microscopy. Nat Biomed Eng 2017;1. https://doi.org/10.1038/s41551-016-0027.

76. Miyagi Y, Shima F, Sasaki T. Brain shift: an error factor during implantation of deep brain stimulation electrodes. J Neurosurg 2007;989–97. https://doi.org/10.3171/jns-07/11/0989.

77. Li Z, Zhang JG, Ye Y, et al. Review on Factors Affecting Targeting Accuracy of Deep Brain Stimulation Electrode Implantation between 2001 and 2015. Stereotact Funct Neurosurg 2016;351–62. https://doi.org/10.1159/000449206.

78. Manfield JH, Yu KKH. Real-time ultrasound-guided external ventricular drain placement: technical note. Neurosurg Focus 2017;43(5):E5.

79. Padayachy LC, Fieggen G. Intraoperative Ultrasound-Guidance in Neurosurgery. World Neurosurg 2014;e409–11. https://doi.org/10.1016/j.wneu.2013.09.052.

80. Moiyadi AV, Unsgård G. Navigable ultrasound, 3D ultrasound and fusion imaging in neurosurgery. In: Francesco P, Luigi S, Alberto M, et al, editors. Intraoperative Ultrasound (IOUS) in Neurosurgery: From Standard B-mode to Elastosonography. Cham, Springer: International Publishing; 2016. p. 135–45.

81. Fomenko A, Serletis D. Robotic stereotaxy in cranial neurosurgery: a qualitative systematic review. Neurosurgery 2018;83(4):642–50.

82. Hollon TC, Pandian B, Adapa AR, et al. Near real-time intraoperative brain tumor diagnosis using stimulated Raman histology and deep neural networks. Nat Med 2020;26(1):52–8.

83. Ahluwalia M, Barnett GH, Deng D, et al. Laser ablation after stereotactic radiosurgery: a multicenter prospective study in patients with metastatic brain tumors and radiation necrosis. J Neurosurg 2018; 130(3):804–11.

84. Bander ED, Jones Samuel H, Pisapia D, et al. Tubular brain tumor biopsy improves diagnostic yield for subcortical lesions. J Neurooncol 2019; 141(1):121–9.

85. Eberlin LS, Norton I, Orringer D, et al. Ambient mass spectrometry for the intraoperative molecular diagnosis of human brain tumors. Proc Natl Acad Sci U S A 2013;1611–6. https://doi.org/10.1073/pnas.1215687110.

86. Eissa A, Zoeir A, Sighinolfi MC, et al. "Real-time" assessment of surgical margins during radical prostatectomy: state-of-the-art. Clin Genitourin Cancer 2019. https://doi.org/10.1016/j.clgc.2019.07.012.

Techniques for Open Surgical Resection of Brain Metastases

Joshua L. Wang, MD*, J. Bradley Elder, MD

KEYWORDS

- Brain tumors • Neoplasm metastasis • Craniotomy • Surgical resection • Technique

KEY POINTS

- Surgical resection is a primary treatment modality for newly diagnosed or recurrent brain metastases from radiation-resistant or intermediate primary cancers.
- Tumor location and relationship to eloquent structures dictate the approach trajectory, and selected surgical adjuncts help maximize resection while minimizing neurologic deficits.
- En bloc resection is associated with improved overall survival, local recurrence rates, intraoperative hemostasis, and decreased postoperative neurologic complications, compared with piecemeal resection.
- Preoperative mapping with functional MRI and diffusion tensor imaging and intraoperative mapping and monitoring with electrophysiologic techniques aid preservation of normal neurologic function.

BACKGROUND

Brain metastases are the most common intracranial tumor, and roughly 25% of all patients with cancer have metastases at autopsy.[1] Brain metastases were recognized as a significant cause of morbidity and mortality early in the twentieth century, but surgical resection was not common given the associated high morbidity and poor postoperative survival.[2] However, surgical technique and neuroanesthesia advancements in the latter half of the twentieth century significantly decreased perioperative complication rates, and currently surgery remains the primary treatment of single or dominant metastases from radiation-resistant or -intermediate primary cancers.

In the early 1990s, two randomized controlled trials demonstrated that for solitary brain metastases, resection versus needle biopsy[3] or no surgery[4] before whole brain radiotherapy (WBRT) led to decreased rates of local recurrence (20% vs 52%), improved overall survival (OS; 40 vs 15 weeks), and more rapid and sustained functional independence (38 vs 8 weeks). In both trials, stable extracranial disease was a positive prognostic factor. Although a similar study by Mintz and colleagues[5] showed no significant benefit in terms of OS of surgical resection plus WBRT compared with WBRT alone, nearly half of these patients had progressive extracranial disease, and this study included patients with Karnofsky Performance Status (KPS) greater than or equal to 50. Based on these three trials, a Cochrane meta-analysis concluded that surgical resection with adjuvant WBRT provided the best outcome for patients with single brain metastases, good performance statuses (KPS $\geq$ 70), and controlled systemic disease.[6]

In patients with multiple brain metastases, several groups have reported that resection of all metastases (up to three) is associated with significantly longer survival when compared with resection of only some brain metastases, and provides similar survival to patients with completely resected single brain metastases.[7,8] In patients with recurrence of brain metastases after initial resection, reoperation has been associated with prolonged survival and improved quality of life, even for those undergoing second reoperation

Department of Neurological Surgery, The Ohio State University Wexner Medical Center, Doan Hall N1004, 410 West 10th Avenue, Columbus, OH 43210, USA
* Corresponding author.
E-mail address: joshua.wang@osumc.edu

Neurosurg Clin N Am 31 (2020) 527–536
https://doi.org/10.1016/j.nec.2020.06.003
1042-3680/20/© 2020 Elsevier Inc. All rights reserved.

for further recurrence, whether the recurrence was local or distant.[9] The factors that affected survival were status of systemic disease, KPS greater than 70, time to recurrence greater than 4 months, age, and primary tumor type.

Given the significant clinical benefits associated with aggressive surgical management of brain metastases established by these early studies, neurosurgeons have refined and developed surgical techniques and operative adjuncts that optimize surgical outcomes. Some techniques help limit potential neurologic morbidity associated with surgery, whereas others make surgery less invasive or more efficient. What follows highlights some of the most common current surgical strategies for resection of brain metastases: from selecting the approach, to intraoperative localization and verification, to mapping and monitoring of eloquent function.

SURGICAL APPROACHES
Craniotomy

Metastatic tumors may arise anywhere within the brain but are most commonly located at the junction of the gray and white matter, where the caliber of the cerebral capillaries no longer permits passage of tumor cells and results in tumor deposition and growth. As such, the surgical approach typically involves a linear or curvilinear incision to allow convexity or posterior fossa craniotomy directly overlying the tumor. Typically, standard neurosurgical approaches, including convexity, pterional, bifrontal, interhemispheric, and suboccipital craniotomies, are selected based on the location of the tumor. Although less frequently used, orbitozygomatic and transsphenoidal craniotomies provide improved access to the skull base. Larger tumors may require curvilinear or S-shaped incisions that allow for a larger craniotomy compared with linear incisions. For superficial tumors, the craniotomy must usually encompass the entire area of the tumor, whereas deep tumors can potentially be accessed through smaller craniotomies because the intracranial operative field widens with increasing distance from the skull (**Fig. 1**).[10] Nuances arise for eloquent and deep-seated lesions.

Minimally invasive (ie, "keyhole") approaches are refinements of conventional craniotomies and are particularly useful for minimizing approach morbidity for deep-seated tumors.[10] In contrast to conventional craniotomies, keyhole craniotomies can be smaller than the lesion itself, which can be fully exposed by subtending the full angles of approach at the extents of the craniotomy. The retrosigmoid craniotomy is the most familiar keyhole for many neurosurgeons: the surface

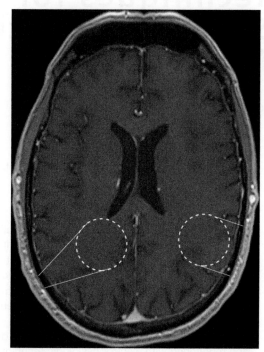

Fig. 1. Two hypothetical masses (*circles*) show the effect of depth on the size of craniotomy required to access and visualize the entire lesion.

opening is modest because of local anatomy, the target is often deep, and full visualization of the cranial nerves from the trochlear nerve to the spinal accessory nerve is obtained by sweeping the angle of view from superior to inferior. Keyhole craniotomies have been safely and successfully used to achieve gross total resection for numerous intrinsic and extrinsic lesions, including brain metastases.[11–15] Rates of gross total resection have been reported in the range of 74% to 87%, even in patients undergoing simultaneous multiple minimally invasive craniotomies.[11–15] Complication rates ranged from 2% to 9%, and most patients demonstrated improvement in their performance statuses postoperatively.[13–15] The use of endoscopes, although not obligatory, may improve extent of resection by accessing residual tumor not visualized by standard operative microscopy.

The supraorbital "eyebrow" craniotomy is a variation of the standard pterional or orbitozygomatic craniotomies that provides access to the frontal pole and subfrontal, suprasellar, and retrosellar regions (Case 1, **Fig. 2**).[16–18] An incision is made in or just above the eyebrow, following the curve of the eyebrow with the option of extending laterally, through which a low frontal craniotomy is made with or without removal of the orbital rim. Care is taken to preserve the supraorbital nerve medially and the frontalis branch of the facial nerve laterally,

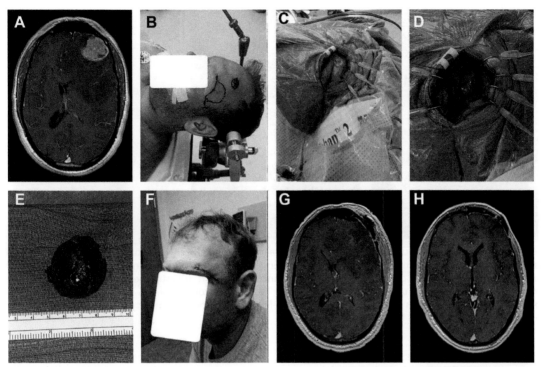

Fig. 2. Eyebrow craniotomy for a patient with metastatic melanoma. (*A*) T1-weighted with gadolinium axial MRI demonstrating a heterogeneously enhancing lesion in the left frontal lobe. (*B*) Positioning of the patient, with the planned curvilinear incision marked inferiorly and C-shaped *dotted line* superiorly marking the planned craniotomy. (*C*) Exposure of the skull. (*D*) The tumor and associated gliotic capsule exposed after craniotomy and dural flap. (*E*) Gross examination of the tumor after en bloc resection. Final pathology demonstrated metastatic melanoma. (*F*) Postoperative follow-up at 2 weeks. T1-weighted with contrast MRI obtained at 1 day (*G*) and 10 months postoperatively (*H*).

and to minimize transecting the temporalis and orbicularis oculi to maximize cosmetic outcome. In a series of 418 patients who underwent eyebrow craniotomies, high patient satisfaction was reported with cosmetic and clinical outcomes.[19]

Case 1: A 38-year-old man with a history of melanoma presented with several episodes of loss of consciousness, falls, and flat affect. MRI of the brain demonstrated a heterogeneously enhancing lesion in the left frontal lobe with significant surrounding edema and mass effect (see **Fig. 2**A). Given the symptomatic presentation, size, and location of the mass, surgical resection via an eyebrow incision was recommended to the patient, who elected to proceed. The patient was positioned supine on the operative table and the planned incision and craniotomy were marked (see **Fig. 2**B). The scalp was reflected superiorly to expose the skull (see **Fig. 2**C), after which the craniotomy was turned, and the dural flap was reflected inferiorly, revealing the tumor and associated gliotic capsule (see **Fig. 2**D). The tumor was extirpated en bloc and final pathology demonstrated metastatic melanoma. The incision demonstrated excellent healing at 2-week follow-

up after surgery (see **Fig. 2**F). MRI performed on the day after surgery demonstrated postoperative changes and gross total resection (see **Fig. 2**G), and there was no evidence of recurrence on MRI 10 months postoperatively (see **Fig. 2**H).

Tubular Retractor

Neurosurgeons have long used retractor systems to maintain adequate visualization of the operative field. Blade retractors are commonly used, but pressure on the brain is uneven and can lead to damage via ischemia or hemorrhage. Cylindrical, or tubular retractor systems (colloquially, "ports") apply even pressure to the walls of the operative corridor, allowing for dilation and maintenance of the operative corridor while minimizing retractor-induced injury, to access deep-seated lesions within the parenchyma or ventricles (**Fig. 3**).[20–23] Use of tubular retractors has been described extensively, with interoperator nuances, although general principles remain the same.[24] Preoperative diffusion tensor imaging (DTI) allows identification of the projecting white matter fibers and selection of a trajectory that results in the least

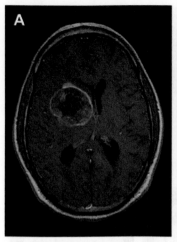 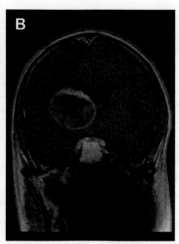 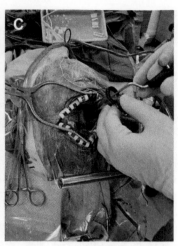

Fig. 3. Intraoperative ultrasound for resection of sarcoma metastasis. Axial (*A*) and coronal (*B*) T1-weighted with gadolinium MRI demonstrating large, heterogeneously enhancing mass with central necrosis located in the basal ganglia, with associated vasogenic edema, mass effect, and midline shift. (*C*) Intraoperative photograph demonstrating placement of port under neuronavigation for resection through a modestly sized craniotomy. The connector for the snake arm is held in the surgeon's left hand and the remainder of the snake arm is visible to the right of the surgeon's hands.

disruption of white matter fascicles, which may not be the shortest intraparenchymal route.[22]

Microscope visualization with tubular retractors is preferred at our institution because of improved field of view and lighting, three-dimensional optics, and clinical experience, which showed improved extent of resection.[24] Endoscopes continue to be used based on operator familiarity and resection is aided with specialized tools, such as side-cutting aspirators.[25,26] Although exoscopes are not yet standard of care at many large neurosurgical centers, they provide much of the same benefits of standard microscopy, such as three-dimensional optics and bimanual operation, and can increase ease of angular adjustment.[27–29]

TUMOR RESECTION

Brain metastases are composed of solid and/or cystic tumor without intervening brain tissue, and correspond to the contrast-enhancing regions observed on computed tomography (CT) or MRI.[30] Although some tumor cells may be infiltrative into the surrounding brain, this is usually less than 5 mm deep.[31] Typically, brain metastases are circumscribed by a rim of gliotic tissue that separates the tumor from the surrounding brain. Dissection within this plane allows for safe resection.

En Bloc

En bloc resection of brain metastases is associated with decreased likelihood of developing leptomeningeal disease (LMD) at any point after surgery. In a clinical study of 542 patients with supratentorial brain metastases who underwent surgical resection, the rate of developing LMD was significantly lower with en bloc resection (3% of 351 patients) compared with piecemeal resection (9% of 191 patients).[32] Similarly, in 260 patients with posterior fossa metastases, 6% of 123 patients receiving en bloc resection developed LMD compared with 14% of 137 patients receiving piecemeal resection. In both studies, these findings remained significant after controlling for tumor size, location, and patient characteristics. En bloc resection also improves hemostasis, which reduces operative time and complications for highly vascular tumors, such as renal cell carcinoma. In a study of 1033 patients, en bloc resection was associated with decreased postoperative complications compared with piecemeal removal, including tumors in eloquent regions and larger tumors.[33]

Supratotal

Several studies have evaluated whether "supra-marginal" or "microscopic total" resection improves local recurrence rates of brain metastases.[31,34–36] In four retrospective studies, an additional 5 mm of surrounding, normal-appearing brain parenchyma was resected in patients following standard gross microsurgical resection. In one study, intraoperative frozen biopsy samples were obtained from the additional resection margin until no tumor cells were

seen.[31] Supramarginal resection was well tolerated in all four studies and could be safely
achieved in eloquent areas with awake craniotomies and intraoperative monitoring.[34] Additionally, survival outcomes suggested improved local
tumor control compared with in-study and historical control subjects.[31,35] Prospective data are
needed to help delineate the role of supramarginal
resection in the management of brain metastases.

Piecemeal

For tumors in eloquent areas, aggressive brain
dissection superficial to the tumor may result in
unacceptable neurologic deficits, and en bloc
resection through a longitudinal corticectomy
may not be feasible. In such cases when the corticectomy must be limited in size, the tumor is typically resected from the inside out in a piecemeal
fashion. Ultrasonic aspirators may assist in tumor
debulking while minimizing retraction and manipulation of normal brain tissue and have been associated with low rates of surgical morbidity.[37]
Deep-seated tumors resected through a tubular
retractor also represent challenges for achieving
en bloc removal given the small working diameter
of the port and increased likelihood of eloquent
location, such as basal ganglia and thalamus,
and piecemeal resection is often required.

Multiple Tumors

In the past, multiple brain metastases were
considered a relative contraindication to surgery
because of presumed poor survival of these patients, and initial studies regarding surgical resection focused on patients with solitary brain
metastases. Subsequent studies showed resection of the dominant lesion in the setting of multiple
brain metastases can be considered to provide
symptomatic relief, but at present there is no
consensus on surgical treatment of oligometastatic disease (up to three lesions).[7,38–40] Several
retrospective studies have matched oligometastatic with solitary metastatic patients and found
no significant differences in OS between patients
receiving resection of all oligometastatic disease
and those receiving resection of their solitary
metastasis, with OS ranging from 14 to
17 months.[7,38–40] However, patients with only
partially resected oligometastatic disease had
significantly shorter OS.[7] Those patients with
KPS greater than or equal to 70, less than 65 years
of age, and controlled extracranial disease
benefitted the most from resection of all oligometastatic central nervous system disease.[38–40] Prospective studies are needed to elucidate the role
of resection of multiple brain metastases and

clarify associated variables, such as whether to
stage craniotomies in this setting.

SURGICAL ADJUNCTS

Techniques and technologies that aid in optimizing
surgical resection of brain metastases have
improved clinical outcomes. Penetration of these
technologies in neurosurgery for brain metastases
ranges from the virtually ubiquitous, such as neuronavigation, to uncommon, such as three-
dimensional ultrasound.

Fluorescence

Although the use of 5-aminolevulenic acid (5-ALA)
has been shown to improve extent of resection
and progression-free survival in glioma surgery,
brain metastases do not display consistent 5-
ALA fluorescence (only 41% in a series of 84 metastases), and a recent study showed its use did
not correlate with improved survival outcomes.[41]
Median OS in 84 patients receiving 5-ALA for
resection of their solitary brain metastases was
15 months, comparable with historical control
subjects. There was no difference in local recurrence rates between tumors that displayed 5-
ALA-induced fluorescence and those that did not.
   In a study of 95 patients with brain metastases,
intraoperative fluorescein was safe and associated
with improved rates of gross total resection (83%)
compared with historical control subjects, but data
regarding survival outcomes were not published.[42]

Neuronavigation

Advancements in stereotaxy technology have
largely replaced frame-based stereotactic navigation with frameless systems that register preoperative (or intraoperative) cross-sectional imaging
reconstructed into a three-dimensional model
with facial landmarks or surface fiducials, with
registration accuracy of 2 to 4 mm regardless of
fiducial use.[43] These "neuronavigation" systems
are particularly useful for planning skin incision,
craniotomy, and trajectory to the lesion. However,
unless updated with intraoperative imaging, navigation systems do not account for changes in
anatomy caused by brain shift, which is caused
by loss of cerebrospinal fluid, osmotic agents,
manipulation of normal brain tissue, and resection
of tumor. Although no outcomes data exist
regarding neuronavigation solely for brain metastases, early data in glioblastoma resection demonstrated significantly improved extent of resection
without significantly prolonging operative time.[44]

Intraoperative Imaging

Intraoperative imaging modalities, such as CT, ultrasound, and MRI, are used to identify tumor in real time and possibly update the navigation system. Intraoperative ultrasound is widely used and is the least expensive and least obtrusive option with rapid and repeatable use. Given the high density of tumor cells in comparison with normal brain tissue, brain metastases are often hyperechoic on ultrasound and easily distinguishable from the surrounding anatomy (Case 2, **Fig. 4**). As resection proceeds, ultrasound is used to evaluate extent of resection, and navigated three-dimensional ultrasound is used to update neuronavigation systems to account for brain shift.[45,46] In multiple trials, use of intraoperative ultrasound increased extent of resection and postoperative KPS.[47]

Case 2: A 60-year-old man with a history of esophageal carcinoma treated with chemoradiation presented with several weeks of migraine-like headaches and lethargy. Preoperative MRI demonstrated a heterogeneously enhancing cystic/solid metastasis with associated vasogenic edema in the right parieto-occipital lobe (see **Fig. 4**A, B). After the craniotomy was performed, intraoperative ultrasound identified the predominantly hyperechoic mass, clarified the appropriate gyrus for corticotomy and trajectory toward the tumor, and verified complete resection of the tumor with layering of intraoperative blood products (see **Fig. 4**C). At 2-month follow-up, the patient reported resolution of his symptoms and was neurologically intact. Follow-up imaging demonstrated postsurgical changes without residual or recurrent enhancing residual tumor.

Intraoperative MRI (iMRI) systems have become more widespread in their use but are still limited by cost. These iMRI systems can update frameless navigation systems, assess extent of resection, and identify surgical complications. However, the additional workflow associated with these systems is not as convenient as intraoperative ultrasound.[48,49] Because most brain metastases are well-circumscribed, the use of iMRI in neurosurgical oncology has usually focused on glioma. In a study of 163 patients, iMRI was associated with increased extent of resection in all enhancing lesions, including gross total resection in 73% of metastases.[49]

Intraoperative CT systems, whether portable or on a sliding gantry, have workflow and applicability advantages over iMRI, but are limited by their soft tissue definition. As such, intraoperative CT is most useful for tumors invading the skull base and for CT angiography of vascular lesions.[50]

Intraoperative Brain Mapping

For tumors in eloquent areas of the brain, mapping of critical functions, such as motor or language, is performed preoperatively and intraoperatively. Functional MRI and DTI can identify important cortical foci and white matter tracts, respectively.[51,52] However, as with frameless stereotaxy, these imaging modalities are limited by their susceptibility to brain shift intraoperatively.

Neurophysiologic techniques for intraoperative monitoring use cortical responses to peripheral inputs and direct stimulation of the cortex with recording of the motor response peripherally. Somatosensory evoked potentials are used to identify the central sulcus and thus the primary motor and somatosensory cortices. A strip electrode placed on the cortical surface records electrical stimulation provided to the contralateral median, ulnar, or posterior tibial nerves (Case 3, **Fig. 5**). Because sensory evoked potentials are negative and motor evoked potentials (MEPs) are positive, the central sulcus is identified between two adjacent leads that demonstrate "phase reversal."

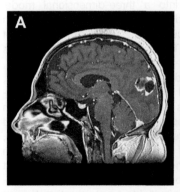
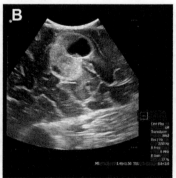
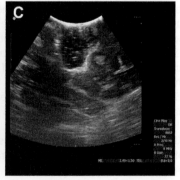

Fig. 4. Patient with history of esophageal cancer presenting with headaches and lethargy. Preoperative sagittal T1-weighted (*A*) pregadolinium and (*B*) postgadolinium MRIs. (*B*) Representative B-mode image of intraoperative ultrasonographic localization preresection. (*C*) Postresection ultrasonographic verification image.

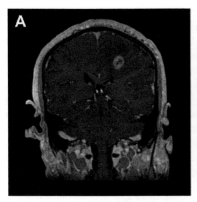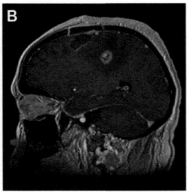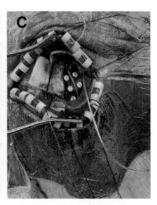

Fig. 5. Intraoperative monitoring and phase reversal for resection of a sarcoma met deep to the precentral gyrus. T1-weighted with gadolinium preoperative MRI (*A*, coronal; *B*, sagittal). (*C*) Intraoperative monitoring and mapping with phase-reversal and white matter mapping.

Intraoperative identification of the motor and sensory cortices aids in selecting the surgical corridor.

Case 3: A 41-year-old man with a history of previously resected left frontal sarcoma metastasis presented with progressive right-sided weakness. He was found to have a new left frontal mass deep to the precentral gyrus on MRI (see **Fig. 5**A, B). Given the anatomic location of the tumor, intraoperative monitoring and mapping with phase reversal and white matter mapping were used to identify the primary motor cortex and guide surgical trajectory, and guide tumor resection to preserve motor function (see **Fig. 5**C). After craniotomy and opening the dura, the 2 × 4 electrode grid was placed on the cortex and advanced under the dura. Identification of phase reversal, which was confirmed with multiple electrode grid positions, located the central sulcus. White matter mapping (not shown) performed during dissection toward the tumor and during tumor resection clarified the proximity of the descending motor fibers in the corona radiate in relation to the tumor. At 6 weeks postoperatively, the patient's strength had improved significantly, and follow-up imaging demonstrated only postoperative changes with no residual enhancement.

Mapping can also be performed using direct cortical and subcortical stimulation. MEPs are measured following cortical stimulation using peripherally placed electrodes or direct visualization of movement in an extremity, depending on the type of anesthesia.[53] Similarly, stimulation of subcortical motor white matter pathways can also elicit motor responses, but are generally less reliable than cortical stimulation.[54] For deep-seated lesions, such white matter mapping may confirm preoperative DTI and influence the surgical trajectory. For motor mapping, awake craniotomy may increase the sensitivity and specificity of direct cortical stimulation.

There is a lack of concordance in the literature regarding the optimal and safest surgical management of eloquent brain metastases. For motor strip tumors, several groups posit that intraoperative monitoring and mapping using somatosensory evoked potentials and MEPs under general anesthesia (with or without preoperative mapping) improves extent of resection while minimizing neurologic complications,[55–57] although MEPs do have an associated false-negative rate.[58] Surgery for tumors involving language areas has potential for severe neurologic morbidity, and awake mapping of language centers is considered. Eight studies demonstrated safety and feasibility of awake craniotomy in a total of 135 patients with brain metastases located in motor or speech areas, with 76% of patients demonstrating improvement or stability of neurologic function immediately postoperatively.[59,60] Of the 24% with worsening postoperative neurologic symptoms, most (96%) experienced long-term improvement in neurologic function. In a retrospective study of 49 patients with intrinsic brain tumors located in the primary motor cortex, there was no difference in long-term functional outcome or extent of resection in patients undergoing awake versus asleep craniotomies.[61] In the absence of high-quality prospective data, selection of awake versus asleep craniotomies depends on surgeon preference, anesthesia familiarity, quality of preoperative and intraoperative mapping and monitoring, and individual patient selection. Techniques for awake speech mapping are well described in glioblastoma literature.

SUMMARY

Brain metastases remain a leading cause of morbidity and mortality for patients with cancer, but options for surgical management continue to expand. Advances in techniques and technologies have allow the modern neurosurgeon to resect tumors that were once deemed unresectable, either because of their depth or their proximity to eloquent brain. Keyhole approaches and tubular retractors decrease approach morbidity and improve patient satisfaction. Preoperative and intraoperative mapping and monitoring allow for maximal resection with minimal neurologic compromise. Until systemic therapies become viable options, continued advances in surgical strategies are needed to optimize outcomes for patients with brain metastases.

DISCLOSURE

The authors have nothing to disclose.

REFERENCES

1. Ostrom QT, Wright CH, Barnholtz-Sloan JS. Brain metastases: epidemiology. Handb Clin Neurol 2018;149:27–42.
2. Grant FC. Concerning intracranial malignant metastases: their frequency and the value of surgery in their treatment. Ann Surg 1926;84(5):635–46.
3. Patchell RA, Tibbs PA, Walsh JW, et al. A randomized trial of surgery in the treatment of single metastases to the brain. N Engl J Med 1990; 322(8):494–500.
4. Vecht CJ, Haaxma-Reiche H, Noordijk EM, et al. Treatment of single brain metastasis: radiotherapy alone or combined with neurosurgery? Ann Neurol 1993;33(6):583–90.
5. Mintz AH, Kestle J, Rathbone MP, et al. A randomized trial to assess the efficacy of surgery in addition to radiotherapy in patients with a single cerebral metastasis. Cancer 1996;78(7):1470–6.
6. Hart MG, Grant R, Walker M, et al. Surgical resection and whole brain radiation therapy versus whole brain radiation therapy alone for single brain metastases. Cochrane Database Syst Rev 2005;(1): CD003292.
7. Bindal RK, Sawaya R, Leavens ME, et al. Surgical treatment of multiple brain metastases. J Neurosurg 1993;79(2):210–6.
8. Iwadate Y, Namba H, Yamaura A. Significance of surgical resection for the treatment of multiple brain metastases. Anticancer Res 2000;20(1B):573–7.
9. Bindal RK, Sawaya R, Leavens ME, et al. Reoperation for recurrent metastatic brain tumors. J Neurosurg 1995;83(4):600–4.
10. Garrett M, Consiglieri G, Nakaji P. Transcranial minimally invasive neurosurgery for tumors. Neurosurg Clin N Am 2010;21(4):595–605, v.
11. Raza SM, Garzon-Muvdi T, Boaehene K, et al. The supraorbital craniotomy for access to the skull base and intraaxial lesions: a technique in evolution. Minim invasive Neurosurg 2010;53(1):1–8.
12. Gazzeri R, Nishiyama Y, Teo C. Endoscopic supraorbital eyebrow approach for the surgical treatment of extraaxial and intraaxial tumors. Neurosurg Focus 2014;37(4):E20.
13. Baker CM, Glenn CA, Briggs RG, et al. Simultaneous resection of multiple metastatic brain tumors with multiple keyhole craniotomies. World Neurosurg 2017;106:359–67.
14. Eroglu U, Shah K, Bozkurt M, et al. Supraorbital keyhole approach: lessons learned from 106 operative cases. World Neurosurg 2019. https://doi.org/10.1016/j.wneu.2018.12.188.
15. Phang I, Leach J, Leggate JRS, et al. Minimally invasive resection of brain metastases. World Neurosurg 2019;130:e362–7.
16. Reisch R, Perneczky A. Ten-year experience with the supraorbital subfrontal approach through an eyebrow skin incision. Neurosurgery 2005;57(4 Suppl):242–55 [discussion: 242–55].
17. Ormond DR, Hadjipanayis CG. The supraorbital keyhole craniotomy through an eyebrow incision: its origins and evolution. Minim Invasive Surg 2013;2013:296469.
18. Ditzel Filho LF, McLaughlin N, Bresson D, et al. Supraorbital eyebrow craniotomy for removal of intraaxial frontal brain tumors: a technical note. World Neurosurg 2014;81(2):348–56.
19. Reisch R, Marcus HJ, Hugelshofer M, et al. Patients' cosmetic satisfaction, pain, and functional outcomes after supraorbital craniotomy through an eyebrow incision. J Neurosurg 2014;121(3):730–4.
20. Kelly PJ, Goerss SJ, Kall BA. The stereotaxic retractor in computer-assisted stereotaxic microsurgery. Technical note. J Neurosurg 1988;69(2):301–6.
21. Plaha P, Livermore LJ, Voets N, et al. Minimally invasive endoscopic resection of intraparenchymal brain tumors. World Neurosurg 2014;82(6):1198–208.
22. Eliyas JK, Glynn R, Kulwin CG, et al. Minimally invasive transsulcal resection of intraventricular and periventricular lesions through a tubular retractor system: multicentric experience and results. World Neurosurg 2016;90:556–64.
23. Newman WC, Engh JA. Stereotactic-guided dilatable endoscopic port surgery for deep-seated brain tumors: technical report with comparative case series analysis. World Neurosurg 2019;125: e812–9.
24. Hong CS, Prevedello DM, Elder JB. Comparison of endoscope- versus microscope-assisted resection of deep-seated intracranial lesions using a minimally invasive port retractor system. J Neurosurg 2016; 124(3):799–810.
25. Kassam AB, Engh JA, Mintz AH, et al. Completely endoscopic resection of intraparenchymal brain tumors. J Neurosurg 2009;110(1):116–23.

26. McLaughlin N, Ditzel Filho LF, Prevedello DM, et al. Side-cutting aspiration device for endoscopic and microscopic tumor removal. J Neurol Surg B Skull Base 2012;73(1):11–20.

27. Habboub G, Sharma M, Barnett GH, et al. A novel combination of two minimally invasive surgical techniques in the management of refractory radiation necrosis: technical note. J Clin Neurosci 2017;35: 117–21.

28. Bakhsheshian J, Strickland BA, Jackson C, et al. Multicenter investigation of channel-based subcortical trans-sulcal exoscopic resection of metastatic brain tumors: a retrospective case series. Oper Neurosurg (Hagerstown) 2019;16(2):159–66.

29. Gassie K, Alvarado-Estrada K, Bechtle P, et al. Surgical management of deep-seated metastatic brain tumors using minimally invasive approaches. J Neurol Surg A Cent Eur Neurosurg 2019;80(3): 198–204.

30. Sawaya R, Bindal RK, Lang FF, et al. Metastatic brain tumors. In: Kaye AH, Laws RR, editors. Brain tumors: an encyclopedic approach. 3rd edition. London: Elsevier Saunders; 2011. p. 864–92.

31. Yoo H, Kim YZ, Nam BH, et al. Reduced local recurrence of a single brain metastasis through microscopic total resection. J Neurosurg 2009;110(4): 730–6.

32. Suki D, Hatiboglu MA, Patel AJ, et al. Comparative risk of leptomeningeal dissemination of cancer after surgery or stereotactic radiosurgery for a single supratentorial solid tumor metastasis. Neurosurgery 2009;64(4):664–74 [discussion: 674–6].

33. Patel AJ, Suki D, Hatiboglu MA, et al. Impact of surgical methodology on the complication rate and functional outcome of patients with a single brain metastasis. J Neurosurg 2015;122(5):1132–43.

34. Kamp MA, Dibue M, Niemann L, et al. Proof of principle: supramarginal resection of cerebral metastases in eloquent brain areas. Acta Neurochir (Wien) 2012;154(11):1981–6.

35. Kamp MA, Rapp M, Slotty PJ, et al. Incidence of local in-brain progression after supramarginal resection of cerebral metastases. Acta Neurochir (Wien) 2015;157(6):905–10 [discussion: 910–1].

36. Pessina F, Navarria P, Cozzi L, et al. Role of surgical resection in patients with single large brain metastases: feasibility, morbidity, and local control evaluation. World Neurosurg 2016;94:6–12.

37. Henzi S, Krayenbuhl N, Bozinov O, et al. Ultrasonic aspiration in neurosurgery: comparative analysis of complications and outcome for three commonly used models. Acta Neurochir (Wien) 2019;161(10): 2073–82.

38. Pollock BE, Brown PD, Foote RL, et al. Properly selected patients with multiple brain metastases may benefit from aggressive treatment of their intracranial disease. J Neurooncol 2003;61(1):73–80.

39. Paek SH, Audu PB, Sperling MR, et al. Reevaluation of surgery for the treatment of brain metastases: review of 208 patients with single or multiple brain metastases treated at one institution with modern neurosurgical techniques. Neurosurgery 2005; 56(5):1021–34 [discussion: 1021–34].

40. Salvati M, Tropeano MP, Maiola V, et al. Multiple brain metastases: a surgical series and neurosurgical perspective. Neurol Sci 2018;39(4):671–7.

41. Kamp MA, Fischer I, Buhner J, et al. 5-ALA fluorescence of cerebral metastases and its impact for the local-in-brain progression. Oncotarget 2016;7(41): 66776–89.

42. Hohne J, Hohenberger C, Proescholdt M, et al. Fluorescein sodium-guided resection of cerebral metastases: an update. Acta Neurochir (Wien) 2017; 159(2):363–7.

43. Pfisterer WK, Papadopoulos S, Drumm DA, et al. Fiducial versus nonfiducial neuronavigation registration assessment and considerations of accuracy. Neurosurgery 2008;62(3 Suppl 1):201–7 [discussion: 207–8].

44. Wirtz CR, Albert FK, Schwaderer M, et al. The benefit of neuronavigation for neurosurgery analyzed by its impact on glioblastoma surgery. Neurol Res 2000;22(4):354–60.

45. Hammoud MA, Ligon BL, elSouki R, et al. Use of intraoperative ultrasound for localizing tumors and determining the extent of resection: a comparative study with magnetic resonance imaging. J Neurosurg 1996;84(5):737–41.

46. Lindner D, Trantakis C, Renner C, et al. Application of intraoperative 3D ultrasound during navigated tumor resection. Minim invasive Neurosurg 2006; 49(4):197–202.

47. de Lima Oliveira M, Picarelli H, Menezes MR, et al. Ultrasonography during surgery to approach cerebral metastases: effect on Karnofsky index scores and tumor volume. World Neurosurg 2017;103: 557–65.

48. Garcia-Baizan A, Tomas-Biosca A, Bartolome Leal P, et al. Intraoperative 3 Tesla magnetic resonance imaging: our experience in tumors. Radiologia 2018; 60(2):136–42.

49. Livne O, Harel R, Hadani M, et al. Intraoperative magnetic resonance imaging for resection of intraaxial brain lesions: a decade of experience using low-field magnetic resonance imaging, Polestar N-10, 20, 30 systems. World Neurosurg 2014; 82(5):770–6.

50. Schichor C, Terpolilli N, Thorsteinsdottir J, et al. Intraoperative computed tomography in cranial neurosurgery. Neurosurg Clin N Am 2017;28(4): 595–602.

51. Heilbrun MP, Lee JN, Alvord L. Practical application of fMRI for surgical planning. Stereotact Funct Neurosurg 2001;76(3–4):168–74.

52. Witwer BP, Moftakhar R, Hasan KM, et al. Diffusion-tensor imaging of white matter tracts in patients with cerebral neoplasm. J Neurosurg 2002;97(3):568–75.

53. Berger MS, Ojemann GA. Intraoperative brain mapping techniques in neuro-oncology. Stereotact Funct Neurosurg 1992;58(1–4):153–61.

54. Skirboll SS, Ojemann GA, Berger MS, et al. Functional cortex and subcortical white matter located within gliomas. Neurosurgery 1996;38(4):678–84 [discussion: 684–5].

55. Krieg SM, Schaffner M, Shiban E, et al. Reliability of intraoperative neurophysiological monitoring using motor evoked potentials during resection of metastases in motor-eloquent brain regions: clinical article. J Neurosurg 2013;118(6):1269–78.

56. Krieg SM, Picht T, Sollmann N, et al. Resection of motor eloquent metastases aided by preoperative nTMS-based motor maps-comparison of two observational cohorts. Front Oncol 2016;6:261.

57. Sanmillan JL, Fernandez-Coello A, Fernandez-Conejero I, et al. Functional approach using intraoperative brain mapping and neurophysiological monitoring for the surgical treatment of brain metastases in the central region. J Neurosurg 2017;126(3):698–707.

58. Obermueller T, Schaeffner M, Shiban E, et al. Intraoperative neuromonitoring for function-guided resection differs for supratentorial motor eloquent gliomas and metastases. BMC Neurol 2015;15:211.

59. Chua TH, See AAQ, Ang BT, et al. Awake craniotomy for resection of brain metastases: a systematic review. World Neurosurg 2018;120:e1128–35.

60. Groshev A, Padalia D, Patel S, et al. Clinical outcomes from maximum-safe resection of primary and metastatic brain tumors using awake craniotomy. Clin Neurol Neurosurg 2017;157:25–30.

61. Magill ST, Han SJ, Li J, et al. Resection of primary motor cortex tumors: feasibility and surgical outcomes. J Neurosurg 2018;129(4):961–72.

Laser Ablation for Cerebral Metastases

Evan Luther, MD[a,b,*], Samuel Mansour, BS[c], Nikolas Echeverry, BS[c], David McCarthy, MSc[a,b], Daniel G. Eichberg, MD[a,b], Ashish Shah, MD[a,b], Ahmed Nada, MD[a,b], Katherine Berry, MD[a,b], Michael Kader, MD[a,b], Michael Ivan, MD[a,b,d], Ricardo Komotar, MD[a,b,d]

KEYWORDS

- Brain metastasis • Laser interstitial thermal therapy • Laser ablation • Metastases • Brain tumor
- Neuro-oncology • Oncology • Minimally invasive surgery

KEY POINTS

- Laser interstitial thermal therapy is an effective salvage therapy for treatment refractory brain metastases.
- Local progression-free survival and overall survival rates varied widely among studies but seem to be comparable with radiation therapy and/or craniotomy for recurrent brain metastases.
- Complication rates are low with only 5.26% risk of developing any permanent neurologic sequelae.
- Future prospective, randomized studies are necessary to determine if laser interstitial thermal therapy is an effective primary therapy for brain metastases.

INTRODUCTION

Laser interstitial thermal therapy (LITT) is a minimally invasive surgical alternative for neuro-oncology patients deemed poor candidates for open resection. The technology delivers laser light through a stereotactically navigated fiber optic probe to create thermal damage, leading to cellular death within the target lesion. Although LITT has become increasingly used as an adjunct treatment for gliomas, dural-based lesions, and even radiation necrosis, most neuro-oncologic studies evaluating the use of LITT have focused on the treatment of cerebral metastases.[1–3] A systematic review of the available literature is provided to concisely summarize the current indications, results, and limitations of laser ablation in cerebral metastases. A brief overview of the technology and case examples are also provided.

SYSTEMATIC REVIEW OF THE AVAILABLE LITERATURE

The systematic review was performed in accordance with the PRISMA guidelines. Relevant articles were found via the following electronic databases: MEDLINE (PubMed), Cochrane Central Register of Controlled Trials (CENTRAL), and the Cochrane Database of Systematic Reviews.

Eligibility Criteria and Study Selection

Only peer-reviewed articles evaluating the use of LITT in the management of metastatic lesions to the brain published after January 1, 2000 were included. Articles in which subjects undergoing LITT for brain metastases were only a subgroup of a larger cohort were also included as long as the majority of the results for brain metastases could be interpreted separately from their

[a] Department of Neurosurgery, University of Miami Miller School of Medicine, Miami, FL, USA; [b] Department of Neurological Surgery, University of Miami/Jackson Health System, Lois Pope Life Center, 2nd Floor, 1095 Northwest 14th Terrace, Miami, FL 33136, USA; [c] Florida Atlantic University Charles E. Schmidt College of Medicine, 777 Glades Road, Boca Raton, FL 33431, USA; [d] Sylvester Comprehensive Cancer Center, University of Miami Health System, Miami, FL, USA

* Corresponding author. Department of Neurological Surgery, University of Miami/Jackson Health System, Lois Pope Life Center, 2nd Floor, 1095 Northwest 14th Terrace, Miami, Fl 33136.
E-mail address: evan.luther@jhsmiami.org

Neurosurg Clin N Am 31 (2020) 537–547
https://doi.org/10.1016/j.nec.2020.06.004
1042-3680/20/© 2020 Elsevier Inc. All rights reserved.

nonmetastatic counterparts. Case reports and studies in which LITT was used exclusively for lesions other than brain metastases were excluded. Studies not written in English, not performed on human subjects, and review articles that did not include their own patient subset were all excluded. The PRISMA flowchart is shown in **Fig. 1**.

Data Collection Process

The following search string was used to identify relevant articles: (LITT) OR ("laser interstitial thermal therapy") OR ("stereotactic laser ablation") AND (metastases OR metastatic OR metastasis). The language (English) and publication date (01/

01/2000–12/31/2020) filters were used in all searches. The search yielded 213 articles and 7 additional articles were located using the references of the articles initially located via the database search. After duplicate articles were removed, 198 remained. After further screening and elimination of irrelevant articles, 14 were found to meet all the inclusion criteria and were included in this qualitative analysis.

Data Analysis

The 14 articles were critically evaluated and the data regarding LITT for metastatic lesions were compiled. Variables included study size, patient

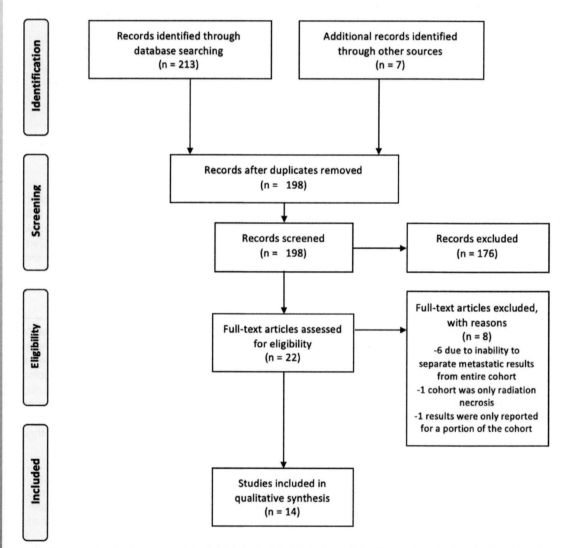

Fig. 1. PRISMA flowchart of the systematic review. Data added to the PRISMA template. (*Adapted from* Moher D, Liberati A, Tetzlaff J, Altman DG, The PRISMA Group [2009]. Preferred Reporting Items for Systematic Reviews and Meta-Analyses: The PRISMA Statement. PLoS Med 6(7):e1000097) under the terms of the Creative Commons Attribution License.)

demographics, size/location, extent of ablation, patient outcomes, and periprocedural complications. The results of these variables were compiled and reported as either a sum total, a percentage of the pooled results, or a weighted average, as applicable. Included articles did not uniformly report every variable evaluated in this analysis and, as such, the reported results are based on aggregate data from the subgroup of articles in which the variable in question was both available and consistent.

Study Demographics, Indications for Laser Interstitial Thermal Therapy, and Ablation Volumes

In total, 228 cases of LITT were reported for the treatment of cerebral metastases. In the subset of articles for which the total number of patients was available, 156 patients underwent 203 LITT procedures. Demographic data for each study including patient age, gender, lesion size, extent of ablation, and primary indication for LITT is available in **Table 1**.[1,4–16] Ten articles reported the mean patient age and the weighted average age within this subset was 58.86 years. Eleven articles reported patient sex, of which 68.92% were female.

The most frequently stated primary indication for performing LITT was prior treatment failure (98.25% of all lesions). Other primary indications for LITT included patient preference (1.32%) and LITT as an initial treatment (0.44%). Other secondary indications for LITT included lesions deemed as poor surgical or radiation candidates (10.09%) or a deep-seated location (14.92%). The criteria for poor surgical candidates, deep or inoperable lesions, and recurrent or refractory disease were not universally congruent throughout the included studies. However, prior treatment failure was frequently defined as previously failed stereotactic radiosurgery (SRS) or craniotomy and most studies defined a poor surgical candidate based on advanced age and the presence of multiple medical comorbidities that would preclude the patient from undergoing a large surgery under general anesthesia. Deep or inoperable lesions were most frequently defined as an area deemed inappropriate for open surgical resection owing to either close proximity to eloquent areas, deep brain structures, or crossing hemispheres or lobes. LITT as an initial treatment, defined as LITT before standard of care, typically occurred because of the study design.

Lesion-Specific Data

The median pre-LITT lesion size and extent of ablation were available for a majority of the included studies and can be found in **Table 1**. The average median preoperative lesion size and extent of ablation were 16.22 cm^3 and 97.04%, respectively. Data regarding lesion location and primary pathology were available in 11 of the included articles. Therefore, the rest of the analysis in this section is restricted to this subgroup. Lesion locations were categorized as either lobar, deep, or within the posterior fossa. Approximately 80% of all lobar lesions were in the frontal, temporal, and parietal lobes and all of the deep lesions were found in either the thalamus or basal ganglia. Posterior fossa lesions comprised 18.45% of all brain metastases treated with LITT. The 3 most common primary pathologies for the metastatic lesions were lung and breast cancer followed by melanoma. Specific data regarding lesion locations and primary pathology types can be found in **Table 2**.

Post-Laser Interstitial Thermal Therapy Lesion Progression, Overall Survival, and Follow-Up

The median overall survival and time to local disease recurrence for brain metastases treated with LITT were provided in only a minority of the included studies and were not uniformly reported when available. As a result, it was not possible to accurately calculate aggregate outcomes data across all the studies. The median length of follow-up was available in 9 studies. The average median follow-up for this subset of patients was 12.12 months. Details regarding patient outcomes can be found in **Table 3**.

Laser Interstitial Thermal Therapy Perioperative Adverse Events

Perioperative adverse events were available for every included study and are displayed in **Table 4**. The overall perioperative adverse event rate across all studies was 18.42%. However, the majority of these adverse events resolved over time resulting in an overall complication rate at last follow-up of only 5.26%. The most frequently experienced adverse event was a new postoperative neurologic deficit or complaint. Some were as serious as aphasia or paresis, whereas others were as benign as a headache; the majority resolved with expectant and/or medical management regardless of severity. Other less common adverse events included symptomatic cerebral edema, postablation seizures, intracranial hemorrhage, infection, hydrocephalus, probe misplacement, metabolic derangements, and cerebrospinal fluid leak.

Table 1
Demographic data, lesion size and extent of ablation

Study, Year	No. of Patients	No. of Lesions	Mean Age (y), (IQR)	No. of Females	Primary Indication for LITT	Median Preoperative Lesion Size (cm³), (Range)	Median EOA (%), (IQR)
Carpentier et al,[14] 2008	4	6	58.25 (50–73)	3	Prior treatment failure	N/A	N/A
Carpentier et al,[8] 2011	7	15	54[a]	N/A	Prior treatment failure	N/A	N/A
Hawasli et al,[10] 2013	5	5	59 (57–61)	3	Prior treatment failure	6.6 (5.2–9.9)	100 (98.3–100.0)
Ali et al,[5] 2016	23	26	59.13 (51.0–68.5)	16	Prior treatment failure	4.9 (0.4–28.9)	87.4 (73.9–97.5)
Wright et al,[13] 2016	1	1	63[a]	0	Prior treatment failure	14.2[a]	92[a]
Kamath et al,[11] 2017	N/A	25	N/A	N/A	Prior treatment failure	N/A	94[a]
Beechar et al,[6] 2018	36	50	N/A	20	Prior treatment failure	5.05 (0.54–23.31)	N/A
Borghei-Razavi et al,[7] 2018	3	3	68 (65.5–73.0)	1	Patient preference	2.01 (1.05–13.26)	100 (100–100)
Maraka et al,[12] 2018	1	1	N/A	N/A	Initial treatment	101.48[a]	100[a]
Eichberg et al,[9] 2018	4	4	54.25 (46.25–62.5)	1	Prior treatment failure	2.55 (1.1–7.2)	100 (97.05–100.00)
Shah et al,[1] 2019	36	45	60 (27–75)	30	Prior treatment failure	4.3 (0.6–28.0)	100 (88–100)
Ahluwalia et al,[4] 2019	20	20	N/A	14	Prior treatment failure	N/A	N/A
Traylor et al,[16] 2019	8	8	60.88 (36–79)	7	Prior treatment failure	4.91 (0.33–7.52)	100 (100–100)
Eichberg et al,[15] 2019	8	19	53.75 (26–69)	7	Prior treatment failure	N/A	N/A

N/A signifies either that the variable was not reported, unable to be separated from the rest of the study cohort, or reported in a matter incongruent with the majority of the other studies.

Abbreviations: EOA, extent of ablation; IQR, interquartile range.
[a] IQR/range unavailable or unable to be reported for the subset in question

Table 2
Lesion locations and primary pathology

	Location	No. of Lesions	% Total	Pathology	No. of Lesions	% Total
Lobar	Frontal	65	38.7	Lung	56	33.5
	Parietal	20	11.9	Breast	48	28.7
	Temporal	16	9.5	Melanoma	29	17.4
	Occipital	14	8.3	Colorectal	10	6
	Parieto-occipital	5	3	Gynecologic	6	3.6
	Frontoparietal	4	2.4	Sarcoma	5	3
	Insular	2	1.2	Bladder	2	1.2
	Cingulate	1	0.6	Esophagus	2	1.2
Deep	Thalamus	7	4.2	Renal	2	1.2
	Basal ganglia	3	1.8	Prostate	1	0.6
Posterior fossa		31	18.5	Other[a]	6	3.6

[a] Other signifies either a carcinoma of unknown origin or that the study did not specify the primary tumor origin.

SURGICAL PROCEDURE FOR LASER ABLATION

LITT is a minimally invasive neuro-oncologic technique that uses focused laser light, delivered through a fiber optic probe housed within a sterile catheter, to thermally ablate a variety of intracranial lesions (**Fig. 2**).[1,2] The trajectory of the catheter is planned using stereotactic neuronavigation and is typically selected so that the fiber traverses the longest axis of the lesion while avoiding injury to any critical anatomic structures. A multiarticulated precision aiming device, or PAD, is then positioned over the entry site along the planned trajectory to provide support as the catheter is advanced into the lesion (**Fig. 3**). Using a stab incision, a small burr hole is then made through the skull. The laser probe is subsequently inserted through the PAD and then advanced stereotactically through the burr hole along the designated trajectory into the lesion.[1,2] The probe is then fixed into position

Table 3
Patient outcomes and follow-up

Study	Median Time to Local Recurrence (mo)	Median Overall Survival (mo)	Median Length of Follow-up (mo), (IQR)
Carpentier et al,[14] 2008	3	N/A	3
Carpentier et al,[8] 2011	3.8[a]	17.4[a]	N/A
Hawasli et al,[10] 2013	2.85	4.2	4.2 (1.9–5.8)
Ali et al,[5] 2016	N/A	N/A	5.05 (3.32–10.90)
Wright et al,[13] 2016	–	–	13.07[b]
Kamath et al,[11] 2017	N/A	17.2	9.8[b]
Beechar et al,[6] 2018	10.5	N/A	1.82 (0.25–4.50)[c]
Borghei-Razavi et al,[7] 2018	7.5	N/A	N/A
Maraka et al,[12] 2018	N/A	N/A	N/A
Eichberg et al,[9] 2018	–	–	10.5 (9.25–14.25)
Shah et al,[1] 2019	55.9	16.9	7.6 (3.4–17.2)
Ahluwalia et al,[4] 2019	N/A	N/A	N/A
Traylor et al,[16] 2019	N/A	N/A	N/A
Eichberg et al,[15] 2019	9	N/A	54 (23.4–49.4)

N/A signifies either that the variable was not reported, unable to be separated from the rest of the study cohort, or reported in a matter incongruent with the majority of the other studies.
Abbreviations: IQR, interquartile range; –, no event occurred during the follow-up period.
[a] Values reported as a mean.
[b] Values reported as median only without IQR.
[c] Values reported as median and range.

Table 4
LITT perioperative adverse events

| Study | Adverse Events (n, %) | Complication Type | | | | | | No. at Last Follow-Up |
		Neurologic	Edema	Seizure	ICH	Infection	Other[a]	
Carpentier et al,[14] 2008	0 (0)	–	–	–	–	–	–	–
Carpentier et al,[8] 2011	4 (26.67)	2	–	–	1	–	1	–
Hawasli et al,[10] 2013	2 (40)	2	–	–	–	–	–	–
Ali et al,[5] 2016	5 (19.23)	3	1	–	–	–	1	1
Wright et al,[13] 2016	1 (100)	1	–	–	–	–	–	1
Kamath et al,[11] 2017	5 (20)	1	1	2	–	–	1	1
Beechar et al,[6] 2018	16 (32)	16	–	–	–	–	–	7
Borghei-Razavi et al,[7] 2018	1 (33.33)	1	–	–	–	–	–	–
Maraka et al,[12] 2018	1 (100)	–	1	–	–	–	–	–
Eichberg et al,[9] 2018	0 (0)	–	–	–	–	–	–	–
Shah et al,[1] 2019	2 (4.44)	–	–	1	–	1	–	–
Ahluwalia et al,[4] 2019	3 (15)	2	–	–	1	–	–	2
Traylor et al,[16] 2019	0 (0)	–	–	–	–	–	–	–
Eichberg et al,[15] 2019	2 (10.53)	–	–	–	–	1	1	–

Abbreviation: ICH, intracranial hemorrhage.
[a] In descending order, the other complications are as follows: probe misplacement, transient hydrocephalus, hyponatremia, and transient cerebrospinal fluid leak.

with a bone anchor to prevent any future dislodgement (**Fig. 4**). Intraoperative MRI is then used to ensure proper placement of the laser probe. Once the catheter is confirmed to be intralesional, the system is activated, allowing the probe to deliver near-infrared laser light to generate temperatures sufficient to coagulate tumor foci. **Fig. 5** displays a cross-sectional view of the catheter during ablation. The bone anchor provides coaxial stability and the cap lock limits any further longitudinal probe movement. The catheter has 2 channels with the inner channel containing the fiber optic core and the outer channel containing a continuously circulating coolant to prevent unwanted damage to the tissues along the catheter trajectory. The fiber optic core is attached to a diffuser at the tip of the probe that allows the laser light to be concentrically delivered to the lesion. Real-time MRI thermography is concurrently performed to ensure the lesion receives adequate thermal exposure while simultaneously preventing injury to the normal surrounding parenchyma (**Fig. 6**).[2]

Generating temperatures of 40°C to 90°C at the site of the lesion, the lasers are fired in pulsatile doses of 10 to 15 W each in intervals lasting from 30 seconds to 3 minutes with a total ablation time of 10 to 30 minutes.[2] Pulsatile thermal dosing is essential because prolonged administration at therapeutic temperatures has been shown to lead to coagulative necrosis of the adjacent normal parenchyma.[17] At the level of the tissue, absorption of the laser light results in heat production, which is then distributed throughout the

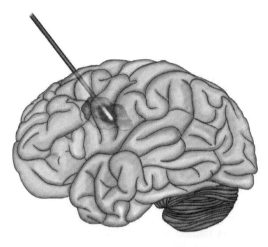

Fig. 2. Illustration demonstrating placement of the LITT catheter into a deep-seated intracranial lesion.

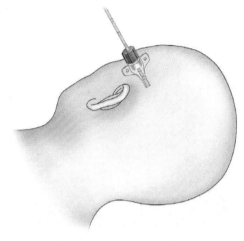

Fig. 4. LITT catheter secured to the skull with a plastic bone anchor after precision aiming device-assisted placement of the fiber optic probe.

lesion and is further facilitated by local blood flow.[18] At temperatures of 42°C to 45°C, cells become highly susceptible to thermal damage and further increases in temperature can result in cell death at much shorter time intervals.[2] Additionally, if temperatures surpass 60°C, rapid coagulation necrosis can occur from the induction of mitochondrial and nuclear damage.[19] Intraprocedural LITT temperatures are typically restricted to less than 90°C at the probe tip and less than 50°C at the periphery of the ablation zone because

temperatures of more than 100°C have been shown to lead to irreversible damage to the surrounding extralesional brain and place the patient at greater risk of developing tissue vaporization, which can decrease the effectiveness of the ablation and potentially cause elevated intracranial pressures.[2] Continuous cooling of the portions of

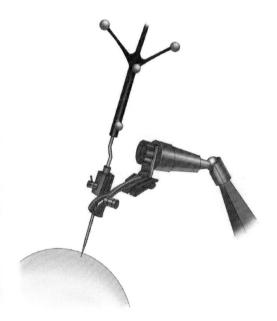

Fig. 3. Precision aiming device and neuronavigation wand positioned along the planned trajectory for the LITT catheter.

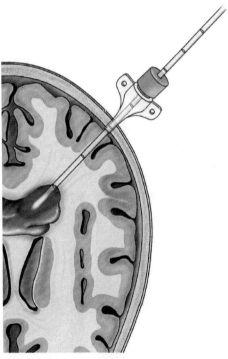

Fig. 5. Cross-sectional view of the LITT catheter during ablation.

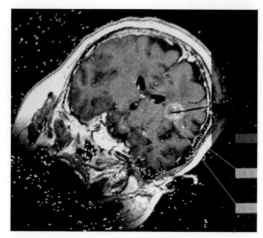

Fig. 6. Intraprocedural MR thermography provides a real-time heat map of the concentric tissues surrounding the probe.

the probe not in direct contact with the target lesion further decrease the possibility of iatrogenic thermal injury of healthy brain tissue.[2] Once the entirety of the planned ablation zone reaches 50°C, ablation is considered complete and the probe is removed. The wound is typically closed with a single absorbable suture. Postoperatively, a repeat MRI is frequently performed to confirm the extent of the ablation.[20,21]

Available Laser Interstitial Thermal Therapy Platforms

Two LITT platforms have been approved by the US Food and Drug Administration for intracranial use and are commercially available: the Neuroblate Laser Ablation System (Monteris, Inc., Minneapolis, MN) and the Visualase Thermal Therapy System (Medtronic, Inc., Dublin, Ireland). Both systems function very similarly and can be integrated with most MRIs. The main differences between the 2 systems are that the Neuroblate

system produces a 12 W, 1064 nm beam and is cooled using CO_2 gas, whereas the Visualase system operates at 15 W, 980 nm, and uses circulating saline for cooling.[2]

Case Example

A 70-year-old woman with a past medical history of metastatic ovarian cancer to the left cerebellum underwent surgical excision followed by SRS to the resection cavity. Fifteen months later, the patient developed recurrence of the lesion on surveillance MRI (**Fig. 7**A). Owing to her radiation history, she was not eligible for repeat radiosurgery, given the lesion's proximity to the brainstem. Given the location and history of prior craniotomy, the patient was treated with LITT. A total ablation was achieved (**Fig. 7**B) and the patient has remained recurrence free at last follow-up over 6 years after the procedure.

DISCUSSION
Current Applications of Laser Interstitial Thermal Therapy in Brain Metastases

Although SRS and/or craniotomy have been considered the first line of therapy for metastatic brain tumors, LITT has been increasingly used over the last decade as either a primary therapy or an alternative to repeat resection or radiation for these lesions.[2] SRS-associated complications, including the development of radiation necrosis, have been observed in approximately 14% of patients at 1 year and this risk is known to only increase with further radiation treatments.[3,22–25] Furthermore, craniotomy is not always a viable alternative when the risk of neurologic injury or a perioperative adverse event is thought to be high. Comparatively, LITT offers more direct access to most noncortical intracranial lesions and, as such, does not confer as high of a risk of secondary damage to the healthy surrounding parenchyma when compared with open surgical

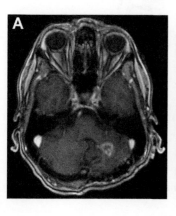
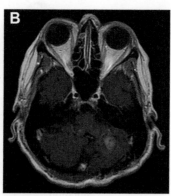

Fig. 7. (*A*) T1-weighted MRI demonstrating recurrent ovarian metastasis in the left cerebellum. (*B*) Post-LITT T1-weighted MRI demonstrating total lesional ablation.

resection or repeat SRS.[2,26] For brain metastases, LITT is most frequently used in lesions that are resistant to, or recur after, initial treatment.[7,10–12] Lesion locations deemed inaccessible via open surgery is another common indication for using LITT, with surgical inaccessibility typically defined as either close proximity to deep or eloquent structures or because open resection conferred unacceptably high morbidity.[2,3] The majority of metastatic lesions treated with LITT were lobar; more specifically, frontal with deep and posterior fossa ablations accounting for only a small percentage of the lesions reported. This likely represents surgical selection bias. Because the trajectory of the LITT catheter must avoid any important anatomic structures, surgeons will likely only offer LITT to patients in which a safe trajectory can be selected. This finding, coupled with the fact that brain metastases tend to occur more often at the cortical grey–white interface, likely explains why lobar lesions were more commonly ablated than deep or posterior fossa lesions.

Laser Interstitial Thermal Therapy for Radiation Necrosis

Although this review did not focus on the use of LITT in radiation necrosis, an overview of the topic is warranted given that it is often seen as a long-term complication of SRS in brain metastases. Briefly, radiation necrosis is a non-neoplastic inflammatory process that is thought to occur secondary to persistent free radical formation after radiation-induced cellular death. It can occur months to years after a single radiation treatment and can be very difficult to manage. Currently, treatments for radiation necrosis are limited, with either surgical resection or corticosteroids considered the mainstays of treatment. However, given the risks associated with both surgical intervention and prolonged steroid use, their efficacy is limited.[2] Interestingly, in patients with radiation necrosis, LITT has shown to cause long-term decreases in lesion size and symptomatology.[2,27–31] Given that patients with metastatic disease are often sicker and less able to handle the rigors of open surgery, LITT offers a viable alternative to resection of the radiation necrosis lesion.[1]

Perioperative Adverse Events Associated with Laser Interstitial Thermal Therapy in Cerebral Metastases

Among the studies reviewed, we found an overall perioperative adverse event rate of 18.42% with the majority (~66.67%) being composed of new-onset neurologic deficits or complaints. The severity of the neurologic symptoms ranged from aphasia or paresis to headaches and imbalance. Symptomatic cerebral edema and postoperative seizures were the second most frequently reported adverse events after LITT. More than two-thirds of these adverse events resolved over time, leading to an overall complication rate of 5.26% at the last follow-up. Although the upfront risk of LITT may be greater than that seen in radiation therapy, the overall complication rate seems to be similar to that seen in craniotomy for recurrent metastatic disease. This finding suggests that LITT can be a safe and effective alternative to radiation or resection in the management of treatment-refractory metastases.[3,32–39] This can be especially true when the patient has already received high cumulative radiation doses or craniotomy is considered exceptionally high risk.

Overall Survival and Local Disease Progression in Laser Interstitial Thermal Therapy: Brain Metastases

The median overall survival ranged from 4.2 to 16.9 months in the available studies for patients undergoing LITT for cerebral metastases. However, it should be noted that the majority of the included studies did not provide enough necessary data to calculate a true aggregate median overall survival.[1,11] Despite this fact, the range of median overall survival seems to be comparable with those seen in craniotomy or radiation therapy.[22,40] This finding may support assertions by previous studies that suggest that LITT is similarly efficacious in providing overall survival benefit when compared with typical treatment measures.[2]

Unfortunately, the median time to local disease recurrence could not be calculated across all the included studies because insufficient data were available; a majority of the articles did not stratify local recurrence rates by pathologic diagnosis. The median time to local recurrence ranged from 2.85 to 55.9 months in the available results. This large variability in local progression free survival is likely the result of 2 different yet dependent variables: pre-LITT lesion size and extent of ablation. Several studies have now demonstrated that total ablations increase time to local recurrence in lesions treated with LITT.[4,31] However, larger lesions are more difficult to completely ablate and thus require more thermal energy to do so. This increase in energy requirements may ultimately lead to adverse effects and clinical progression of the lesion, despite undergoing complete ablation.[41] Further studies are necessary to determine how to optimize energy delivery to lesional tissue via LITT.

Limitations

Given the highly variable reporting of various outcome measures, the time to local disease recurrence and overall survival could not be compiled to calculate meaningful aggregate results across the cohorts. Furthermore, because the majority of the included articles were case-control studies or retrospective analyses, inclusion criteria were not universally consistent, which can thus introduce significant selection bias. As a result, further research in the form of prospective, randomized, controlled trials are necessary to produce enough adequate data to truly compare LITT with traditional first-line therapies.

SUMMARY

LITT is an effective therapy for the management of recurrent or refractory metastatic brain tumors, but is still considered a salvage therapy when repeat radiation or craniotomy is thought to confer too much risk. Although LITT carries slightly more upfront risk than SRS, it still can provide a minimally invasive option for various surgically inaccessible lesions. Further trials are needed to assess the relative efficacy of LITT in the management of cerebral lesions compared with standard therapies.

ACKNOWLEDGMENTS

The authors thank Roberto Suazo for creating the figures displayed in this article.

DISCLOSURE

M. Ivan, MD is a consultant for Medtronic. The other authors have nothing to disclose.

REFERENCES

1. Shah AH, Semonche A, Eichberg DG, et al. The role of laser interstitial thermal therapy in surgical neuro-oncology: series of 100 consecutive patients. Neurosurgery 2019. https://doi.org/10.1093/neuros/nyz424.

2. Sharma M, Balasubramanian S, Silva D, et al. Laser interstitial thermal therapy in the management of brain metastasis and radiation necrosis after radiosurgery: an overview. Expert Rev Neurother 2016; 16(2):223–32.

3. Sneed PK, Mendez J, Vemer-van den Hoek JG, et al. Adverse radiation effect after stereotactic radiosurgery for brain metastases: incidence, time course, and risk factors. J Neurosurg 2015;123(2):373–86.

4. Ahluwalia M, Barnett GH, Deng D, et al. Laser ablation after stereotactic radiosurgery: a multicenter prospective study in patients with metastatic brain tumors and radiation necrosis. J Neurosurg 2018; 130(3):804–11.

5. Ali MA, Carroll KT, Rennert RC, et al. Stereotactic laser ablation as treatment for brain metastases that recur after stereotactic radiosurgery: a multiinstitutional experience. Neurosurg Focus 2016; 41(4):E11.

6. Beechar VB, Prabhu SS, Bastos D, et al. Volumetric response of progressing post-SRS lesions treated with laser interstitial thermal therapy. J Neurooncol 2018;137(1):57–65.

7. Borghei-Razavi H, Koech H, Sharma M, et al. Laser interstitial thermal therapy for posterior fossa lesions: an initial experience. World Neurosurg 2018; 117:e146–53.

8. Carpentier A, McNichols RJ, Stafford RJ, et al. Laser thermal therapy: real-time MRI-guided and computer-controlled procedures for metastatic brain tumors. Lasers Surg Med 2011;43(10):943–50.

9. Eichberg DG, VanDenBerg R, Komotar RJ, et al. quantitative volumetric analysis following magnetic resonance-guided laser interstitial thermal ablation of cerebellar metastases. World Neurosurg 2018; 110:e755–65.

10. Hawasli AH, Bagade S, Shimony JS, et al. Magnetic resonance imaging-guided focused laser interstitial thermal therapy for intracranial lesions: single-institution series. Neurosurgery 2013;73(6):1007–17.

11. Kamath AA, Friedman DD, Hacker CD, et al. MRI-guided interstitial laser ablation for intracranial lesions: a large single-institution experience of 133 cases. Stereotact Funct Neurosurg 2017;95(6): 417–28.

12. Maraka S, Asmaro K, Walbert T, et al. Cerebral edema induced by laser interstitial thermal therapy and radiotherapy in close succession in patients with brain tumor. Lasers Surg Med 2018;50(9): 917–23.

13. Wright J, Chugh J, Wright CH, et al. Laser interstitial thermal therapy followed by minimal-access transsulcal resection for the treatment of large and difficult to access brain tumors. Neurosurg Focus 2016;41(4):E14.

14. Carpentier A, McNichols RJ, Stafford RJ, et al. Real-time magnetic resonance-guided laser thermal therapy for focal metastatic brain tumors. Neurosurgery 2008;63(1 Suppl 1):ONS21–8 [discussion: ONS28-29].

15. Eichberg DG, Menaker SA, Jermakowicz WJ, et al. Multiple iterations of magnetic resonance-guided laser interstitial thermal ablation of brain metastases: single surgeon's experience and review of the literature. Oper Neurosurg (Hagerstown) 2019. https://doi.org/10.1093/ons/opz375.

16. Traylor JI, Patel R, Habib A, et al. Laser interstitial thermal therapy to the posterior fossa: challenges and nuances. World Neurosurg 2019;132:e124–32.

17. Missios S, Bekelis K, Barnett GH. Renaissance of laser interstitial thermal ablation. Neurosurg Focus 2015;38(3):E13.

18. Jaunich MRS, Kim K, Mitra K, et al. Bio-heat transfer analysis during short pulse laser irradiation of tissues. Int J Heat Mass Transfer 2008;51(23–24):5511–21.

19. Thomsen S. Pathologic analysis of photothermal and photomechanical effects of laser-tissue interactions. Photochem Photobiol 1991;53(6):825–35.

20. Allahdini F, Amirjamshidi A, Reza-Zarei M, et al. Evaluating the prognostic factors effective on the outcome of patients with glioblastoma multiformis: does maximal resection of the tumor lengthen the median survival? World Neurosurg 2010;73(2):128–34 [discussion: e116].

21. Carpentier A, Chauvet D, Reina V, et al. MR-guided laser-induced thermal therapy (LITT) for recurrent glioblastomas. Lasers Surg Med 2012;44(5):361–8.

22. Aiyama H, Yamamoto M, Kawabe T, et al. Complications after stereotactic radiosurgery for brain metastases: incidences, correlating factors, treatments and outcomes. Radiother Oncol 2018;129(2):364–9.

23. Jagannathan J, Petit JH, Balsara K, et al. Long-term survival after gamma knife radiosurgery for primary and metastatic brain tumors. Am J Clin Oncol 2004;27(5):441–4.

24. Kano H, Shuto T, Iwai Y, et al. Stereotactic radiosurgery for intracranial hemangioblastomas: a retrospective international outcome study. J Neurosurg 2015;122(6):1469–78.

25. Minniti G, Clarke E, Lanzetta G, et al. Stereotactic radiosurgery for brain metastases: analysis of outcome and risk of brain radionecrosis. Radiat Oncol 2011;6:48.

26. Ashraf O, Patel NV, Hanft S, et al. Laser-induced thermal therapy in neuro-oncology: a review. World Neurosurg 2018;112:166–77.

27. Rao MS, Hargreaves EL, Khan AJ, et al. Magnetic resonance-guided laser ablation improves local control for postradiosurgery recurrence and/or radiation necrosis. Neurosurgery 2014;74(6):658–67 [discussion: 667].

28. Torres-Reveron J, Tomasiewicz HC, Shetty A, et al. Stereotactic laser induced thermotherapy (LITT): a novel treatment for brain lesions regrowing after radiosurgery. J Neurooncol 2013;113(3):495–503.

29. Fabiano AJ, Alberico RA. Laser-interstitial thermal therapy for refractory cerebral edema from post-radiosurgery metastasis. World Neurosurg 2014;81(3–4):652.e1-4.

30. Rahmathulla G, Recinos PF, Valerio JE, et al. Laser interstitial thermal therapy for focal cerebral radiation necrosis: a case report and literature review. Stereotact Funct Neurosurg 2012;90(3):192–200.

31. Luther E, McCarthy D, Shah A, et al. Radical laser interstitial thermal therapy ablation volumes increase progression-free survival in biopsy-proven radiation necrosis. World Neurosurg 2020;136:e646–59.

32. Chua TH, See AAQ, Ang BT, et al. Awake craniotomy for resection of brain metastases: a systematic review. World Neurosurg 2018;120:e1128–35.

33. Fang C, Zhu T, Zhang P, et al. Risk factors of neurosurgical site infection after craniotomy: a systematic review and meta-analysis. Am J Infect Control 2017;45(11):e123–34.

34. Abode-Iyamah KO, Chiang HY, Winslow N, et al. Risk factors for surgical site infections and assessment of vancomycin powder as a preventive measure in patients undergoing first-time cranioplasty. J Neurosurg 2018;128(4):1241–9.

35. Abu Hamdeh S, Lytsy B, Ronne-Engstrom E. Surgical site infections in standard neurosurgery procedures- a study of incidence, impact and potential risk factors. Br J Neurosurg 2014;28(2):270–5.

36. Chiang HY, Kamath AS, Pottinger JM, et al. Risk factors and outcomes associated with surgical site infections after craniotomy or craniectomy. J Neurosurg 2014;120(2):509–21.

37. Davies BM, Jones A, Patel HC. Implementation of a care bundle and evaluation of risk factors for surgical site infection in cranial neurosurgery. Clin Neurol Neurosurg 2016;144:121–5.

38. Jimenez-Martinez E, Cuervo G, Hornero A, et al. Risk factors for surgical site infection after craniotomy: a prospective cohort study. Antimicrob Resist Infect Control 2019;8:69.

39. Schipmann S, Akalin E, Doods J, et al. When the infection hits the wound: matched case-control study in a neurosurgical patient collective including systematic literature review and risk factors analysis. World Neurosurg 2016;95:178–89.

40. Kennion O, Holliman D. Outcome after craniotomy for recurrent cranial metastases. Br J Neurosurg 2017;31(3):369–73.

41. Alattar AA, Bartek J Jr, Chiang VL, et al. Stereotactic laser ablation as treatment of brain metastases recurring after stereotactic radiosurgery: a systematic literature review. World Neurosurg 2019;128:134–42.

Pathological Features of Brain Metastases

Saber Tadros, MD[a],*, Abhik Ray-Chaudhury, MD, MBBS[b]

KEYWORDS

- Brain metastases • Pathogenesis • Pathology • Immunohistochemistry • Molecular • Marker
- Cytology • Diagnosis

KEY POINTS

- Metastases are the most common intracranial tumors in adults and are spread via the hematogenous route to the central nervous system (CNS). Discovery of lymphatics in the brain may offer new insights into the metastasis pathogenesis. Brain microenvironment and intrinsic cancer properties play different roles in the process.
- Metastases are found generally near the gray-white junction with prevalence at certain brain sites. Some primary sites have a predilection for specific compartments. They typically appear as multiple masses, but metastases from breast, colon, and renal cell carcinoma are more often single.
- Leptomeningeal carcinomatosis and miliary brain metastases are rare forms of brain metastasis, and cerebrospinal fluid (CSF) is the sine qua non of diagnosis.
- Differentiating metastasis from primary brain tumor is not always a straightforward diagnosis.

INTRODUCTION

One of the 8 hallmarks of cancer as defined by Hanahan and Weinberg[1] is activating invasion and metastasis. A common site of metastasis for many types of solid tumor is the brain. Statistically, brain metastases are the most common intracranial tumors in adults. Autopsies and demographics studies showed that in patients with systemic malignancies, brain metastases occur in 10% to 30% of adults and 6% to 10% of children.[2–5] Noteworthy, most of the autopsy series are outdated. The incidence shows an increasing trend in the recent years, which may be due to improved detection of small metastases and improved systemic therapy for the solid tumors whereby the brain serves as a "safe haven" from chemotherapies that do not cross the blood-brain barrier (BBB).[2,4,6–8]

On the other hand, primary brain tumors rarely metastasize to extraneural sites,[9–11] either after surgical intervention like craniotomy or shunt or in absence of previous surgeries.[12–15] It was hypothesized that the lack of a lymphatic system in the brain, the presence of the BBB, and the lack of direct connection between the subarachnoid space and blood or lymphatic vessels may account for the rarity of glioma metastases.[16]

PATHOGENESIS

The World Health Organization 2016 classification of tumors defines metastatic tumors of the central nervous system (CNS) as tumors that originate outside the CNS and spread via the hematogenous route or invade the CNS from adjacent anatomic structures. Recently, it has been described for the first time that lymphatic vessels exist in the brain[17–19] and subsequent studies showed a functional role for brain lymphatics in aging and Alzheimer disease.[20–23] These discoveries may generate new investigations of various CNS disorders, including metastatic disease. In view of these recent discoveries, one can speculate that the dural lymphatic vascular system could encompass immune cell trafficking, thereby

a Laboratory of Pathology, National Cancer Institute, 10 Center Drive, Building 10, Room 3N248, Bethesda, MD 20814, USA; b Surgical Neurology Branch, National Cancer Institute, 10 Center Drive, Building 10, Room 3D-03, MSC1414, Bethesda, MD 20892-3704, USA
* Corresponding author.
E-mail address: tadross2@nih.gov

Neurosurg Clin N Am 31 (2020) 549–564
https://doi.org/10.1016/j.nec.2020.06.005

explaining why primary brain tumors rarely metastasize into cervical lymph nodes.

Paget[24] started a theory in 1889 that metastasis is dependent on the interactions between "seeds" (or the cancer cells) and the "soil" (or the host microenvironment). Then, Fidler described that successful metastatic colonization could occur only at certain organ sites.[25,26] Fidler's findings reignited interest in Paget's question of why tumor cells emerge within specific organs. Although the organ specificity observed in metastasis (known as organotropism) remains one of the most intriguing unanswered questions in cancer research, there are some features that make the brain an attractive territory for metastasis. First, the protective advantage of brain isolation that BBB offers makes it more vulnerable in the face of metastatic diseases. Few studies provided some insight into the evolution of BBB vascular permeability during cancer metastasis.[27,28] Second, tumors induce the formation of microenvironments in distant organs that are conducive to the survival and outgrowth of tumor cells before their arrival at these sites (premetastatic niches). Not enough research has explored the microenvironment of brain metastasis, but there is evidence of metabolic reprogramming of stromal cells in breast cancer metastasis to the brain.[29,30]

Speaking of the hallmarks of cancer, inducing angiogenesis is another hallmark of cancer because tumors require nutrients and oxygen as well as a pathway to evacuate metabolic wastes and carbon dioxide.[1] However, reports of tumors growing without the formation of new vessels are found in the literature since the earliest days of tumor description. In 1996, nonangiogenic tumors in lungs were described for the first time. Nonangiogenic tumors are tumors whereby the only blood vessels present are those originating from normal tissue.[31–34] The organs most commonly described to host nonangiogenic tumors, both for primary tumors and for metastatic lesions, are the lung, liver, and brain. Pezzella and his colleagues[31] summarized 4 different growth patterns seen in both primary and metastatic brain tumors.[35] One pattern is where single cells or small clusters of cells spread into the brain parenchyma without coming into contact with the preexisting vessels and without inducing formation of new vessels. Another pattern is the "cooptive" pattern, in which the cancer cells advance by coopting the normal vessels (perivascular cuffing) (**Fig. 1**D). In the putative angiogenic pattern, the tumor cells induce new vessel formation. Although a small number of tumors are purely nonangiogenic, many others contain both angiogenic and nonangiogenic areas. It appears that brain influences the nonangiogenic

growth of the tumors. Interestingly, nonangiogenic metastases have also been described in lymph nodes.[36]

In addition to the role of the microenvironment, "the soil," in the metastasis pathologic condition, cancer cells, "the seeds," have intrinsic features that facilitate their implantation. Today, next-generation sequencing (NGS) fortunately has provided a huge insight into the genetic landscape of malignancy with emphasis on the genetic heterogeneity of the primary tumors through cancer evolution. The presence of clonal diversity is expected to provide a rich repertoire of alterations that could be adaptive under the alterations in the tumor environment or metastatic colonization of distant sites. Recent studies of the tumor heterogeneity and tumor evolution showed that metastases share driver gene mutation with minimal heterogeneity,[37–39] an observation that could be explained by many factors like neutral evolution, tumor growth dynamics, or because of the available resources in the organ hosting the metastasis, a phenomenon that is observed in bacterial evolution.

Other intrinsic cancer cell properties were investigated, and data suggested some role of different genes and pathways in regulating metastases' colonization and in directing the organotropism.[40–43] In addition, the exosomes from tumor cells, namely, exosomal integrins α6β4 and α6β1, integrin αvβ5, and integrin β3, fuse preferentially with lung fibroblasts and epithelial cells, liver Kupffer cells, and brain endothelial cells, respectively.[44]

GENERAL ASPECTS

Because most brain metastases are of hematogenous origin, the distribution of the metastasis correlates with the blood supply of the brain. The middle cerebral artery is the largest and most complex of cerebral vessels with a series of bifurcations at its distal divisions. This anatomic complexity provides mechanical disadvantage for the moving secondaries resulting in lodging at one of its territories that is the most commonly afflicted, especially at the border zones with the posterior cerebral artery.[45–47] In light of the facts that regulation of cerebrovascular circulation is coupled to the high metabolic demand of the neuronal tissue and metastases are found generally in the cortex near the gray-white junction, the new insights into the understanding of the neurovascular unit might discover the link between the metabolic changes associated with the metastasis and prevalence of the metastasis at certain brain sites.

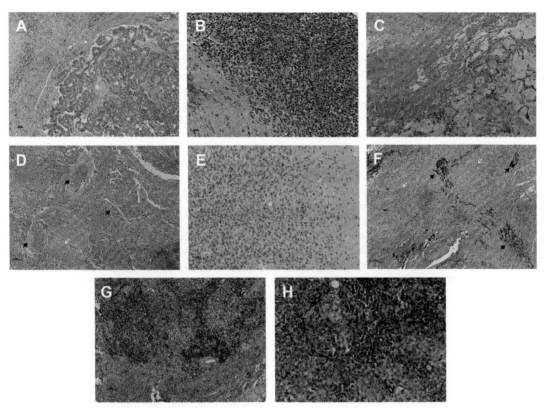

Fig. 1. (*A*) Metastatic lung adenocarcinoma to cerebellum of a 37-year-old woman. Notice the well-defined brain/tumor interface. Tumor shows glandular differentiation, which suggested epithelioid neoplasm. Tumor is positive for AE1/AE3. Then, staining for CK7+/CK20− suggested lung origin, which prompted TTF1 staining that confirms the lung origin. Subsequent CT scan for chest/abdomen/pelvis showed lung mass. (*B*) Metastatic small cell lung carcinoma to right frontal lobe of 67-year-old man. Notice the well-defined brain/tumor interface. Tumor cells show focal nuclear molding characteristic for small cell carcinoma. Tumor stains positive for CAM5.2, which suggested carcinomatous process. Synaptophysin positivity showed the neuroendocrine nature of the lesion. CK7+/CK20− pointed to lung origin, and TTF1 confirmed it. (*C*) Metastatic colorectal carcinoma to left temporal lobe of a 73-year-old woman. The tumor compresses surrounding brain tissue, forming a pseudocapsule. Tumor shows mucin-producing glands, suggesting adenocarcinoma. The patient had a prior history of both lung and colorectal carcinomas. Tumor positivity to CK20 and CDX2 favored colorectal origin over lung origin. (*D*) Metastatic duct carcinoma of the breast to the left frontal lobe of a 47-year-old woman. Tumor is formed of sheets of malignant epithelioid cells with poor attempts of tubular formation. Notice the angiocentric growth of tumor cells (*black arrow*) sparing uninvolved brain parenchyma in between (*white arrow*). Because of the suspicion of breast carcinoma morphologically, ER, PR, HER2 positivity in addition to GATA3 staining confirmed breast origin. (*E*) Poorly differentiated neoplasm in the occipital lobe of a 79-year-old man. This tumor showed vague tumor/brain interface suggesting metastasis. There is no glandular or papillary formation suggesting adenocarcinoma, but there is some nuclear molding favoring small cell carcinoma. Synaptophysin and TTF1 are positive, favoring small cell lung carcinoma. However, the tumor shows heterogeneous morphology with areas of small cell phenotype and large pleomorphic cells, so more IHC were attempted. GFAP, S100 (gliomas markers), and keratins (carcinoma markers) were negative. BRAF V600E mutation analysis (for melanoma) was negative. Finally, methylation classifier favors glioblastoma. TTF1 could be positive in glioblastoma. (*F*) Metastatic melanoma to right infratentorial region of a 13-year-old girl. The patient has a history of uveal melanoma. The tumor exhibits spindle cell morphology (*white arrow*) with heavily pigmented areas (*black arrow*). (*G, H*) CPC in the left parietal lobe of a 4-year-old boy. Note the vaguely defined mass of sheets of epithelioid cells. The patient's age is very important in this case (H&E staining).

The most common primary tumors responsible for brain metastases are carcinomas and include lung, breast, kidney, and colorectal cancers, and melanoma, whereas Hodgkin lymphoma, prostate carcinoma, ovarian carcinoma, esophagus, and oropharynx and nonmelanoma skin cancers rarely metastasize to the brain. Furthermore, some primary sites have a predilection for specific compartments. Breast carcinomas frequently give rise to dural and leptomeningeal metastases, sparing the brain parenchyma. Renal cell carcinoma (RCC) is the most frequent metastasis to the choroid plexus. In children, the most common sources of brain metastases are sarcomas, neuroblastoma, and germ cell tumors.[2–5,7]

Although brain metastases typically appear as multiple masses, they are single in 20% to 30% of patients. Metastases from breast, colon, and RCC are more often single, whereas lung cancers and malignant melanoma have a greater tendency to produce multiple metastases.[47]

Generally, 80% of melanoma brain metastases are supratentorial, whereas 15% are infratentorial or leptomeningeal, and 5% are in the brainstem.[48] In a study of 335 patients from China with a total of 2046 metastatic lesions, the cerebellum (56%) of patients, right parietal lobe (54%), right frontal lobe (47%), and left frontal lobe (45%) were the regions with the highest incidence of brain metastasis. Different distribution was observed with different pathologic types.[49]

Biopsy should be performed when the diagnosis of brain metastases is in doubt. Biopsy is particularly important in patients with a single lesion. The importance of biopsy was demonstrated in a study in which 6 patients of 54 patients with a single lesion were proven to have second primary tumors or inflammatory or infectious processes.[50]

SPECIAL ASPECTS
Leptomeningeal Carcinomatosis

Leptomeningeal carcinomatosis is a rare complication that is diagnosed in approximately 5% of patients with metastatic cancer.[51–53] Coexisting brain metastases are present in 50% to 80% of patients.[54–58] Meningeal carcinomatosis is caused by the spread of cancer cells to the leptomeninges. Spread to the cerebrospinal fluid (CSF) rapidly disseminates over the entirety of the CNS. The molecular mechanisms underlying leptomeningeal carcinomatosis is not well understood, but a recent study showed that complement component 3 (C3) was upregulated in 4 leptomeningeal metastatic models, and C3 is essential for this process. In addition, the study showed that interruption of C3a receptor signaling blocks leptomeningeal metastasis in mice.[59]

Metastasis via Perineural Route

Perineural tumor invasion is one of the mechanisms by which cancer cells extend beyond their primary site of development. It is either anterograde or retrograde, and mostly, there is no skip lesions.[60] In an experimental study, inoculation of myeloma and sarcoma tumor cells into the subcutaneous tissue of BALB/c mice resulted in perineural angiogenesis around the nerves adjacent to the deposit of tumor cells.[61] It was shown that the Schwann cells facilitate cancer progression through cancer cell dispersion, promoting epithelial mesenchymal transformation.[62,63] In pancreatic cancer, CX3CR1 expression is involved in the perineural invasion and dissemination of neoplastic cells along pancreatic nerves.[64]

A distinctive feature of head and neck tumors is the perineural tumor spread and perineural invasion.[65] Spread toward the skull base and CNS occurs in less than 5% of head and neck carcinoma.[66,67] Perineural tumor spread in head and neck is most often caused by squamous cell carcinoma with 3% to 14% incidence of intracranial perineural extension.[65–69] The most frequently affected nerves are the trigeminal and facial nerves. Other common malignancies with perineural spread include adenoid cystic carcinoma and nasopharyngeal carcinoma.

Tumor-to-Tumor Metastasis

In 1930, Fried[70] published autopsy results that showed metastatic inoculation of a meningioma by a bronchiogenic carcinoma. This phenomenon of tumor-to-tumor metastasis involves hematogenous spread of a malignancy to the parenchyma of an anatomically distant tumor, whereas collision tumors represent 2 distinct malignancies arising within the same organ and growing into one another. The most common host "recipient" tumor for a metastasis is pituitary adenoma or meningioma, with breast and lung malignancies being the common metastatic "donors."[71] Rare combinations of primary and recipient tumors were reported, such as melanoma metastasis to central neurocytoma,[72] hematopoietic neoplasms to meningiomas.[73] In von Hippel-Lindau disease, RCC can metastasize to hemangioblastomas (**Fig. 2**).[74,75]

Metastasis by Ophthalmic Tumors

Melanocytic tumors are the most common primary neoplasms of the uvea, and unlike the cutaneous melanoma metastases from uveal melanoma, occur primarily to the liver.[76,77]

Retinoblastoma is the most common primary intraocular tumor of childhood that arises from the retina. Retinoblastoma spreads to the CSF and then to brain and spinal cord via invasion through the optic disc into the optic nerve.[78] Retinoblastoma can also spread to the brain through hematogenous spread. One major related disease observed is trilateral retinoblastoma. It is a rare

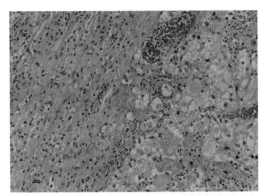

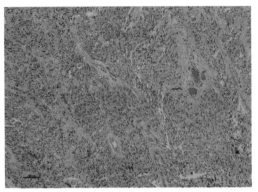

Fig. 2. Metastatic clear cell RCC to hemangioblastoma in a 42-year-old man diagnosed with Von Hippel-Lindau disease and presented with ataxia. No history of RCC was known at the time of the resection. Classical hemangioblastoma (*left*) is positive for inhibin and negative for PAX8 and AE1/AE3 IHC. RCC (*right*) that is positive for AE1/AE3 and PAX8 and negative for inhibin IHC (H&E staining).

Fig. 3. Metastatic ependymoma to right frontotemporal lobe in a 29-year-old man with prior resected ependymoma in the spinal cord. Methylation-based tumor profiling and NGS showed it is myxopapillary ependymoma.

condition in children with germline mutation in the *RB1* gene that presents with either unilateral or bilateral retinoblastoma and an intracranial midline neuroblastic tumor, usually in the pineal gland or in the supra/parasellar region.[79]

Intracranial Retrograde Dissemination

Retrograde intracranial dissemination is one of the ways that spinal tumors can spread to the brain. There are a few reported cases of myxopapillary ependymomas metastasized to the brain[80–82] (**Fig. 3**). High-grade ependymomas were also reported to have metastasized to the brain from the spinal cord.[83]

Special Clinicopathological Scenarios

Pulmonary cancers are the most common primaries that metastasized to the brain. Usually most of nonpulmonary cancers first metastasize to the lungs before forming secondaries in the brain. Although these lung metastases can remain clinically silent, the brain masses typically cause symptoms that usually result in medical attention. Less commonly, metastases to the CNS can bypass the lungs, especially those reaching the posterior fossa.

Patients with clinical history of non–small cell lung cancer (NSCLC) are living several years because of the advancement of therapies, allowing more time for brain metastases to develop as well as for adverse effects of prior therapies for brain metastases to emerge. Because newer targeted therapies against the epidermal growth factor receptor (EGFR) and anaplastic lymphoma kinase (ALK) have demonstrated far greater

intracranial efficacy, definitive assessment of the brain resection specimen for these markers is needed if the final diagnosis is adenocarcinoma.[84–86] Noteworthy, some data have suggested patients with *c-ROS* oncogene 1-positive NSCLC have lower rates of brain metastases than those with *ALK* rearrangements.[87,88]

Next to lung cancer, breast cancer is the second most common cancer associated with brain metastases in the United States.[89,90] The brain is frequently reported as the first site of relapse in women with human epidermal growth factor receptor 2 (HER2)-positive breast cancer treated with trastuzumab.[91,92] Patients with HER2-positive or estrogen receptor (ER)-positive disease appear to have a prolonged survival.[93] For the difference in the prognosis and the management of these patients, it is incumbent on the pathologist to provide this information for the oncologists.

In the past, metastatic melanoma to the brain contributed to death of most patients.[94,95] Recently, these patients' prognosis has been substantially improved by major advances in neuroimaging and improved options for the neurosurgical and radiotherapeutic management of brain metastases. Assessment for *BRAF V600* mutation, PD-L1 expression is necessary for guiding to BRAF or MEK inhibitor therapy and immunotherapy.

Adenocarcinoma of the brain of unknown primary after a complete staging evaluation could be seen occasionally in patients. In most of these patients, other metastatic sites manifest within a relatively short time.[96] The approach currently is resection of the solitary lesion if there is no evidence of additional metastasis elsewhere.[97] Although quite rare, germ cell tumors have high affinity for the brain as a brain metastasis of unknown primary. They are very responsive to chemotherapy, and their identification is of great value. A recent history of pregnancy may be a clue especially in women with metastatic choriocarcinoma.[98–100]

Hippocampal Metastasis

Whole-brain radiotherapy (WBRT) is one of the most commonly delivered treatments of patients with multiple brain metastases.[101,102] Several retrospective studies of patients receiving WBRT have suggested a relationship between the radiation dose to the hippocampus and neurocognitive decline.[103] As a result, the hippocampal avoidance-WBRT approach was proposed. The hippocampal avoidance-WBRT approach could partially reduce neurocognitive impairment, but it may be risky for the development of hippocampal metastasis in small cell lung cancer.[104] Interestingly, it does not seem to increase the risk of hippocampal metastasis in breast cancer.[105]

METASTASES MORPHOLOGY
Gross Appearance

Brain metastases typically appear as rounded, well-circumscribed masses. Superficial cortical metastasis may invade the leptomeninges and form a plaque. Subependymal ones may spread along the ventricular lining. "Miliary brain metastases," also termed "carcinomatous encephalitis," are an extremely rare form of brain metastasis.[106–108]

Leptomeningeal carcinomatosis involvement is commonly seen as diffuse opacification and thickening of the leptomeninges, as minute whitish nodules particularly at the base of the brain (basilar cisterns or posterior fossa), and the sylvian fissures, as bulky tumor following neoplastic invasion of the leptomeninges with associated inflammation, as CSF flow obstruction causing hydrocephalus, invasion of the cranial nerves, or in some cases, the brain has normal appearance grossly.[109] Dissemination along the ventricles may occur. The cytologic examination of the CSF is the sine qua non of diagnosis of leptomeningeal carcinomatosis.

Metastases are usually soft on the cut surface. Necrosis is focal or diffuse. Areas of hemorrhage are frequently seen that can present clinically as intracranial hemorrhage.[110] Several tumors have a characteristic gross appearance. Melanomas could present as pigmented lesions, and mucous-secreting adenocarcinomas will have a mucoid appearance. Choriocarcinoma, lung cancers, and RCCs have a tendency to be hemorrhagic.[110]

Microscopy

Histologic features of the metastases are usually similar to their primary lesions, but there may be less differentiation. For starters, epithelial structures are scarce in the normal CNS (choroid plexus, pituitary gland anterior, and intermediate lobes) so any epithelioid lesion should arise the suspicion for metastatic carcinoma. Second, although the pattern of infiltration is often helpful in distinguishing a metastatic tumor from primary CNS tumor (eg, diffuse glioma), occasionally cases of Glioblastoma (GBM) can demonstrate a pushing margin and/or invasion via Virchow-Robin spaces rather than a single-cell infiltration pattern that define the infiltrating gliomas. Local invasion along Virchow-Robin spaces is commonly seen in metastases of small cell lung carcinomas and melanomas. On the other hand, metastasis can exhibit infiltrative "pseudogliomatous" growth pattern.[111,112]

Brain metastases elicit several reactive changes in the parenchyma. Astrocytosis is often present surrounding the metastatic nodules. Microglial activation may occur around areas of necrosis. Neovascularization with some degree of vascular endothelial "glomeruloid" proliferation could be seen, but not of the extent seen in GBM.

Ancillary Tests

Many panels of immunohistochemical markers (IHC) were established to identify the primaries, summarized in (see **Figs. 1, 5,** and **6**).[113–117] Although IHC is usually informative in differentiation between metastasis and primary CNS neoplasm, it is important to remember that cytokeratin (AE1/AE3) cross-reacts with Glial fibrillary acidic protein (GFAP). Moreover, S100 is commonly positive in metastatic melanomas and gliomas. Some immunostaining is lost or significantly decreased on previously frozen tissue,[118] and none of these IHC results have been prospectively evaluated for accuracy in identifying the primary site.

Regardless, when the IHC profile fails to suggest the primary site, molecular cancer classifier assays could be used to classify the tumor.[119–124] The use of gene expression–based signatures for classifying tumor tissue of origin has been increasingly used at this molecular era.[125–127] Recently, methylation-based classification of CNS tumors was proved to have substantial impact on diagnostic precision compared with standard method (**Fig. 4**),[128] and DNA methylation-based assay was shown to be a useful approach to unmask

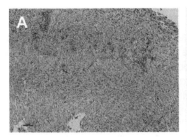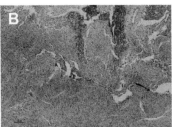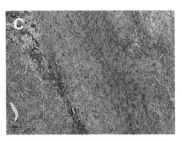

Fig. 4. (*A*) Undifferentiated sarcoma in a cerebellum of a 19-year-old man. Methylation-based tumor profiling and NGS failed to classify the tumor as primary brain tumor or conventional sarcoma. (*B*) Osteosarcoma in the right frontal lobe of a 58-year-old man. Methylation-based tumor profiling and NGS favored glioblastoma. (*C*) Osteosarcoma in the left frontal lobe of a 56-year-old man with synchronous osteosarcoma of sinonasal region (H&E staining).

the original primary tumor site of cancer of unknown primary cases.[129,130]

Imaging

It is exceptionally important for diagnosing brain lesions to determine the lesion location, especially when the neoplastic process is in question. The first denominator is whether the lesion is dura-based or intra-axial, followed by developing differential diagnosis based on specific locales. Many regional CNS vulnerabilities to particular tumor types are evident. For example, metastatic carcinomas have a predilection to intra-axial location within the cerebral hemispheres, whereas ependymomas frequently affect the spinal cord in adults.

Contrast-enhanced MRI is the preferred imaging study for the diagnosis of brain metastases, which was proved to be superior to double-dose delayed computerized tomography (CT) scan.[131] Brain metastases can be hypointense, isointense, or hyperintense on T1- and T2-weighted images. Contrast enhancement is nearly universal. Occasionally, very thin-walled cystic metastases will not enhance or only enhance minimally. The presence of multiple lesions, localization at the junction of the gray and white matter, circumscribed margins, and large amounts of vasogenic edema compared with the size of the lesion are features that can help differentiate brain metastases from other CNS lesions.[132]

Newer modalities, such as echo planar imaging, spectroscopy, PET, and single-photon emission computed tomography also may prove to be useful.[133]

DIFFERENTIAL DIAGNOSIS

Although there are many features, as discussed earlier, that can help differentiate metastasis from primary brain tumor, there are a few differential diagnoses worth highlighting.

In Von Hippel-Lindau syndrome, patients are predisposed for hemangioblastoma and clear cell RCC that can metastasize to the brain. Both tumors share the clear cytoplasm histology. Immunostaining for PAX 8 and inhibin proteins are helpful tools to separate them because RCC is positive in the former and hemangioblastoma for the latter (see **Fig. 2**). Oligodendroglioma can show clear cytoplasm and might be considered in the differential diagnosis. Olig-2-positive cells that are cytokeratin negative would be supportive for oligodendroglioma diagnosis.

Choroid plexus carcinoma (CPC) originates from the choroid plexus epithelium and shows typical carcinoma features. It is usually limited to young children and is extremely rare in adults[134] (see **Fig. 1**G). Unfortunately, most of the available markers for CPC are nonspecific. Another rare tumor that is characterized by a papillary and solid area and stain positive for keratins is papillary tumor of the pineal region.[135]

Anaplastic ependymomas always remain circumscribed masses, rarely invade the adjacent brain tissue, and can mimic embryonal tumors or small round blue cell tumors. In contrast to metastasis, ependymomas are strongly GFAP positive and cytokeratin negative.

Medulloblastoma has many morphologic variants, including desmoplastic medulloblastoma with extensive nodularity, and large cell/anaplastic medulloblastoma. Age and posterior fossa location are critical factors to consider when contemplating the diagnostic range of small round blue cell tumors in the CNS. Metastatic neuroblastoma, retinoblastoma, or lymphoma would not enter differential diagnosis except in exceptional clinical scenarios. Hematopoietic markers should identify the lymphoma.

Meningiomas display a wide range of histologic variants that might bring some challenges diagnostically. Meningothelial/transitional, clear cell, secretory, and papillary variants can mimic metastatic carcinoma. EMA and somatostatin receptor often aid in confirming diagnosis of meningioma.

Excluding metastatic melanoma is mandatory before diagnosing any of the primary CNS melanocytic neoplasms (see **Fig. 6**). Clinical correlation is extremely necessary in such situations. Some other primary tumors could show melanization phenomenon. These lesions include schwannoma, paraganglioma, medulloblastoma, and a few gliomas[136,137] (**Fig. 5**).

Germ cell tumors of the CNS could be part of multicentric germ cell neoplasia with independent intracranial and gonadal or mediastinal primaries.[138–140] Studying clonal origin would be helpful to determine the origin of the intracranial teratoma as primary, synchronous, and metachronous tumors. Exquisitely, a primary intracranial teratoma in a fetus of a mother who was diagnosed with independent ovarian teratoma was reported.[141]

CEREBROSPINAL FLUID CYTOLOGY

Since 1904, when a French neurologist described malignant cells in the CSF, CSF examination became an important component in the diagnosis of brain metastasis.[142]

Malignant cells are easily identified in the CSF, and in most cases, the patient is known to have malignancy.[143,144] However, in 10% of patients with positive CSF for malignancy, there is no known primary tumor.[145] In such cases of positive CSF for malignancy with no history of cancer, likely primaries are lung, stomach, melanoma, and lymphoma.

SERUM TUMOR MARKERS

The classic serum tumor markers, such as carcinoembryonic antigen, cancer antigen (CA) 19-9, CA 15-3, and CA 125, are not useful as either diagnostic or prognostic tests. However, they are often elevated in the serum of patients with

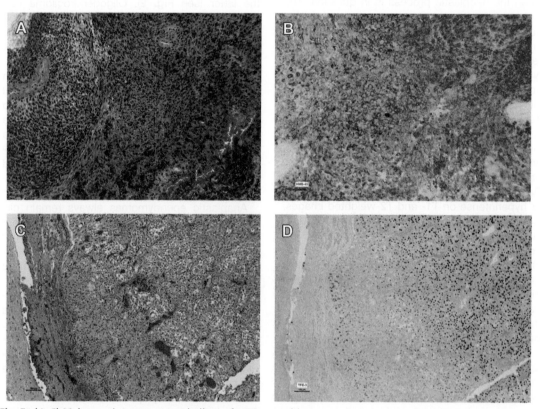

Fig. 5. (*A*, *B*) Melanocytic tumor at cerebellum of a 57-year-old woman. Because it is a heavily pigmented tumor (HMB-45 positive), the differential diagnosis included metastatic pigmented epithelioid melanocytoma from the skin, metastatic melanoma, and brain melanocytoma. CT showed concerning liver nodule. No ocular melanoma was detected. Although the patient had no history of skin melanoma, metastatic melanoma possibility could not be excluded. *BRAF V600E* negativity and comparative genomic hybridization helped to exclude metastatic melanoma, and diagnosis of melanocytoma was established [A: H&E staining, B: HMB-45 IHC]. (*C,D*) Metastatic alveolar soft part sarcoma to left frontal lobe of a 66-year-old man. Tumor cells stain positive for TFE-3. The patient had a right thigh mass resection 5 years earlier that proved to be alveolar soft part sarcoma [C: H&E staining, D: TFE-3 IHC].

adenocarcinoma, and the only use for them currently is in following the response to therapy for individual tumors through serial measurement. Some other serum markers are more specific, such as calcitonin, which can be used to screen for recurrence and estimate prognosis in medullary thyroid cancer. Prostate-specific antigen (PSA) use is common, but its value is controversial. Some new concepts, including PSA density and velocity, have emerged to refine the test interpretation, although these have not been widely adopted. Some of the proteins secreted by germ cell tumors provide high sensitivity for the presence of certain histologic components in the tumor. Human chorionic gonadotropin level is elevated in embryonal carcinomas, choriocarcinomas, mixed germ cell tumors, seminomas, and some dysgerminomas. Alpha-fetoprotein is present in yolk sac tumors, embryonal cell carcinomas, mixed germ cell tumors, and some immature teratomas. However, their utility is for monitoring response to treatment and detecting recurrence and not for initial diagnosis.

In the modern era, liquid biopsies from plasma, in contrast to tissue biopsies that are the gold standard for cancer diagnosis, are emerging as screening and staging tools. Sequencing of plasma cell-free DNA (cfDNA) is one of the most promising tools that could be helpful as less invasive circulating tumor markers.

In 1948, fragments of cell-free nucleic acids in human blood were discovered,[146] and after decades, it was reported that cfDNA levels increased in the serum of patients with cancer.[147] Later, it was demonstrated that some cfDNA in the plasma of patients with cancer originates from cancer cells,[148] and they carry similar mutations of the primary tumor.[149–152] Mutations in cfDNA are specific markers for cancer, so the term "circulating tumor DNA" was coined. Vastly, most cfDNA molecules are heavily fragmented; however, this fragmentation is not random, as shown in recent study.[153]

In a similar vein, detection of circulating tumor cells (CTCs) starts to find its way to the clinical practice as a tumor marker. CTCs/circulating tumor microemboli (CTMs) are malignant cells that depart from cancerous lesions and shed into the bloodstream. Analysis of messenger RNAs and long noncoding RNAs of CTCs could be used as a noninvasive liquid biopsy. Detection of CTCs in blood samples of patients with metastatic breast cancer has been shown to be a predictor of progression-free survival and overall survival, but using it for monitoring of patients remains controversial.[154,155] Subsequent data have shown the potential benefits of CTC detection in other cancer types, like melanoma, prostatic cancer, colonic cancer, and sarcomas.[156–159] In addition, analysis of tumor-derived exosomes is a new active area of research to help diagnosing and follow-up for tumor progression, although more work is needed to validate its use.

PATHOLOGIST SURGEON INTERFACE

To accomplish the task of establishing the diagnosis of brain metastasis, the pathologist assesses multiple aspects of certain lesions to reach the final diagnosis. Clinical information regarding the location of the tumor is of great value. Multifocal masses are more likely to be metastatic than primary tumor. Diffuse leptomeningeal MRI enhancement is a very rare presentation of a glial tumor and is increasingly seen with metastasis. A history of malignancy elsewhere always prompts scrutiny before diagnosing a second tumor, unless the patient has a known syndrome causing multiple neoplasms.

The first interpretation usually is done on stained slides from frozen (intraoperative consult) section. In adults, lesions with epithelioid, papillary, or glandular differentiation always point to metastatic epithelioid neoplasms. Apart from small cell variant of carcinomas, carcinoma cells are relatively large with an increase in the nuclear size (3–5 times of red blood cell size), pleomorphic nuclei, coarsely clumped chromatin, and often prominent nucleoli. Mitotic figures and tumor cell necrosis are usually common. Sampling the tumor/brain parenchyma interface is necessary to assess the tumor infiltration because a sharp border of normal parenchyma with the neoplasm suggests metastasis instead of glioblastoma or lymphoma. The metastatic tumors might lose the architecture pattern of carcinoma and form sheets of neoplastic epithelioid cells. In such a condition, differential diagnosis includes melanoma, lymphoma, and glioblastoma. Sometimes, it is impossible to distinguish a melanoma from carcinoma during an intraoperative consult. A more confident diagnosis is usually based on formalin-fixed, paraffin-embedded (FFPE) sections.

FFPE sections are used for more ancillary tests to confirm diagnosis and investigate specific targets for therapy. IHC provides valuable information about the nature of the lesion. There are many approaches to the interpretation of IHC analysis when it is used for statistical analysis. A comprehensive PubMed search showed at least 7 different methods of IHC data interpretation, such as qualitative scoring and combinative semiquantitative scoring.[160] However, using IHC in clinical settings is more an art than a science. Pathologists cannot rely on IHC results

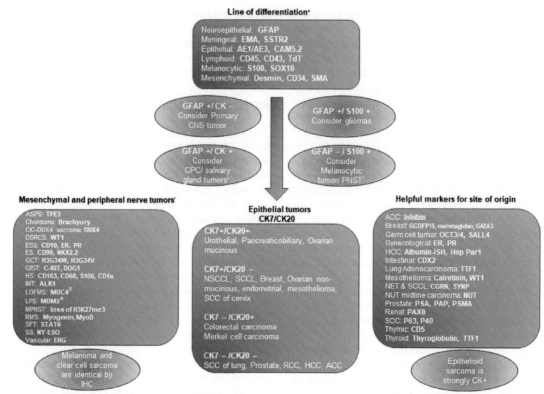

Line of differentiation[a]

Neuroepithelial: GFAP
Meningeal: EMA, SSTR2
Epithelial: AE1/AE3, CAM5.2
Lymphoid: CD45, CD43, TdT
Melanocytic: S100, SOX10
Mesenchymal: Desmin, CD34, SMA

GFAP +/ CK –
Consider Primary
CNS tumor

GFAP +/ S100 +
Consider gliomas

GFAP +/ CK +
Consider
CPC/ salivary
gland tumors[b]

GFAP – / S100 +
Consider
Melanocytic
tumor/ PNST[c]

Mesenchymal and peripheral nerve tumors[f]

ASPS: TFE3
Chordoma: Brachyury
CIC-DUX4 sarcoma: DUX4
DSRCS: WT1
ESS: CD10, ER, PR
ES: CD99, NKX2.2
GCT: H3G34W, H3G34V
GIST: C-KIT, DOG1
HS: CD163, CD68, S100, CD1a
IMT: ALK1
LGFMS: MUC4[d]
LPS: MDM2[e]
MPNST: loss of H3K27me3
RMS: Myogenin, MyoD
SFT: STAT6
SS: NY-ESO
Vascular: ERG

Melanoma and
clear cell sarcoma
are identical by
IHC

**Epithelial tumors
CK7/CK20**

CK7+/CK20+
Urothelial, Pancreaticobiliary, Ovarian
mucinous

CK7+/CK20 –
NSCCL, SCCL, Breast, Ovarian non-
mucinous, endometrial, mesothelioma,
SCC of cervix

CK7 – /CK20+
Colorectal carcinoma
Merkel cell carcinoma

CK7 – /CK20 –
SCC of lung, Prostate, RCC, HCC, ACC

Helpful markers for site of origin

ACC: Inhibin
Breast: GCDFP15, mammaglobin, GATA3
Germ cell tumor: OCT3/4, SALL4
Gynecological: ER, PR
HCC: Albumin-ISH, Hep Par1
Intestinal: CDX2
Lung Adenocarcinoma: TTF1
Mesothelioma: Calretinin, WT1
NET & SCCL: CGRN, SYNP
NUT midline carcinoma: NUT
Prostate: PSA, PAP, PSMA
Renal: PAX8
SCC: P63, P40
Thymic: CD5
Thyroid: Thyroglobulin, TTF1

Epithelioid
sarcoma is
strongly CK+

Fig. 6. Stepwise approach of brain metastasis immunophenotype.[a] It is recommended always to use 2 markers for each line of differentiation. [b] CPC is focally positive for GFAP. Salivary gland carcinoma with ductal component is GFAP positive. [c] MPNST usually loses S100 expression. [d] MUC4 is positive in 20% of meningiomas. [e] MDM2 is expressed in many sarcomas and nonspecific. [f] Some of the listed tumors required gene fusions testing for confirmation (CIC-DUX4 sarcoma, DSRCS, ES, IMT, clear cell sarcoma). ACC, adrenocortical carcinoma; ASPS, alveolar soft part sarcoma; CPC, choroid plexus carcinoma; DSRCS, desmoplastic small round cell sarcoma; ES, ewing sarcoma; ESS, endometrial stromal sarcoma; GCT, giant cell tumor; GIST, gastrointestinal stromal tumor; HCC, hepatocellular carcinoma; HS, histiocytic sarcoma; IMT, inflammatory myofibroblastic tumor; LGFMS, low-grade fibromyxoid sarcoma; LPS, liposarcoma; MPNST, malignant peripheral nerve sheet tumor; NET, neuroendocrine tumor; NSCCL:, non-small cell carcinoma of lung; RCC, renal cell carcinoma; RMS:, rhabdomyoasrcoma; SCC, squamous cell carcinoma; SCCL, small cell carcinoma of the lung; SFT, solitary fibrous tumor; SS, Synovial sarcoma.

independently from histologic impression on hematoxylin and eosin–stain slides. Immunophenotype of the tumors is very complex, but there are some commonly used markers that can stratify the tumors globally. Cytokeratin cocktail (AE1/AE3, CAM5.2) and GFAP combination can be helpful to separate primary glial tumor from metastatic carcinoma. S100 and SOX10 are good markers to highlight melanocytic lesions like melanoma. CD43, CD45 and TdT would be positive in most of the hematopoietic neoplasms. Generally, when the initial impression is a carcinomatous lesion, a CK7 and CK20 combination has been shown to be helpful to suggest the site of primary origin of a wide range of carcinomas. Then, there are many other markers that support certain sites of origin (as in **Fig. 6**) after the initial assessment by CK7/CK20, but, if the initial impression is a sarcomatous lesion, a panel of desmin, CD34,

smooth muscle actin, and S100 usually helps to guide diagnosis of mesenchymal tumors. Eventually, the final diagnosis requires integration of anatomic, histologic, and immunophenotypical features of the lesion and sometimes the molecular findings as well.

SUMMARY

Brain metastases have historically been approached as end-stage disease with uniform poor clinical outcomes regardless of the primary tumor type. Nevertheless, with the emergence of precision medicine and the feasibility of various treatment interventions, accurate classification of the metastases based not only on morphologic features but also on molecular and immunologic features becomes imperative. Moreover, newer disease-specific prognostic factors, such as

EGFR mutation and ALK rearrangement, in metastatic lung cancer have been incorporated in the modern decision making. In addition, the available material from metastases, such as biopsies or excisions, might unmask important targeted molecular abnormalities that were hidden in the primary tumor because of tumor heterogeneity. Finally, response determination, which is solely based on imaging with its inherited limitations,[161] might require in the future pathologic assessment as a more definitive method.

DISCLOSURE

The authors have nothing to disclose.

REFERENCES

1. Hanahan D, Weinberg RA. Hallmarks of cancer: the next generation. Cell 2011;144(5):646–74.
2. Gavrilovic IT, Posner JB. Brain metastases: epidemiology and pathophysiology. J Neurooncol 2005; 75(1):5–14.
3. Graus F, Walker RW, Allen JC. Brain metastases in children. J Pediatr 1983;103(4):558–61.
4. Johnson JD, Young B. Demographics of brain metastasis. Neurosurg Clin N Am 1996;7(3):337–44.
5. Lassman AB, DeAngelis LM. Brain metastases. Neurol Clin 2003;21(1):1–23, vii.
6. Sundermeyer ML, Meropol NJ, Rogatko A, et al. Changing patterns of bone and brain metastases in patients with colorectal cancer. Clin Colorectal Cancer 2005;5(2):108–13.
7. Bouffet E, Doumi N, Thiesse P, et al. Brain metastases in children with solid tumors. Cancer 1997; 79(2):403–10.
8. Smedby KE, Brandt L, Bäcklund ML, et al. Brain metastases admissions in Sweden between 1987 and 2006. Br J Cancer 2009;101(11):1919–24.
9. Schweitzer T, Vince GH, Herbold C, et al. Extraneural metastases of primary brain tumors. J Neurooncol 2001;53(2):107–14.
10. Hoffman HJ, Duffner PK. Extraneural metastases of central nervous system tumors. Cancer 1985;56(7 Suppl):1778–82.
11. Lun M, Lok E, Gautam S, et al. The natural history of extracranial metastasis from glioblastoma multiforme. J Neurooncol 2011;105(2):261–73.
12. Ricard JA, Cramer SW, Charles R, et al. Infratentorial glioblastoma metastasis to bone. World Neurosurg 2019;131:90–4.
13. Stephens S, Tollesson G, Robertson T, et al. Diffuse midline glioma metastasis to the peritoneal cavity via ventriculo-peritoneal shunt: case report and review of literature. J Clin Neurosci 2019;67:288–93.
14. Xu K, Khine KT, Ooi YC, et al. A systematic review of shunt-related extraneural metastases of primary central nervous system tumors. Clin Neurol Neurosurg 2018;174:239–43.
15. Hulbanni S, Goodman PA. Glioblastoma multiforme with extraneural metastases in the absence of previous surgery. Cancer 1976;37(3):1577–83.
16. Beauchesne P. Extra-neural metastases of malignant gliomas: myth or reality? Cancers 2011;3(1): 461–77.
17. Louveau A, Smirnov I, Keyes TJ, et al. Structural and functional features of central nervous system lymphatic vessels. Nature 2015;523(7560):337–41.
18. Aspelund A, Antila S, Proulx ST, et al. A dural lymphatic vascular system that drains brain interstitial fluid and macromolecules. J Exp Med 2015; 212(7):991–9.
19. Antila S, Karaman S, Nurmi H, et al. Development and plasticity of meningeal lymphatic vessels. J Exp Med 2017;214(12):3645–67.
20. Da Mesquita S, Louveau A, Vaccari A, et al. Functional aspects of meningeal lymphatics in ageing and Alzheimer's disease. Nature 2018;560(7717): 185–91.
21. Louveau A, Herz J, Alme MN, et al. CNS lymphatic drainage and neuroinflammation are regulated by meningeal lymphatic vasculature. Nat Neurosci 2018;21(10):1380–91.
22. Ma Q, Ineichen BV, Detmar M, et al. Outflow of cerebrospinal fluid is predominantly through lymphatic vessels and is reduced in aged mice. Nat Commun 2017;8(1):1434.
23. Da Mesquita S, Fu Z, Kipnis J. The meningeal lymphatic system: a new player in neurophysiology. Neuron 2018;100(2):375–88.
24. Paget S. The distribution of secondary growths in cancer of the breast. Lancet 1889;133:571–3.
25. Fidler IJ, Nicolson GL. Organ selectivity for implantation survival and growth of B16 melanoma variant tumor lines. J Natl Cancer Inst 1976;57(5):1199–202.
26. Hart IR, Fidler IJ. Role of organ selectivity in the determination of metastatic patterns of B16 melanoma. Cancer Res 1980;40(7):2281–7.
27. Benoit P, Michelet FX, Benoit JP, et al. [Clinical study of the indications for the use of the new anti-inflammatory irrigating solution, Hexo-imotryl]. Rev Odontostomatol Midi Fr 1971;29(1):56–63.
28. Percy DB, Ribot EJ, Chen Y, et al. In vivo characterization of changing blood-tumor barrier permeability in a mouse model of breast cancer metastasis: a complementary magnetic resonance imaging approach. Invest Radiol 2011;46(11): 718–25.
29. Fong MY, Zhou W, Liu L, et al. Breast-cancer-secreted miR-122 reprograms glucose metabolism in premetastatic niche to promote metastasis. Nat Cell Biol 2015;17(2):183–94.
30. Li L, Kang L, Zhao W, et al. miR-30a-5p suppresses breast tumor growth and metastasis through

inhibition of LDHA-mediated Warburg effect. Cancer Lett 2017;400:89–98.

31. Pezzella F, Pastorino U, Tagliabue E, et al. Non-small-cell lung carcinoma tumor growth without morphological evidence of neo-angiogenesis. Am J Pathol 1997;151(5):1417–23.

32. Evidence for novel non-angiogenic pathway in breast-cancer metastasis. Breast Cancer Progression Working Party. Lancet 2000;355(9217):1787–8.

33. Küsters B, Leenders WPJ, Wesseling P, et al. Vascular endothelial growth factor-A(165) induces progression of melanoma brain metastases without induction of sprouting angiogenesis. Cancer Res 2002;62(2):341–5.

34. Vermeulen PB, Colpaert C, Salgado R, et al. Liver metastases from colorectal adenocarcinomas grow in three patterns with different angiogenesis and desmoplasia. J Pathol 2001;195(3):336–42.

35. Donnem T, Reynolds AR, Kuczynski EA, et al. Non-angiogenic tumours and their influence on cancer biology. Nat Rev Cancer 2018;18(5):323–36.

36. Naresh KN, Nerurkar AY, Borges AM. Angiogenesis is redundant for tumour growth in lymph node metastases. Histopathology 2001;38(5):466–70.

37. Reiter JG, Makohon-Moore AP, Gerold JM, et al. Minimal functional driver gene heterogeneity among untreated metastases. Science 2018; 361(6406):1033–7.

38. Sottoriva A, Kang H, Ma Z, et al. A Big Bang model of human colorectal tumor growth. Nat Genet 2015; 47(3):209–16.

39. Williams MJ, Werner B, Heide T, et al. Quantification of subclonal selection in cancer from bulk sequencing data. Nat Genet 2018;50(6):895–903.

40. Müller A, Homey B, Soto H, et al. Involvement of chemokine receptors in breast cancer metastasis. Nature 2001;410(6824):50–6.

41. Zhou W, Fong MY, Min Y, et al. Cancer-secreted miR-105 destroys vascular endothelial barriers to promote metastasis. Cancer cell 2014;25(4):501–15.

42. Cox TR, Rumney RMH, Schoof EM, et al. The hypoxic cancer secretome induces pre-metastatic bone lesions through lysyl oxidase. Nature 2015; 522(7554):106–10.

43. Kaplan RN, Riba RD, Zacharoulis S, et al. VEGFR1-positive haematopoietic bone marrow progenitors initiate the pre-metastatic niche. Nature 2005; 438(7069):820–7.

44. Hoshino A, Costa-Silva B, Shen T-L, et al. Tumour exosome integrins determine organotropic metastasis. Nature 2015;527(7578):329–35.

45. Gibo H, Carver CC, Rhoton AL, et al. Microsurgical anatomy of the middle cerebral artery. J Neurosurg 1981;54(2):151–69.

46. Tanriover N, Rhoton AL, Kawashima M, et al. Microsurgical anatomy of the insula and the sylvian fissure. J Neurosurg 2004;100(5):891–922.

47. Delattre JY, Krol G, Thaler HT, et al. Distribution of brain metastases. Arch Neurol 1988;45(7): 741–4.

48. Sloan AE, Nock CJ, Einstein DB. Diagnosis and treatment of melanoma brain metastasis: a literature review. Cancer Control 2009;16(3):248–55.

49. Wang G, Xu J, Qi Y, et al. Distribution of brain metastasis from lung cancer. Cancer Manag Res 2019;11:9331–8.

50. Patchell RA, Tibbs PA, Walsh JW, et al. A randomized trial of surgery in the treatment of single metastases to the brain. N Engl J Med 1990;322(8):494–500.

51. Kaplan JG, DeSouza TG, Farkash A, et al. Leptomeningeal metastases: comparison of clinical features and laboratory data of solid tumors, lymphomas and leukemias. J Neurooncol 1990; 9(3):225–9.

52. Kesari S, Batchelor TT. Leptomeningeal metastases. Neurol Clin 2003;21(1):25–66.

53. Bruno MK, Raizer J. Leptomeningeal metastases from solid tumors (meningeal carcinomatosis). Cancer Treat Res 2005;125:31–52.

54. Clarke JL, Perez HR, Jacks LM, et al. Leptomeningeal metastases in the MRI era. Neurology 2010; 74(18):1449–54.

55. Lara-Medina F, Crismatt A, Villarreal-Garza C, et al. Clinical features and prognostic factors in patients with carcinomatous meningitis secondary to breast cancer. Breast J 2012;18(3):233–41.

56. Umemura S, Tsubouchi K, Yoshioka H, et al. Clinical outcome in patients with leptomeningeal metastasis from non-small cell lung cancer: Okayama Lung Cancer Study Group. Lung Cancer 2012;77(1):134–9.

57. Morris PG, Reiner AS, Szenberg OR, et al. Leptomeningeal metastasis from non-small cell lung cancer: survival and the impact of whole brain radiotherapy. J Thorac Oncol 2012;7(2):382–5.

58. Raizer JJ, Hwu W-J, Panageas KS, et al. Brain and leptomeningeal metastases from cutaneous melanoma: survival outcomes based on clinical features. Neuro Oncol 2008;10(2):199–207.

59. Boire A, Zou Y, Shieh J, et al. Complement component 3 adapts the cerebrospinal fluid for leptomeningeal metastasis. Cell 2017;168(6):1101–13.e13.

60. Panizza B, Warren TA, Solares CA, et al. Histopathological features of clinical perineural invasion of cutaneous squamous cell carcinoma of the head and neck and the potential implications for treatment. Head Neck 2014;36(11):1611–8.

61. Warner TF, Krueger RG. Perineural angiogenesis in mice bearing subcutaneous tumours. Br J Exp Pathol 1978;59(3):282–7.

62. Deborde S, Omelchenko T, Lyubchik A, et al. Schwann cells induce cancer cell dispersion and invasion. J Clin Invest 2016;126(4):1538–54.

63. Shan C, Wei J, Hou R, et al. Schwann cells promote EMT and the Schwann-like differentiation of salivary adenoid cystic carcinoma cells via the BDNF/TrkB axis. Oncol Rep 2016;35(1):427–35.

64. Marchesi F, Locatelli M, Solinas G, et al. Role of CX3CR1/CX3CL1 axis in primary and secondary involvement of the nervous system by cancer. J Neuroimmunol 2010;224(1–2):39–44.

65. Amit M, Eran A, Billan S, et al. Perineural spread in noncutaneous head and neck cancer: new insights into an old problem. J Neurol Surg B Skull Base 2016;77(2):86–95.

66. Gupta A, Veness M, De'Ambrosis B, et al. Management of squamous cell and basal cell carcinomas of the head and neck with perineural invasion. Australas J Dermatol 2016;57(1):3–13.

67. Singh N, Eskander A, Huang S-H, et al. Imaging and resectability issues of sinonasal tumors. Expert Rev Anticancer Ther 2013;13(3):297–312.

68. Karia PS, Morgan FC, Ruiz ES, et al. Clinical and incidental perineural invasion of cutaneous squamous cell carcinoma: a systematic review and pooled analysis of outcomes data. JAMA Dermatol 2017;153(8):781–8.

69. Stambuk HE. Perineural tumor spread involving the central skull base region. Semin Ultrasound CT MR 2013;34(5):445–58.

70. Fried BM. Metastatic inoculation of a meningioma by cancer cells from a bronchiogenic carcinoma. Am J Pathol 1930;6(1):47–52, 1.

71. Takei H, Powell SZ. Tumor-to-tumor metastasis to the central nervous system. Neuropathology 2009;29(3):303–8.

72. Brown HM, McCutcheon IE, Leeds NE, et al. Melanoma metastatic to central neurocytoma: a novel case of tumor-to-tumor metastasis. J Neurooncol 2003;61(3):209–14.

73. Widdel L, Kleinschmidt-DeMasters BK, Kindt G. Tumor-to-tumor metastasis from hematopoietic neoplasms to meningiomas: report of two patients with significant cerebral edema. World Neurosurg 2010;74(1):165–71.

74. Jarrell ST, Vortmeyer AO, Linehan WM, et al. Metastases to hemangioblastomas in von Hippel-Lindau disease. J Neurosurg 2006;105(2):256–63.

75. Ingold B, Wild PJ, Nocito A, et al. Renal cell carcinoma marker reliably discriminates central nervous system haemangioblastoma from brain metastases of renal cell carcinoma. Histopathology 2008;52(6):674–81.

76. Seedor RS, Eschelman DJ, Gonsalves CF, et al. An outcome assessment of a single institution's longitudinal experience with uveal melanoma patients with liver metastasis. Cancers 2020;12(1):117.

77. Jochems A, van der Kooij MK, Fiocco M, et al. Metastatic uveal melanoma: treatment strategies and survival-results from the Dutch Melanoma Treatment Registry. Cancers 2019;11(7):1007.

78. Ueda T, Koga Y, Yoshikawa H, et al. Survival and ocular preservation in a long-term cohort of Japanese patients with retinoblastoma. BMC Pediatr 2020;20(1):37.

79. de Jong MC, Kors WA, de Graaf P, et al. Trilateral retinoblastoma: a systematic review and meta-analysis. Lancet Oncol 2014;15(10):1157–67.

80. Plans G, Brell M, Cabiol J, et al. Intracranial retrograde dissemination in filum terminale myxopapillary ependymomas. Acta Neurochir (Wien) 2006; 148(3):343–6 [discussion: 6].

81. Fonseca L, Cicuendez M, Martínez-Ricarte F, et al. A rare case of an intramedullary metastasis of a myxopapillary ependymoma. Surg Neurol Int 2019;10:83.

82. Kittel K, Gjuric M, Niedobitek G. Metastasis of a spinal myxopapillary ependymoma to the inner auditory canal. HNO 2001;49(4):298–302 [in German].

83. Nagańska E, Matyja E, Zabek M, et al. Disseminated spinal and cerebral ependymoma with unusual histological pattern: clinicopathological study of a case with retrograde tumor spread. Folia Neuropathol 2000;38(3):135–41.

84. Johung KL, Yeh N, Desai NB, et al. Extended survival and prognostic factors for patients with ALK-rearranged non-small-cell lung cancer and brain metastasis. J Clin Oncol 2016;34(2):123–9.

85. Zhang I, Zaorsky NG, Palmer JD, et al. Targeting brain metastases in ALK-rearranged non-small-cell lung cancer. Lancet Oncol 2015;16(13): e510–21.

86. Shin D-Y, Na II, Kim CH, et al. EGFR mutation and brain metastasis in pulmonary adenocarcinomas. J Thorac Oncol 2014;9(2):195–9.

87. Gainor JF, Tseng D, Yoda S, et al. Patterns of metastatic spread and mechanisms of resistance to crizotinib in ROS1-positive non-small-cell lung cancer. JCO Precis Oncol 2017;2017. https://doi.org/10.1200/PO.17.00063.

88. Patil T, Smith DE, Bunn PA, et al. The incidence of brain metastases in stage IV ROS1-rearranged non-small cell lung cancer and rate of central nervous system progression on crizotinib. J Thorac Oncol 2018;13(11):1717–26.

89. Barnholtz-Sloan JS, Sloan AE, Davis FG, et al. Incidence proportions of brain metastases in patients diagnosed (1973 to 2001) in the Metropolitan Detroit Cancer Surveillance System. J Clin Oncol 2004;22(14):2865–72.

90. Schouten LJ, Rutten J, Huveneers HAM, et al. Incidence of brain metastases in a cohort of patients with carcinoma of the breast, colon, kidney, and lung and melanoma. Cancer 2002;94(10):2698–705.

91. Yin W, Jiang Y, Shen Z, et al. Trastuzumab in the adjuvant treatment of HER2-positive early breast cancer patients: a meta-analysis of published randomized controlled trials. PloS One 2011;6(6). e21030-e.

92. Pestalozzi BC, Holmes E, de Azambuja E, et al. CNS relapses in patients with HER2-positive early breast cancer who have and have not received adjuvant trastuzumab: a retrospective substudy of the HERA trial (BIG 1-01). Lancet Oncol 2013; 14(3):244–8.

93. Sperduto PW, Kased N, Roberge D, et al. Summary report on the graded prognostic assessment: an accurate and facile diagnosis-specific tool to estimate survival for patients with brain metastases. J Clin Oncol 2012;30(4):419–25.

94. Sampson JH, Carter JH, Friedman AH, et al. Demographics, prognosis, and therapy in 702 patients with brain metastases from malignant melanoma. J Neurosurg 1998;88(1):11–20.

95. Carlino MS, Fogarty GB, Long GV. Treatment of melanoma brain metastases: a new paradigm. Cancer J 2012;18(2):208–12.

96. Rades D, Kühnel G, Wildfang I, et al. Localised disease in cancer of unknown primary (CUP): the value of positron emission tomography (PET) for individual therapeutic management. Ann Oncol 2001;12(11):1605–9.

97. Salvati M, Cervoni L, Raco A. Single brain metastases from unknown primary malignancies in CT-era. J Neurooncol 1995;23(1):75–80.

98. Johnson K, Brunet B. Brain metastases as presenting feature in 'burned out' testicular germ cell tumor. Cureus 2016;8(4):e551.

99. Lo AC, Hodgson D, Dang J, et al. Intracranial germ cell tumors in adolescents and young adults: a 40-year multi-institutional review of outcomes. Int J Radiat Oncol Biol Phys 2020;106(2):269–78.

100. Feldman DR, Lorch A, Kramar A, et al. Brain metastases in patients with germ cell tumors: prognostic factors and treatment options–an analysis from the global germ cell cancer group. J Clin Oncol 2016; 34(4):345–51.

101. Chao JH, Phillips R, Nickson JJ. Roentgen-ray therapy of cerebral metastases. Cancer 1954;7(4):682–9.

102. Brown PD, Ahluwalia MS, Khan OH, et al. Whole-brain radiotherapy for brain metastases: evolution or revolution? J Clin Oncol 2018;36(5):483–91.

103. Chang EL, Wefel JS, Hess KR, et al. Neurocognition in patients with brain metastases treated with radiosurgery or radiosurgery plus whole-brain irradiation: a randomised controlled trial. Lancet Oncol 2009;10(11):1037–44.

104. Korkmaz Kirakli E, Oztekin O. Is hippocampal avoidance during whole-brain radiotherapy risky for patients with small-cell lung cancer? Hippocampal metastasis rate and associated risk factors. Technol Cancer Res Treat 2017;16(6):1202–8.

105. Sun B, Huang Z, Wu S, et al. Incidence and relapse risk of intracranial metastases within the perihippocampal region in 314 patients with breast cancer. Radiother Oncol 2016;118(1):181–6.

106. Madow L, Alpers BJ. Encephalitic form of metastatic carcinoma. AMA Arch Neurol Psychiatry 1951; 65(2):161–73.

107. Iguchi Y, Mano K, Goto Y, et al. Miliary brain metastases from adenocarcinoma of the lung: MR imaging findings with clinical and post-mortem histopathologic correlation. Neuroradiology 2007; 49(1):35–9.

108. Ogawa M, Kurahashi K, Ebina A, et al. Miliary brain metastasis presenting with dementia: progression pattern of cancer metastases in the cerebral cortex. Neuropathology 2007;27(4):390–5.

109. Francolini M, Sicurella L, Rizzuto N. Leptomeningeal carcinomatosis mimicking Creutzfeldt-Jakob disease: clinical features, laboratory tests, MRI images, EEG findings in an autopsy-proven case. Neurol Sci 2013;34(4):441–4.

110. Nutt SH, Patchell RA. Intracranial hemorrhage associated with primary and secondary tumors. Neurosurg Clin N Am 1992;3(3):591–9.

111. Baumert BG, Rutten I, Dehing-Oberije C, et al. A pathology-based substrate for target definition in radiosurgery of brain metastases. Int J Radiat Oncol Biol Phys 2006;66(1):187–94.

112. Neves S, Mazal PR, Wanschitz J, et al. Pseudogliomatous growth pattern of anaplastic small cell carcinomas metastatic to the brain. Clin Neuropathol 2001;20(1):38–42.

113. Drlicek M, Bodenteich A, Urbanits S, et al. Immunohistochemical panel of antibodies in the diagnosis of brain metastases of the unknown primary. Pathol Res Pract 2004;200(10):727–34.

114. Perry A, Parisi JE, Kurtin PJ. Metastatic adenocarcinoma to the brain: an immunohistochemical approach. Hum Pathol 1997;28(8):938–43.

115. Oien KA. Pathologic evaluation of unknown primary cancer. Semin Oncol 2009;36(1):8–37.

116. Becher MW, Abel TW, Thompson RC, et al. Immunohistochemical analysis of metastatic neoplasms of the central nervous system. J Neuropathol Exp Neurol 2006;65(10):935–44.

117. Park S-Y, Kim B-H, Kim J-H, et al. Panels of immunohistochemical markers help determine primary sites of metastatic adenocarcinoma. Arch Pathol Lab Med 2007;131(10):1561–7.

118. Edgerton ME, Roberts SA, Montone KT. Immunohistochemical performance of antibodies on previously frozen tissue. Appl Immunohistochem Mol Morphol 2000;8(3):244–8.

119. Monzon FA, Lyons-Weiler M, Buturovic LJ, et al. Multicenter validation of a 1,550-gene expression profile for identification of tumor tissue of origin. J Clin Oncol 2009;27(15):2503–8.

120. Wu AHB, Drees JC, Wang H, et al. Gene expression profiles help identify the tissue of origin for metastatic brain cancers. Diagn Pathol 2010;5:26.

121. Dumur CI, Fuller CE, Blevins TL, et al. Clinical verification of the performance of the pathwork tissue of origin test: utility and limitations. Am J Clin Pathol 2011;136(6):924–33.

122. Erlander MG, Ma X-J, Kesty NC, et al. Performance and clinical evaluation of the 92-gene real-time PCR assay for tumor classification. J Mol Diagn 2011;13(5):493–503.

123. Pillai R, Deeter R, Rigl CT, et al. Validation and reproducibility of a microarray-based gene expression test for tumor identification in formalin-fixed, paraffin-embedded specimens. J Mol Diagn 2011;13(1):48–56.

124. Meiri E, Mueller WC, Rosenwald S, et al. A second-generation microRNA-based assay for diagnosing tumor tissue origin. The oncologist 2012;17(6):801–12.

125. Bloom G, Yang IV, Boulware D, et al. Multi-platform, multi-site, microarray-based human tumor classification. Am J Pathol 2004;164(1):9–16.

126. Buckhaults P, Zhang Z, Chen Y-C, et al. Identifying tumor origin using a gene expression-based classification map. Cancer Res 2003; 63(14):4144–9.

127. Ramaswamy S, Tamayo P, Rifkin R, et al. Multiclass cancer diagnosis using tumor gene expression signatures. Proc Natl Acad Sci U S A 2001;98(26): 15149–54.

128. Capper D, Jones DTW, Sill M, et al. DNA methylation-based classification of central nervous system tumours. Nature 2018;555(7697):469–74.

129. Moran S, Martínez-Cardús A, Sayols S, et al. Epigenetic profiling to classify cancer of unknown primary: a multicentre, retrospective analysis. Lancet Oncol 2016;17(10):1386–95.

130. Orozco JIJ, Knijnenburg TA, Manughian-Peter AO, et al. Epigenetic profiling for the molecular classification of metastatic brain tumors. Nat Commun 2018;9(1):4627.

131. Davis PC, Hudgins PA, Peterman SB, et al. Diagnosis of cerebral metastases: double-dose delayed CT vs contrast-enhanced MR imaging. AJNR Am J Neuroradiol 1991;12(2):293–300.

132. Loeffler JS, Patchell RA, Sawaya R. Treatment of metastatic cancer. In: DeVita VT Jr, Hellman S, Rosenberg SA, editors. Cancer: Principles and Practice of Oncology. 5th ed. Philadelphia: Philadelphia: Lippincott–Raven Publishers; 1997.

133. Schaefer PW, Budzik RF, Gonzalez RG. Imaging of cerebral metastases. Neurosurg Clin N Am 1996; 7(3):393–423.

134. Due-Tønnessen B, Helseth E, Skullerud K, et al. Choroid plexus tumors in children and young adults: report of 16 consecutive cases. Childs Nerv Syst 2001;17(4–5):252–6.

135. Fèvre Montange M, Vasiljevic A, Bergemer Fouquet A-M, et al. Histopathologic and ultrastructural features and claudin expression in papillary tumors of the pineal region: a multicenter analysis. Am J Surg Pathol 2012;36(6):916–28.

136. Brat DJ, Giannini C, Scheithauer BW, et al. Primary melanocytic neoplasms of the central nervous systems. Am J Surg Pathol 1999;23(7):745–54.

137. Küsters-Vandevelde HVN, Küsters B, van Engen-van Grunsven ACH, et al. Primary melanocytic tumors of the central nervous system: a review with focus on molecular aspects. Brain Pathol 2015;25(2):209–26.

138. Hashimoto T, Sasagawa I, Ishigooka M, et al. Down's syndrome associated with intracranial germinoma and testicular embryonal carcinoma. Urol Int 1995;55(2):120–2.

139. Surcel HM, Tapaninaho S, Herva E. Cytotoxic CD4+ T cells specific for Francisella tularensis. Clin Exp Immunol 1991;83(1):112–5.

140. Eom KS, Kim JM, Kim TY. Mixed germ cell tumors in septum pellucidum after radiochemotherapy of suprasellar germinoma: de novo metachronous or recurrent neoplasms? Childs Nerv Syst 2008; 24(11):1355–9.

141. Poremba C, Dockhorn-Dworniczak B, Merritt V, et al. Immature teratomas of different origin carried by a pregnant mother and her fetus. Diagn Mol Pathol 1993;2(2):131–6.

142. Dufour H. Méningite carcinomateuse diffuse avec envahissement de la moelle et de la Racine: cytologie positive et spéciale du liquide céphalorachidien. Rev Neurol 1904;(12):104–6.

143. Lee EQ. Nervous system metastases from systemic cancer. Continuum (Minneapolis, Minn) 2015;21(2 Neuro-oncology):415–28.

144. Chamberlain M, Soffietti R, Raizer J, et al. Leptomeningeal metastasis: a response assessment in neuro-oncology critical review of endpoints and response criteria of published randomized clinical trials. Neuro Oncol 2014;16(9):1176–85.

145. Bigner SH, Johnston WW. The diagnostic challenge of tumors manifested initially by the shedding of cells into cerebrospinal fluid. Acta Cytol 1984;28(1):29–36.

146. Mandel P, Metais P. Les acides nucléiques du plasma sanguin chez l'homme. C R Seances Soc Biol Fil 1948;142(3–4):241–3.

147. Leon SA, Shapiro B, Sklaroff DM, et al. Free DNA in the serum of cancer patients and the effect of therapy. Cancer Res 1977;37(3):646–50.

148. Stroun M, Anker P, Maurice P, et al. Neoplastic characteristics of the DNA found in the plasma of cancer patients. Oncology 1989;46(5):318–22.

149. Sidransky D, Von Eschenbach A, Tsai YC, et al. Identification of p53 gene mutations in bladder cancers and urine samples. Science 1991; 252(5006):706–9.

150. Sidransky D, Tokino T, Hamilton SR, et al. Identification of ras oncogene mutations in the stool of

patients with curable colorectal tumors. Science 1992;256(5053):102–5.

151. Caldas C, Hahn SA, Hruban RH, et al. Detection of K-ras mutations in the stool of patients with pancreatic adenocarcinoma and pancreatic ductal hyperplasia. Cancer Res 1994;54(13):3568–73.

152. Mao L, Hruban RH, Boyle JO, et al. Detection of oncogene mutations in sputum precedes diagnosis of lung cancer. Cancer Res 1994;54(7): 1634–7.

153. Ulz P, Perakis S, Zhou Q, et al. Inference of transcription factor binding from cell-free DNA enables tumor subtype prediction and early detection. Nat Commun 2019;10(1):4666.

154. Cristofanilli M, Hayes DF, Budd GT, et al. Circulating tumor cells: a novel prognostic factor for newly diagnosed metastatic breast cancer. J Clin Oncol 2005;23(7):1420–30.

155. Hayes DF, Cristofanilli M, Budd GT, et al. Circulating tumor cells at each follow-up time point during therapy of metastatic breast cancer patients predict progression-free and overall survival. Clin Cancer Res 2006;12(14 Pt 1):4218–24.

156. Hoshimoto S, Shingai T, Morton DL, et al. Association between circulating tumor cells and prognosis in patients with stage III melanoma with sentinel lymph node metastasis in a phase III international multicenter trial. J Clin Oncol 2012;30(31):3819–26.

157. Goldkorn A, Ely B, Quinn DI, et al. Circulating tumor cell counts are prognostic of overall survival in SWOG S0421: a phase III trial of docetaxel with or without atrasentan for metastatic castration-resistant prostate cancer. J Clin Oncol 2014; 32(11):1136–42.

158. Rahbari NN, Aigner M, Thorlund K, et al. Meta-analysis shows that detection of circulating tumor cells indicates poor prognosis in patients with colorectal cancer. Gastroenterology 2010;138(5): 1714–26.

159. Li X, Seebacher NA, Hornicek FJ, et al. Application of liquid biopsy in bone and soft tissue sarcomas: Present and future. Cancer Lett 2018;439:66–77.

160. Fedchenko N, Reifenrath J. Different approaches for interpretation and reporting of immunohistochemistry analysis results in the bone tissue - a review. Diagn Pathol 2014;9:221.

161. Lin NU, Lee EQ, Aoyama H, et al. Response assessment criteria for brain metastases: proposal from the RANO group. Lancet Oncol 2015;16(6): e270–8.

Whole-Brain Radiation Therapy Versus Stereotactic Radiosurgery for Cerebral Metastases

Haley K. Perlow, MD[a,1], Khaled Dibs, MD[a,1], Kevin Liu, BS[a],
William Jiang, BS[a], Prajwal Rajappa, MD, MS[a,b,c],
Dukagjin M. Blakaj, MD, PhD[a], Joshua Palmer, MD[a],
Raju R. Raval, MD, DPhil[a,*]

KEYWORDS

- WBRT • SRS • Stereotactic radiosurgery • Brain metastases • Radiation
- Whole-brain radiation therapy

KEY POINTS

- There are multiple potential side effects of whole-brain radiation therapy (WBRT), including neurocognitive decline. Hippocampal-avoidance WBRT combined with memantine is a novel way to minimize side effects from treatment.
- The noninferiority of stereotactic radiosurgery (SRS) regarding overall survival combined with its improved side effect profile are the main reasons for the preference for SRS rather than WBRT in patients with limited brain metastases.
- Radiation necrosis and leptomeningeal disease dissemination are uncommon but occur in the setting of SRS, depending on the size, location, and histology of disease. Scheduling radiation therapy preoperatively and/or using multifraction radiotherapy can reduce the rates of these undesired outcomes.
- In the future, combining SRS with immune checkpoint inhibitors (ICIs) can improve patient outcomes. Prospective trials will help understand how to integrate ICIs with SRS treatments.

WHOLE-BRAIN RADIATION THERAPY

Since the mid–twentieth century, whole-brain radiation therapy (WBRT) has been used to treat patients with brain metastases using 2 lateral opposing fields to cover the entire brain parenchyma.[1] When WBRT was first used, patients were only expected to live for a few months after treatment. Therefore, long-term data on the effects of WBRT were scarce. The use of WBRT for brain metastases was further investigated in a study by Patchell and colleagues.[2] They found that treatment with WBRT after surgery led to fewer local and distant recurrences in the brain and fewer neurologic causes of death compared with surgery alone. Treatment with WBRT was also shown to improve functional status.[3] Remission of metastases after treatment depends on tumor volume and histology, with small cell carcinoma and breast cancer shown to be among the most responsive malignancies.[4]

[a] Department of Radiation Oncology, The James Cancer Hospital & Solove Research Institute Ohio State University Wexner Medical Center, 460 West 10th Avenue, Suite D252, Columbus, OH 43210, USA; [b] Department of Neurological Surgery, Nationwide Children's Hospital, Columbus, OH, USA; [c] Department of Pediatrics, Nationwide Children's Hospital, Columbus, OH, USA

[1] These authors made equal contributions.
* Corresponding author.
E-mail address: Raju.Raval@osumc.edu

Neurosurg Clin N Am 31 (2020) 565–573
https://doi.org/10.1016/j.nec.2020.06.006
1042-3680/20/© 2020 Elsevier Inc. All rights reserved.

Current National Comprehensive Cancer Network (NCCN) guidelines outline that WBRT to treat brain metastases is indicated in patients with the following circumstances: (1) limited metastases in the context of disseminated systemic disease with poor or limited systemic treatment options; (2) limited metastases in the context of newly diagnosed or stably systemic disease, although stereotactic radiosurgery (SRS) is preferred; and (3) extensive brain metastases.[5] Current doses for WBRT vary between 20 and 40 Gy delivered in 5 to 20 fractions, but standard regimens include 30 Gy in 10 fractions or 37.5 Gy in 15 fractions. Treating with 20 Gy in 5 fractions can be a good option for patients with a poor prognosis.

The identification of prognostic factors is important when creating subgroups for radiation treatment. Gaspar and colleagues[6] developed a recursive partitioning analysis (RPA) to stratify patients with brain metastases. They determined that patients needed to be separated into 3 classes before determining treatment: class 1 for patients with Karnofsky Performance Status (KPS) greater than or equal to 70 and less than 65 years of age with controlled primary and no extracranial metastases, class 2 for KPS less than 70, and class 3 for all others. Other indexes were also developed.[7,8] The graded prognostic assessment (GPA) is now commonly used because of its prognostic capabilities, lack of subjectivity, and convenience.[8] This index includes age, KPS, number of central nervous system metastases, and presence of extracranial metastases. Initial brain metastasis velocity (cumulative number of brain metastases at the time of SRS divided by time [years] since the initial cancer diagnosis) is another novel algorithm that warrants further evaluation.[9]

The benefits of WBRT are clear in that such treatment reduces the incidence of intracranial relapse and neurologic death.[10,11] However, there are several potentially significant side effects with WBRT. Xerostomia is a frequent side effect that can be reduced by limiting the dose to the parotid gland.[12] Dry eye syndrome is another complication that can be minimized by reducing the dose to the lacrimal gland.[13] One randomized control trial showed that, among patients with up to 3 brain metastases, the use of SRS alone, compared with WBRT and SRS, caused less cognitive deterioration at both 3 months (45.5% vs 94.1%) and 12 months (60% vs 94.4%).[14] Other studies showed similar reductions in learning, quality of life, and memory function for patients receiving WBRT.[15–17] For patients with a poor prognosis, WBRT may not be indicated. The Quality of Life after Treatment for Brain Metastases (QUARTZ) study is a phase 3 randomized trial assessing patients who are ineligible for surgical resection or SRS. WBRT versus dexamethasone and supportive care alone showed no difference in overall survival, quality of life, or the incidence of adverse events.[18]

Radiation-induced cognitive decline can be attributed to vascular injury and demyelination in the hippocampus, which can lead to overactivation of N-methyl-D-aspartate (NMDA) receptors.[19] Memantine, a well-tolerated drug, works as an NMDA receptor antagonist blocking receptors only under conditions of excessive stimulation, with no effect on normal transmission, and memantine can also prevent radiation-induced synaptic remodeling.[20,21] Memantine had already been shown to consistently improve cognition in patients with mild to moderate dementia.[22] In a randomized clinical trial assessing the role of memantine for the prevention of cognitive dysfunction for patients receiving WBRT, the use of memantine during and after WBRT delayed time to cognitive decline and reduced decline in memory, processing speed, and executive function.[23] Donepezil and motexafin gadolinium are other agents that have shown some evidence in reducing radiation-induced cognitive decline but are less commonly used in practice.[24,25]

Hippocampal-avoidance WBRT (HA-WBRT) is a new WBRT technique that can preserve the efficacy of treatment while limiting neurocognitive deficits (**Fig. 1**). RTOG (Radiation Therapy Oncology Group) 0933 was a phase II study of HA-WBRT followed by a cognitive assessment using the Hopkins Verbal Learning Test-Revised Delay Recall.[26] This study found that avoiding the hippocampus during treatment was associated with significant memory preservation. NRG CC001, a phase III trial of WBRT plus memantine with or without hippocampal avoidance, showed the benefits of combining HA-WBRT with memantine.[27] Comparison of HA-WBRT plus memantine with modern SRS techniques will be important in future studies.

STEREOTACTIC RADIOSURGERY

SRS of the brain uses three-dimensional planning to treat small targets with convergent beams or arcs, and the increased precision of this modality can lead to fewer side effects (**Fig. 2**). Early studies showed excellent local tumor control for patients treated with SRS.[28,29] SRS has shown efficacy using multiple treatment delivery modalities, such as helical tomotherapy (TomoTherapy), CyberKnife, Gamma Knife, and LINAC (linear accelerator)-based treatments.[30–35] One study examined

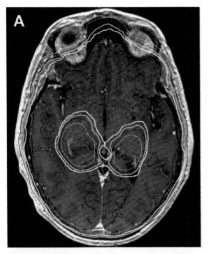 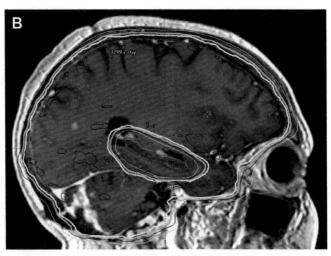

Fig. 1. HA-WBRT. Axial (*A*) and sagittal (*B*) MRI views of a radiation therapy plan using HA-WBRT for a patient with multiple small brain metastases (>15) with a decrease in the isodose lines around the hippocampi (*purple*), with a maximum dose no greater than 16 Gy to these regions, with a prescription dose of 30 Gy (*yellow*) in 10 fractions to the remaining whole brain.

hippocampal sparing when treating multiple brain metastases, and another study examined the databases of 10 institutions that treated patients with Gamma Knife or LINAC-based SRS, with both groups finding equivalent outcomes when comparing these treatment modalities.[36] More recently, proton therapy has been shown to provide similar results to photon therapy.[37] Flexibility of treatment modality has allowed SRS for brain metastases to become widespread even for

facilities without a robotic or cobalt-60–associated treatment machine. SRS is now the standard of care in many instances for patients with brain metastases.

SRS decision making is evolving as radiosurgery literature becomes more robust, and many factors are important to consider before beginning treatment (**Fig. 3**). Total tumor volume was found to be a more effective predictor of overall survival than total number of brain metastases for patients

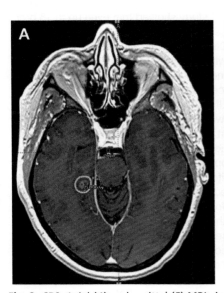 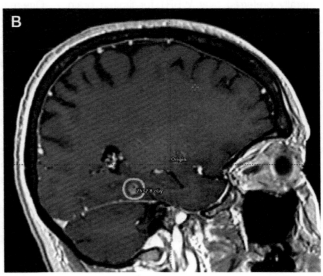

Fig. 2. SRS. Axial (*A*) and sagittal (*B*) MRI views of a LINAC (linear accelerator)-based stereotactic radiation therapy plan using 6-MV (flattening filter free) photons delivered over 3 dynamic conformal arcs to a total dose of 20 Gy in a single fraction using a 2-mm margin on the metastatic lesion.

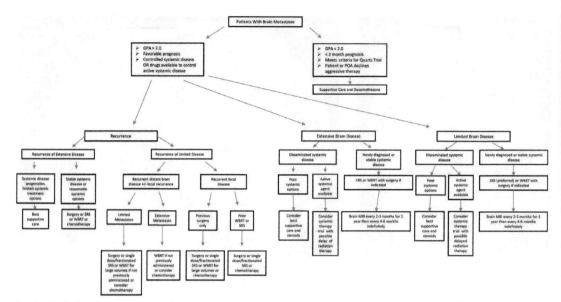

Fig. 3. Radiation treatment decision-making for patients with brain metastases. GPA, graded prognostic assessment; POA, power of attorney.

treated with SRS; with a cutoff of 2 cm^3 used in 1 study.[38] Another study found that a target volume of less than 30 cm^3 was predictive of local tumor control.[39] These studies explain how a range of less than or equal to 15 to 30 cm^3 is used as current standard of practice to determine whether a patient can receive SRS versus more expansive treatment with WBRT. The identification of previously mentioned prognostic factors, including RPA, GPA, and initial brain metastasis velocity, are also important in SRS decision making.[6,8,9]

Current NCCN guidelines state that "SRS is generally preferred over WBRT for limited brain metastases."[5] Before this guideline was in place, multiple studies compared patients who received WBRT and/or SRS for limited brain metastases. In 1 novel study for patients with resected brain metastases treated with either WBRT or SRS, neurocognitive decline was more frequent with the WBRT group.[40] Patients who receive SRS with WBRT versus SRS alone had significant decreases in many quality-of-life and cognitive measures.[14,15] An additional study noted that those who receive SRS with WBRT versus SRS alone have a lower rate of intracranial relapse, and patients receiving SRS alone frequently require additional use of salvage treatment.[11] However, in each of the studies listed earlier, there was no difference in overall survival between WBRT versus SRS. There are multiple trials that are continuing to investigate advances in WBRT and SRS (**Table 1**). The noninferiority of SRS regarding overall survival combined with its improved side effect profile are the main reasons for the current preference toward SRS rather than WBRT in patients with limited brain metastases.

Recently, SRS has been used to treat patients with extensive brain metastases. A prospective study that enrolled patients with up to 10 metastases treated with SRS showed that overall survival did not differ between patients with 2 to 4 tumors and 5 to 10 tumors.[41] Using this same cohort, both mini mental status examinations and post-SRS complication rates were unchanged, thus showing that treating extensive disease with SRS does not lead to increased treatment morbidity.[42] One recent study showed that even up to 15 brain metastases can be treated with no change in survival.[43] Disease-specific studies have been successful with treating extensive brain metastases from kidney cancer and specific non–small cell lung cancer subtypes.[44,45] Single-isocenter multi-target LINAC-based radiotherapy is a time-efficient way to treat multiple brain metastases in a way that maintains similar local control and treatment toxicity compared with multi-isocentric therapy approaches (eg, Gamma Knife or CyberKnife).[46] A phase III trial is currently being conducted by the Canadian Clinical Trials Group/Alliance for Clinical Trials in Oncology comparing SRS with WBRT for patients with 5 to 15 metastases.

Radiation necrosis (RN) and leptomeningeal disease dissemination (LMD) are uncommon but occur in the setting of SRS, and depend on several potential factors. RN can sometimes be diagnosed through MRI. A biopsy or resection might be warranted to confirm the diagnosis or

Table 1
Upcoming and ongoing clinical trials investigating advances in whole-brain radiation therapy and stereotactic radiosurgery

Study	Identifier	Status	Phase	Sponsor	Primary Outcome
Memantine and WBRT With or Without Hippocampal Avoidance	NCT02360215	Active, not recruiting	3	NRG Oncology	Time to neurocognitive failure
SRS Compared with HA-WBRT plus Memantine for 5–15 Metastases	NCT03550391	Recruiting	3	Canadian Cancer Trials Group	Overall survival, neurocognitive progression-free survival
HA-WBRT Plus Simultaneously Integrated Boost vs SRS for Patients with Multiple Brain Metastases	NCT04277403	Not yet recruiting	3	Medical University Innsbruck, Innsbruck, Austria	Intracranial progression-free survival
Pre-Operative or Post-Operative SRS for Patients with Brain Metastases	NCT03741673	Recruiting	3	MD Anderson Cancer Center, Houston, Texas	Leptomeningeal disease-free rate
Neo-Adjuvant vs Post-Operative SRS for Metastatic Brain Metastases	NCT03750227	Recruiting	3	Mayo Clinic, Rochester, Minnesota	Central nervous system composite end point event
Single Fraction vs Fractionated SRS for Patients with Resected Brain Metastases	NCT04114981	Recruiting	3	Alliance for Clinical Trials in Oncology	Surgical bed recurrence-free survival

treat symptomatic patients; however, radiologic diagnosis has proved to be relatively accurate (especially with perfusion imaging) when subsequent surgical specimens are assessed.[47] There are numerous risk factors for RN, including size of lesion, percentage of tumor volume receiving a high dose of radiation, occipital or temporal lesions, and previous WBRT.[47–50] LMD is diagnosed through imaging or a cerebrospinal fluid sample. Risk factors for LMD include colon or breast primary site, number of intracranial metastases at the time of treatment, younger age, and infratentorial tumor location.[51–53] Scheduling radiation therapy preoperatively and hypofractionation have been examined to help mitigate RN and LMD.

SRS can be delivered after surgery to treat brain metastases. Postoperative radiation therapy is more effective than radiotherapy alone because treatment increases functional independence, reduces the incidence of local recurrence, and increases overall survival.[2,54,55] A phase 3 trial confirmed that SRS following complete resection of up to 3 metastases significantly reduces local recurrence compared with observation after surgery.[56] Up to a 2-mm margin around the resection cavity is likely necessary to improve local control.[57] Consensus guidelines have been developed to contour the postoperative cavity, but more clinical data are needed to refine clinical practice.[58]

One retrospective study comparing preoperative and postoperative SRS found no difference in overall survival, local recurrence, or distal brain recurrence; however, postoperative SRS was associated with significantly higher rates of LMD and RN.[59] The investigators argued that preoperative SRS provides advantages for 3 reasons: (1) treating the unresected tumor allows better gross tumor volume delineation and less target uncertainty; (2) the target is more radioresponsive than a hypoxic postsurgical bed; and (3) postsurgical progression, larger cavities, or lack of follow-up may preclude the use of postoperative SRS. However, 1 retrospective study found no relationship between LMD and postoperative SRS.[51] An NRG phase II randomized trial (NRG-BN1605) is currently in development to address the risk of RN and LMD in preoperative SRS versus postoperative SRS.

Hypofractionation is an important technique to optimize SRS in many clinical circumstances. Multiple studies have shown that multifraction SRS (fractionated SRS [FSRS]) more than single-fraction SRS can improve local control while also reducing the risk for RN, especially in larger lesions (>2 cm).[60–62] One institution study suggested that, if the tumor volume receiving 12 Gy was greater than 10 cm^3, the patient would be especially at risk for symptomatic RN and FSRS should be considered.[50] Three to 5 fractions are suggested as an effective therapy for improving local control.[61–64] A phase III Alliance (A071801) trial is currently comparing postoperative single-fraction SRS with FSRS.

FUTURE DIRECTIONS AND CONCLUSION

In the future, combining SRS with immune checkpoint inhibitors (ICIs) has great potential to improve patient outcomes. SRS has already shown stimulatory effects on the immune system.[65] One study used mouse models to show that hypofractionated radiation 7 days before surgery provides more durable anticancer immunity than a short course completed 24 hours before surgery.[66] SRS and ICIs may work synergistically, and, in multiple studies of patients treated for brain metastases, concurrent ICI and SRS delivery was associated with greater reduction in brain lesion diameter versus delayed or nonconcurrent therapy.[67,68] Prospective trials will allow clinicians to better understand how to integrate ICIs into SRS treatments.

With emerging data and new technologies, both radiation oncologists and neurosurgeons now pursue upfront SRS for appropriately selected patients rather than traditional WBRT. WBRT is used less frequently in modern practice, although HA-WBRT is used when clinically indicated. Future clinical trials may incorporate the timing and technique of radiation with new systemic therapies such as targeted inhibitors or immunotherapies.

DISCLOSURE

The authors have nothing to disclose.

REFERENCES

1. Chao JH, Phillips R, Nickson JJ. Roentgen-ray therapy of cerebral metastases. Cancer 1954;7(4): 682–9.
2. Patchell R, Tibbs P, Regine W, et al. Postoperative radiotherapy in the treatment of single metastases to the brain: A randomized trial. JAMA 1998; 280(17):1485–9.
3. Order SE, Hellman S, Von Essen CF, et al. Improvement in quality of survival following whole-brain irradiation for brain metastasis. Radiology 1968;91(1): 149–53.
4. Nieder C, Berberich W, Schnabel K. Tumor-related prognostic factors for remission of brain metastases after radiotherapy. Int J Radiat Oncol Biol Phys 1997;39(1):25.
5. NCCN Guidelines Version 3.2019 Central Nervous System Cancers. Journal of the National Comprehensive Cancer Network 2019.
6. Gaspar L, Scott C, Rotman M, et al. Recursive partitioning analysis (RPA) of prognostic factors in three Radiation Therapy Oncology Group (RTOG) brain metastases trials. Int J Radiat Oncol Biol Phys 1997;37(4):745.
7. Weltman E, Salvajoli JV, Brandt RA, et al. Radiosurgery for brain metastases: a score index for predicting prognosis. Int J Radiat Oncol Biol Phys 2000; 46(5):1155–61.
8. Sperduto PW, Berkey B, Gaspar LE, et al. A new prognostic index and comparison to three other indices for patients with brain metastases: an analysis of 1,960 patients in the RTOG Database. Int J Radiat Oncol Biol Phys 2008;70(2):510–4.
9. Yamamoto M, Aiyama H, Koiso T, et al. Applicability and limitations of a recently-proposed prognostic grading metric, initial brain metastasis velocity, for brain metastasis patients undergoing stereotactic radiosurgery. J Neurooncol 2019;143(3):613–21.
10. Kocher M, Soffietti R, Abacioglu U, et al. Adjuvant whole-brain radiotherapy versus observation after radiosurgery or surgical resection of one to three cerebral metastases: results of the EORTC 22952-26001 study. J Clin Oncol 2011;29(2):134.
11. Aoyama H, Shirato H, Tago M, et al. Stereotactic radiosurgery plus whole-brain radiation therapy vs stereotactic radiosurgery alone for treatment of brain metastases: a randomized controlled trial. JAMA 2006;295(21):2483.

12. Wang K, Pearlstein KA, Moon DH, et al. Assessment of risk of xerostomia after whole-brain radiation therapy and association with parotid dose. JAMA Oncol 2019;5(2):221–8.

13. Wang K, Tobillo R, Mavroidis P, et al. Prospective assessment of patient-reported dry eye syndrome after whole brain radiation. Int J Radiat Oncol Biol Phys 2019;105(4):765–72.

14. Brown PD, Jaeckle K, Ballman KV, et al. Effect of radiosurgery alone vs radiosurgery with whole brain radiation therapy on cognitive function in patients with 1 to 3 brain metastases: a randomized clinical trial. JAMA 2016;316(4):401–9.

15. Chang EL, Wefel JS, Hess KR, et al. Neurocognition in patients with brain metastases treated with radiosurgery or radiosurgery plus whole-brain irradiation: a randomised controlled trial. Lancet Oncol 2009; 10(11):1037–44.

16. Chow E, Davis L, Holden L, et al. Prospective assessment of patient-rated symptoms following whole brain radiotherapy for brain metastases. J Pain Symptom Manage 2005;30(1):18–23.

17. Sun A, Bae K, Gore EM, et al. Phase III trial of prophylactic cranial irradiation compared with observation in patients with locally advanced non-small-cell lung cancer: neurocognitive and quality-of-life analysis. J Clin Oncol 2011;29(3):279–86.

18. Mulvenna P, Nankivell M, Barton R, et al. Dexamethasone and supportive care with or without whole brain radiotherapy in treating patients with non-small cell lung cancer with brain metastases unsuitable for resection or stereotactic radiotherapy (QUARTZ): results from a phase 3, non-inferiority, randomised trial. Lancet 2016;388(10055):2004–14.

19. Monje LM, Palmer LT. Radiation injury and neurogenesis. Curr Opin Neurol 2003;16(2):129–34.

20. Chen H-S, Pellergrini J, Aggarwal S, et al. Open-channel block of N-methyl-D-aspartate (NMDA) responses by memantine: Therapeutic advantage against NMDA receptor-mediated neurotoxicity. J Neurosci 1992;12(11):4427–36.

21. Duman JG, Dinh J, Zhou W, et al. Memantine prevents acute radiation-induced toxicities at hippocampal excitatory synapses. Neuro Oncol 2018; 20(5):655–65.

22. Orgogozo J-M, Rigaud A-S, Stöffler A, et al. Efficacy and safety of memantine in patients with mild to moderate vascular dementia: a randomized, placebo-controlled trial (MMM 300). Stroke 2002; 33(7):1834–9.

23. Brown PD, Pugh S, Laack NN, et al. Memantine for the prevention of cognitive dysfunction in patients receiving whole-brain radiotherapy: a randomized, double-blind, placebo-controlled trial. Neuro Oncol 2013;15(10):1429–37.

24. Rapp SR, Case LD, Peiffer A, et al. Donepezil for irradiated brain tumor survivors: a phase iii randomized placebo-controlled clinical trial. J Clin Oncol 2015;33(15):1653.

25. Meyers CA, Smith JA, Bezjak A, et al. Neurocognitive function and progression in patients with brain metastases treated with whole-brain radiation and motexafin gadolinium: Results of a randomized phase III trial. J Clin Oncol 2004;22(1):157–65.

26. Gondi V, Pugh SL, Tome WA, et al. Preservation of memory with conformal avoidance of the hippocampal neural stem-cell compartment during whole-brain radiotherapy for brain metastases (RTOG 0933): a phase II multi-institutional trial. J Clin Oncol 2014;32(34):3810.

27. Gondi V, Deshmukh S, Brown PD, et al. NRG Oncology CC001: A phase III trial of hippocampal avoidance (HA) in addition to whole-brain radiotherapy (WBRT) plus memantine to preserve neurocognitive function (NCF) in patients with brain metastases (BM). J Clin Oncol 2019;37(15_suppl): 2009.

28. Hussain A, Brown PD, Stafford SL, et al. Stereotactic radiosurgery for brainstem metastases: Survival, tumor control, and patient outcomes. Int J Radiat Oncol Biol Phys 2007;67(2):521–4.

29. Gerosa M, Nicolato A, Foroni R, et al. Analysis of long-term outcomes and prognostic factors in patients with non-small cell lung cancer brain metastases treated by gamma knife radiosurgery. J Neurosurg 2005;102(Suppl):75.

30. Uematsu M, Fukui T, Shioda A, et al. A dual computed tomography linear accelerator unit for stereotactic radiation therapy: A new approach without cranially fixated stereotactic frames. Int J Radiat Oncol Biol Phys 1996;35(3):587–92.

31. Lunsford DL. Image-guided Robotic Radiosurgery. Neurosurgery 1999;44(6):1306–7.

32. Chang DS, Main PW, Martin CD, et al. An analysis of the accuracy of the cyberknife: a robotic frameless stereotactic radiosurgical system. Neurosurgery 2003;52(1):140–7.

33. Lutz W, Winston KR, Maleki N. A system for stereotactic radiosurgery with a linear accelerator. Int J Radiat Oncol Biol Phys 1988;14(2):373–81.

34. Gerosa M, Nicolato A, Foroni R, et al. Gamma knife radiosurgery for brain metastases: a primary therapeutic option. J Neurosurg 2002;97(5 Suppl): 515–24.

35. Flickinger JC, Kondziolka D, Dade Lunsford L, et al. A multi-institutional experience with stereotactic radiosurgery for solitary brain metastasis. Int J Radiat Oncol Biol Phys 1994;28(4):797–802.

36. Zhang I, Antone J, Li J, et al. Hippocampal-sparing and target volume coverage in treating 3 to 10 brain metastases: A comparison of Gamma Knife, single-isocenter VMAT, CyberKnife, and TomoTherapy stereotactic radiosurgery. Pract Radiat Oncol 2017; 7(3):183–9.

37. Atkins KM, Pashtan IM, Bussière MR, et al. Proton stereotactic radiosurgery for brain metastases: a single-institution analysis of 370 patients. Int J Radiat Oncol Biol Phys 2018;101(4):820–9.

38. Baschnagel AM, Meyer KD, Chen PY, et al. Tumor volume as a predictor of survival and local control in patients with brain metastases treated with Gamma Knife surgery. J Neurosurg 2013;119(5):1139.

39. Kondziolka D, Kano H, Harrison GL, et al. Stereotactic radiosurgery as primary and salvage treatment for brain metastases from breast cancer. Clinical article. J Neurosurg 2011;114(3):792–800.

40. Brown PD, Ballman KV, Cerhan JH, et al. Postoperative stereotactic radiosurgery compared with whole brain radiotherapy for resected metastatic brain disease (NCCTG N107C/CEC·3): a multicentre, randomised, controlled, phase 3 trial. Lancet Oncol 2017; 18(8):1049–60.

41. Yamamoto M, Serizawa T, Shuto T, et al. Stereotactic radiosurgery for patients with multiple brain metastases (JLGK0901): a multi-institutional prospective observational study. Lancet Oncol 2014;15(4): 387–95.

42. Yamamoto M, Serizawa T, Higuchi Y, et al. A multi-institutional prospective observational study of stereotactic radiosurgery for patients with multiple brain metastases (JLGK0901 study update): irradiation-related complications and long-term maintenance of mini-mental state examination scores. Int J Radiat Oncol Biol Phys 2017;99(1):31–40.

43. Hughes RT, Masters AH, McTyre ER, et al. Initial SRS for patients with 5 to 15 brain metastases: results of a multi-institutional experience. Int J Radiat Oncol Biol Phys 2019;104(5):1091–8.

44. Wowra B, Siebels M, Muacevic A, et al. Repeated gamma knife surgery for multiple brain metastases from renal cell carcinoma. J Neurosurg 2002;97(4): 785–93.

45. Robin PT, Camidge DR, Stuhr KK, et al. Excellent Outcomes with Radiosurgery for Multiple Brain Metastases in ALK and EGFR Driven Non–Small Cell Lung Cancer. J Thorac Oncol 2018;13(5):715–20.

46. Palmer JD, Sebastian NT, Chu J, et al. Single-isocenter multitarget stereotactic radiosurgery is safe and effective in the treatment of multiple brain metastases. Adv Radiat Oncol 2020;5(1):70–6.

47. Doré M, Martin S, Delpon G, et al. Stereotactic radiotherapy following surgery for brain metastasis: Predictive factors for local control and radionecrosis. Cancer Radiother 2017;21(1):4–9.

48. Korytko T, Radivoyevitch T, Colussi V, et al. 12 Gy gamma knife radiosurgical volume is a predictor for radiation necrosis in non-AVM intracranial tumors. Int J Radiat Oncol Biol Phys 2006;64(2): 419–24.

49. Blonigen BJ, Steinmetz RD, Levin L, et al. Irradiated volume as a predictor of brain radionecrosis after linear accelerator stereotactic radiosurgery. Int J Radiat Oncol Biol Phys 2010;77(4):996–1001.

50. Minniti G, Clarke E, Lanzetta G, et al. Stereotactic radiosurgery for brain metastases: analysis of outcome and risk of brain radionecrosis. Radiat Oncol 2011;6(1):48.

51. Huang A, Huang K, Page B, et al. Risk factors for leptomeningeal carcinomatosis in patients with brain metastases who have previously undergone stereotactic radiosurgery. J Neurooncol 2014;120(1):163–9.

52. Atalar B, Modlin LA, Choi CYH, et al. Risk of leptomeningeal disease in patients treated with stereotactic radiosurgery targeting the postoperative resection cavity for brain metastases. Int J Radiat Oncol Biol Phys 2013;87(4):713–8.

53. Ojerholm E, Lee JYK, Thawani JP, et al. Stereotactic radiosurgery to the resection bed for intracranial metastases and risk of leptomeningeal carcinomatosis. J Neurosurg 2014;121(sS):75.

54. Patchell RA, Tibbs PA, Walsh JW, et al. A randomized trial of surgery in the treatment of single metastases to the brain. N Engl J Med 1990; 322(8):494–500.

55. Soltys SG. Stereotactic radiosurgery of the postoperative resection cavity for brain metastases. Int J Radiat Oncol Biol Phys 2008;70(1):187–93.

56. Mahajan A, Ahmed S, McAleer MF, et al. Post-operative stereotactic radiosurgery versus observation for completely resected brain metastases: a single-centre, randomised, controlled, phase 3 trial. Lancet Oncol 2017;18(8):1040–8.

57. Choi CYH, Chang SD, Gibbs IC, et al. Stereotactic radiosurgery of the postoperative resection cavity for brain metastases: prospective evaluation of target margin on tumor control. Int J Radiat Oncol Biol Phys 2012;84(2):336–42.

58. Soliman H, Ruschin M, Angelov L, et al. Consensus contouring guidelines for postoperative completely resected cavity stereotactic radiosurgery for brain metastases. Int J Radiat Oncol Biol Phys 2018; 100(2):436–42.

59. Patel RK, Burri HS, Asher LA, et al. Comparing preoperative with postoperative stereotactic radiosurgery for resectable brain metastases: a multi-institutional Analysis. Neurosurgery 2016;79(2): 279–85.

60. Lehrer EJ, Peterson JL, Zaorsky NG, et al. Single versus multifraction stereotactic radiosurgery for large brain metastases: an international meta-analysis of 24 trials. Int J Radiat Oncol Biol Phys 2019;103(3):618–30.

61. Minniti G, Scaringi C, Paolini S, et al. Single-Fraction Versus Multifraction (3 × 9 Gy) stereotactic radiosurgery for large (>2 cm) brain metastases: a comparative analysis of local control and risk of radiation-induced brain necrosis. Int J Radiat Oncol Biol Phys 2016;95(4):1142–8.

62. Eaton BR, Riviere MJ, Kim S, et al. Hypofractionated radiosurgery has a better safety profile than single fraction radiosurgery for large resected brain metastases. J Neurooncol 2015;123(1):103.

63. Traylor J, Habib A, Patel R, et al. Fractionated stereotactic radiotherapy for local control of resected brain metastases. J Neurooncol 2019;144(2): 343–50.

64. Ahmed KA, Freilich JM, Abuodeh Y, et al. Fractionated stereotactic radiotherapy to the post-operative cavity for radioresistant and radiosensitive brain metastases. J Neurooncol 2014;118(1):179–86.

65. Michael BB, Sunil K, James WH, et al. Immunotherapy and stereotactic ablative radiotherapy (ISABR): a curative approach? Nat Rev Clin Oncol 2016;13(8):516–24.

66. De La Maza L, Wu M, Wu L, et al. Vaccination after accelerated hypofractionated radiation and surgery in a mesothelioma mouse model. Clin Cancer Res 2017;23(18):5502.

67. Kotecha R, Kim JM, Miller JA, et al. The impact of sequencing PD-1/PD-L1 inhibitors and stereotactic radiosurgery for patients with brain metastasis. Neuro Oncol 2019;21(8):1060–8.

68. Chen L, Douglass J, Kleinberg L, et al. Concurrent immune checkpoint inhibitors and stereotactic radiosurgery for brain metastases in non-small cell lung cancer, melanoma, and renal cell carcinoma. Int J Radiat Oncol Biol Phys 2018;100(4):916–25.

Brain Metastasis Recurrence Versus Radiation Necrosis
Evaluation and Treatment

Dennis Lee, MS[a], Robert A. Riestenberg, BS[a], Aden Haskell-Mendoza, MS[a], Orin Bloch, MD[b],*

KEYWORDS

- Brain metastases • Stereotactic radiosurgery • Radiation necrosis • Radionecrosis • Recurrence

KEY POINTS

- Radiation necrosis is a delayed adverse consequence of radiotherapy for brain metastases observed in 5% to 25% of treated patients.
- The primary risk factors for radiation necrosis include radiation dose, treatment volume, and possibly concurrent use of immune checkpoint inhibitors.
- Radiation necrosis must be distinguished from recurrent tumor for proper treatment.
- Numerous advanced imaging studies can help distinguish radiation necrosis from recurrent tumor, but biopsy remains the gold standard.
- Treatment of radiation necrosis includes corticosteroids, antiangiogenic agents (bevacizumab), surgical resection, and stereotactic laser ablation.

INTRODUCTION

Stereotactic radiosurgery (SRS) is the standard of care for patients with limited brain metastases (BMs) who do not need immediate relief of mass-related symptoms.[1] Patients with larger numbers of metastases often still receive whole-brain radiotherapy (WBRT). Even after SRS and/or WBRT, tumors may progress or recur after regression. However, in addition to true tumor progression, patients may develop radiation necrosis (RN) at the site of a previously treated tumor. The ability to differentiate between tumor recurrence and RN is critical, because treatments for each entity vary significantly. Recurrent tumor may be treated with repeat SRS or surgical resection.[2] In contrast, further radiation should be avoided for RN, and craniotomy is rarely necessary because there are alternative noninvasive and minimally invasive options for management of RN-associated symptoms.

This article reviews the pathophysiology and incidence of RN following SRS for BM. It reviews the options available for the diagnosis of RN to differentiate it from tumor recurrence. In addition, it presents noninvasive and invasive treatment options for RN.

PATHOPHYSIOLOGY OF RADIATION NECROSIS

RN is a delayed adverse consequence of radiation therapy. SRS places patients at a high risk of RN compared with conventional fractionated radiotherapy because the radioresistance of healthy cells, afforded by slower cell cycle turnover and preserved DNA repair mechanisms, becomes overwhelmed.[3] Although this risk is minimized

[a] Department of Neurological Surgery, University of California Davis, 4860 Y Street, Suite 3740, Sacramento, CA 95817, USA; [b] Department of Neurological Surgery, University of California, Davis School of Medicine, University of California Davis, 4860 Y Street, Suite 3740, Sacramento, CA 95817, USA
* Corresponding author.
E-mail address: obloch@ucdavis.edu

Neurosurg Clin N Am 31 (2020) 575–587
https://doi.org/10.1016/j.nec.2020.06.007
1042-3680/20/© 2020 Elsevier Inc. All rights reserved.

with optimal treatment planning and field conformality, the risk of RN following SRS remains significant.[4]

Although the precise mechanisms underlying RN remain unclear, the primary inciting event is thought to be vascular endothelial damage.[5–7] Signs of vascular damage are seen within 24 hours of irradiation in animal models, and are accompanied by loss of blood-brain barrier (BBB) integrity and edema.[6–8] CNS radiation in animal models causes endothelial cell swelling, apoptosis, astrocyte hypertrophy, and loss of blood vessels, which result in tissue hypoxia and precede abnormal vascular proliferation and frank necrosis.[7,9,10] It is hypothesized that decreased blood vessel density and edema following radiation contribute to ischemia of the surrounding tissues and lead to the production of hypoxia inducible factor (HIF)-1α and vascular endothelial growth factor (VEGF).[6,11] VEGF then induces disorganized vascular proliferation, which exacerbates edema and promotes further ischemia, with subsequent infarction and necrosis. This hypothesis is supported by pathology studies on radionecrotic lesions resected from humans, where the perinecrotic area is characterized by proliferation of leaky, disorganized vasculature and increased HIF-1α and VEGF expression.[11–14]

Immune activation and inflammation contribute to RN progression by augmenting vascular permeability and edema. In addition to inducing VEGF, HIF-1α is known to activate the C-X-C motif chemokine 12/C-X-C chemokine receptor type 4 (CXCL12/CXCR4) axis. CXCL12/CXCR4 signaling has pleiotropic effects, which include promoting chemotaxis of mononuclear and myeloid cells and nuclear factor-κB activation.[12,15] Histologic specimens from patients resected for refractory RN have prominent macrophage and cluster of differentiation (CD) 4$^+$/CD8$^+$ lymphocyte infiltrates in the perinecrotic area.[11–14] Resected specimens stain positive for tumor necrosis factor (TNF)-α, interleukin (IL)-1α, and IL-6. These cytokines colocalize to hGLUT5 microglia and CD68$^+$ macrophages, and are not seen in lymphocytes, suggesting that myeloid cells are key mediators of inflammation in RN.[12,14] Mouse models have shown TNF-α is upregulated in the acute phase following cranial radiation, and that administration of TNF-α inhibitors reduces the hypoxia, BBB permeability, reactive astrogliosis, and vascular damage otherwise seen following cranial radiation.[10,16] Notably, the immune response characterized in the studies discussed earlier has no defined role for adaptive immunity. Lymphocytes have been observed in the perinecrotic area, but no studies have characterized any lymphocyte cytokine production or cytotoxic effect.

Ultimately, RN is the result of synergy between vascular damage and immune activation resulting in edema, ischemia, and necrosis.[6] This mechanism of pathogenesis suggests 2 targets for therapeutic intervention: immunosuppressive medications, which are unappealing in the setting of cancer treatment, and anti-VEGF therapy, which is discussed later.

INCIDENCE OF RADIATION NECROSIS

Determining the incidence of RN following SRS presents a variety of challenges that result in a large range reported in the literature. It is often difficult to distinguish between the RN and tumor progression on MRI, even with advanced studies.[17,18] Similarly, distinguishing RN from other forms of radiation injury may be difficult: early delayed radiation injury, thought to be caused by transient demyelination from radiation damage to oligodendrocyte progenitor cells, can appear identical to RN on MRI and produce similar symptoms.[18,19] However, early delayed radiation injury is reversible, and subsequent improvement is the rule; changes from radiation necrosis are permanent (**Fig. 1**). Many studies do not distinguish early reversible changes from true RN. In light of these obstacles, biopsy remains the gold standard for diagnosis of RN but is performed in a minority of cases. In addition, the probability of developing RN increases with increasing follow-up.[20–22] Therefore, studies report significantly different rates of RN depending on their length of follow-up and mortality.

With these limitations in mind, the incidence of RN following SRS for BM reported in the literature ranges from 5% to 26% per lesion treated, with symptomatic RN occurring in 3% to 17% of lesions.[20,21,23–25] The median time to RN following SRS is 6 to 11 months.[20,21,23,24,26] Studies of RN actuarial incidence show a substantial increase over time, with an incidence of 15.4% to 17% at 12 months, and 25.5% to 34% at 2 years.[20,22]

Given limited prospective data, the factors that predict RN after SRS have primarily been identified retrospectively. The volume of tumor receiving 10 Gy (V10 Gy) or 12 Gy (V12 Gy) has been consistently found to be the strongest predictor of RN and symptomatic RN.[21–24,27] V12 Gy of 8 to 10 cm^3 has been proposed as a threshold past which the risk of RN increases considerably.[21,22,24] Korytko and colleagues[27] found that V12 Gy greater than 10 cm^3 increased the risk of symptomatic RN from 22.5% to 55.3% in the subgroup of patients treated with Gamma Knife for metastatic disease. Ohtakara and colleagues found that 8.39 cm^3 was the ideal cutoff for

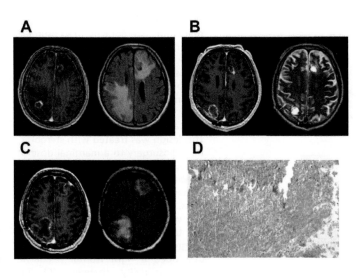

Fig. 1. Radionecrosis following resection and stereotactic radiosurgery for brain metastases. A 65-year-old man with systemically controlled stage IV lung adenocarcinoma and symptomatic oligometastatic disease to the brain. (*A*) T1-weighted postcontrast (*left*) and fluid-attenuated inversion recovery (FLAIR) (*right*) MRI showing the initial lesions with extensive surrounding vasogenic edema. The patient underwent resection of both lesions because of symptomatic mass effect with complete neurologic recovery. (*B*) T1-weighted postcontrast (*left*) and T2-weighted (*right*) MRI 2 weeks after surgery at the time of adjuvant stereotactic radiosurgery. The patient received a marginal dose of 15 Gy to each resection cavity in a single fraction. (*C*) T1-weighted postcontrast (*left*) and FLAIR (*right*) MRI 6 months after SRS showing changes in enhancement and edema associated with clinical symptoms. (*D*) This lesion proved to be radionecrosis on open biopsy, showing minimally cellular, necrotic tissue. The patient was treated with steroids and bevacizumab (biopsied lesion stained with hematoxylin and eosin).

predicting any RN for LINAC-based SRS, whereas Minniti proposed a V12 Gy threshold of 8.5 cm^3 for consideration of hypofractionated SRS, because these lesions had a greater than 10% risk of developing RN at 1 year.[21,22]

Other parameters, such as overall tumor volume and prescription isodose volume, have been shown to be significantly associated with RN.[20,21,23,24] Although volume parameters clearly are important for predicting RN risk, inconsistent conclusions from the literature make it difficult to assign 1 volume criterion that can be relied on to predict RN risk at this time.[4]

Other factors considered as contributors to RN following SRS have more heterogeneous supporting data. These factors include prior or concurrent WBRT, prior SRS, and dose conformality. Although intuitively prior radiation treatment would be expected to increase the risk of RN for any subsequent SRS, it is not always borne out in the literature. Prior or concurrent WBRT and prior SRS have been significant predictors of RN in univariate analysis in only a subset of retrospective studies where they were evaluated.[20,22–26,28] Sneed and colleagues[23] found that prior SRS was the strongest predictor of RN, with a hazard ratio of 3.74 (95% confidence interval, 1.3–10.8) on Cox proportional hazard analysis. However, Fang and colleagues[26] found no effect of prior SRS on development of RN following SRS treatment of melanoma metastases. Clearly, further studies are needed to quantitate the risk of RN in patients

with BMs who have received prior radiation treatment.

Several studies have investigated the contribution of systemic therapies to RN risk. Most have found that conventional chemotherapy is not associated with increased RN.[22,23,28] However, with the expanding use of immune checkpoint inhibitors (ICIs) for cancers that metastasize to the brain, and the potential for local inflammatory responses from immunotherapy, the impact of ICIs on RN risk is of particular interest (**Fig. 2**). Several investigators have raised the possibility that combination of ICIs with SRS may increase the risk of RN, given the proposed role of the immune system in the pathogenesis of RN. Current data suggest that RN occurs following combined SRS and ICI therapy in approximately 10% to 33% of patients treated[26,28–31] and in 2% to 10% of lesions treated[26,32,33] (**Table 1**). Symptomatic RN is reported in 3% to 22% of patients treated with ICIs and SRS.[26,30,31,34,35] These rates have significant overlap with those reported for the general population of patients with BMs receiving SRS. Studies directly comparing patients on ICIs with those not on ICIs report mixed results, with most recent retrospective studies finding trends but no statistically significant increased risk of RN in patients with concurrent ICI therapy receiving SRS[22,23,28,31,36] (see **Table 1**). At this time, concern surrounding increased risk of RN by combining ICI therapy with SRS is not clearly supported by the available data.

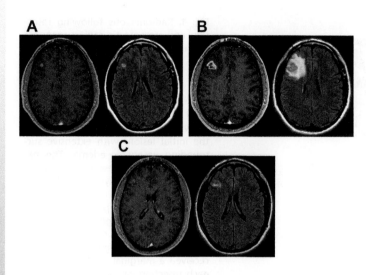

Fig. 2. Inflammatory changes following stereotactic radiosurgery and immunotherapy for brain metastases. A 51-year-old man with a history of metastatic melanoma and asymptomatic brain metastases identified during staging. (*A*) T1-weighted postcontrast (*left*) and FLAIR (*right*) MRI of right frontal metastasis at initial diagnosis. This lesion was treated with stereotactic radiosurgery to a marginal dose of 20 Gy in a single fraction. Following treatment, there was a complete response with total regression of the mass. The patient began systemic therapy with nivolumab 15 months after SRS treatment of extracranial disease progression. Within 3 months, he developed a right frontal headache and personality changes. (*B*) T1-weighted postcontrast (*left*) and FLAIR (*right*) MRI after starting nivolumab, showing inflammatory progression of the right frontal mass, which was treated with bevacizumab for 2 months. (*C*) T1-weighted postcontrast (*left*) and FLAIR (*right*) MRI at 1 year following discontinuation of bevacizumab. At this time, the patient had no evaluable systemic disease and had been off all systemic therapy for more than 1 year.

DIAGNOSTICS

Introduction

Differentiating RN from tumor recurrence/progression is a central challenge in the management of patients with BMs. Distinguishing recurrent tumor from RN is critical because of the vastly different approaches to treatment of each entity. Significant overlap in the radiological features (contrast enhancement, edema, mass effect) of both entities makes distinguishing them using conventional contrast-enhanced MRI (CE-MRI) very difficult. In a meta-analysis of MRI techniques, CE-MRI alone showed a pooled sensitivity and specificity of only 76% and 59% respectively.[37] In addition, both tumor recurrence and RN may have a very similar clinical presentation.

Table 1
Studies of radiation necrosis incidence in patients treated with stereotactic radiosurgery and immune checkpoint inhibitors

Study	Number (Patients/Lesions)	Patients with RN (Any/Symptomatic) (%)	Comparison ICI vs No ICI	Rate of RN (ICI vs No ICI) (%)	Significance
Colaco et al,[28] 2016	180/–	21.7/10.0	Yes	33.3 vs 18.1	*P* = .06
Chen et al,[35] 2018	260/623	–/3.0	Yes	NR	*P* = NS
Fang et al,[26] 2017	137/1094	27/14.6	No	27	All ICI patients
Kaidar-Person et al,[30] 2017	58/–	13.8/10.3	Yes	27.6 vs 0	NR
Patel et al,[31] 2017	54/–	31.5/22.2	Yes	30.0 vs 20.9	*P* = .08
Diao et al,[32] 2018	72/310	8.6/–	Yes	2.3 vs 0[a]	*P* = .22
Martin et al,[29] 2018	480/–	–/20	Yes	20.0 vs 6.8	*P* = .004
Koenig et al,[33] 2019	97/580	17.5/10.3	Yes	6.4 vs 2.0[a]	*P* = .005
Weingarten et al,[34] 2019	57/387	–/7	No	12.3	All ICI patients

Abbreviations: NR, not reported; NS, not significant.
[a] Data is rate per treated lesion.

Biopsy with histopathologic evaluation remains the gold standard to differentiate tumor recurrence from RN. However, stereotactic biopsies can introduce sampling bias, particularly in lesions harboring areas of both recurrent tumor and RN. In addition, biopsies carry all of the common risks associated with a surgical procedure and cannot practically be repeated with regular frequency. Therefore, there has been significant interest in developing cost-effective, noninvasive diagnostic approaches to distinguish recurrent tumor from RN with high sensitivity and specificity. Several imaging techniques have been investigated to improve diagnostic accuracy.

Magnetic Resonance Perfusion

Magnetic resonance perfusion (MRP) is designed to differentiate tumor recurrence from RN on the basis that recurrent tumor is associated with formation of new blood vessels with increased permeability, and thus higher perfusion and blood volume, compared with necrotic tissue characterized by radiation-induced endothelial damage. MRP can be performed using an intravenous contrast agent or with arterial spin labeling. Dynamic susceptibility contrast(DSC) MRI uses a T2* pulse sequence to image a contrast agent as it moves through the cerebrovascular system. In contrast, dynamic contrast-enhanced (DCE) MRI acquires imaging using a T1-based pulse sequence.

Several perfusion parameters are reported in DSC-MRI and DCE-MRI, including relative cerebral blood volume (rCBV), relative peak height, percentage of signal-intensity recovery, and transfer constant. BMs are often highly vascular lesions that tend to show increased rCBV levels, distinguishing them from RN. Mitsuya and colleagues[38] found that a rCBV cutoff of 2.1 provided the highest sensitivity and specificity in differentiating tumor recurrence from RN at 100% and 95.2% respectively. A meta-analysis by Chuang and colleagues[39] also revealed a statistically significant difference in rCBV values derived from tumor recurrence versus RN. However, there remains considerable variability in the sensitivities, specificities, and rCBV cutoffs reported in individual studies.[40,41]

Compared with DSC-MRI, DCE-MRI has better spatial resolution and relative insensitivity to hemorrhage-related susceptibility artifacts. This consideration is important because several malignancies with a predilection to metastasize to the brain, such as melanoma, are known to be hemorrhagic. Morabito and colleagues[42] compared the diagnostic accuracy of DSC with DCE in the differential diagnosis of tumor recurrence from RN. They found that a rCBV cutoff of 1.23 yielded a sensitivity and specificity of 88% and 75% for DSC, compared with 89% and 97% for DCE.

Magnetic Resonance Spectroscopy

Magnetic resonance spectroscopy (MRS) is another method of differentiating tumor recurrence/progression from RN by measuring the relative compositions of various metabolites in a given sample of tissue. Most commonly, these metabolites include choline, creatine, N-acetyl aspartate (NAA), lactate, and lipid. The pattern of these spectral peaks can aid in characterization of specific lesions. Increased choline (Cho)/creatine (Cr) and Cho/NAA ratios are findings that may be associated with tumor recurrence. In general, MRS comes in 2 forms: single-voxel MRS and multivoxel MRS. Although earlier protocols mostly used single-voxel MRS, multivoxel MRS has gained significant traction because of the ability to overcome error from volume averaging and inadequate sampling of heterogeneous lesions associated with single-voxel MRS.

A series of studies in Japan evaluated both single-voxel and/or multivoxel MRS compared with various other techniques in their ability to differentiate RN from brain metastasis recurrence.[43–45] Using single-voxel MRS, the investigators determined that a Cho/Cr threshold of 2.48 measured in whole lesions provided the lowest misdiagnosis rate across all types of lesions that were assessed.[43] Cho/Cr values greater than 2.48 gave a positive predictive value of 88.9% for brain metastasis, whereas a value less than 2.48 gave a positive predictive value of 71.4% for RN. In contrast with Cho/Cr, a Cho/lipid/lactate threshold of 0.3 provided even better performance in differentiating BM from RN, with values greater than 0.3 giving a 94.4% positive predictive value for diagnosing brain metastasis, and values less than 0.3 giving a 100% positive predictive value for diagnosing RN. This study is one of the few that provided histopathologic confirmation of all tested lesions, strengthening its validity. Using the same MRS Cho/Cr cutoff of 2.48 and Cho/lipid cutoff of 0.3 published in their original study, Kimura and colleagues[44,45] showed the accuracy of their proposed threshold values in 2 small follow-up studies with 100% sensitivity and specificity. Despite these promising results, data are only available from a small number of retrospective studies, and more prospective data are necessary to fully use MRS as a sole modality to make treatment decisions for current lesions after SRS.

PET

PET is a nuclear medicine functional imaging technique that evaluates metabolic activity. The rationale behind PET to differentiate tumor recurrence/progression from RN is that the increased metabolism in a growing viable tumor results in increased radiolabeled tracer uptake compared with RN. [^{18}F]-2-fluoro-2-deoxy-D-glucose (FDG) is a glucose analogue used as a standard radiotracer for oncologic PET imaging. Diagnosis of recurrent brain tumors using FDG-PET has been reported in the literature with wide variability, with sensitivity ranging from 40% to 95% and specificity ranging from 50% to 100%.[46–52] In addition, because normal physiologic brain is characterized by high glucose consumption, FDG-PET remains a less than ideal radiotracer in the brain.[49,53] As growing tumors also show increased amino acid uptake, amino acid analogues, such as L-methyl-^{11}C-methionine (MET), O-2-^{18}F-fluoroethyl-L-tyrosine (FET), and 3,4-dihydroxy-6-[18]fluoro-L-phenylalanine (FDOPA), have also been investigated as radiotracers to differentiate tumor recurrence from RN. The improved consistency coupled with the low uptake in normal physiologic brain tissue allowing better tumor-to-background contrast has increased interest in amino acid–derived PET.[54] MET-PET has been shown to differentiate BM recurrence from RN with sensitivities and specificities of 78% to 82% and 75% to 100% respectively.[55–57] Galldiks and colleagues[58] found FET-PET could differentiate recurrence from RN with a sensitivity of 74% and a specificity of 90%, which was further increased to a sensitivity of 95% and specificity of 91% on combined evaluation of time-activity curves with the mean tumor/brain ratio. In addition, besides the improved accuracy, there are other benefits to using FET, which also has a long half-life (110 minutes), precluding the need for an on-site cyclotron.[59]

Studies comparing metabolic PET imaging with advanced MRI techniques, and studies directly comparing different radiolabeled tracers in the same patients, are sparse and inconsistent. Cicone and colleagues[40] reported the overall efficacy of FDOPA-PET as superior to MRP, with sensitivities of 93.3% versus 86.7%, specificities of 90.9% versus 68.2%, and accuracy of 91.9% versus 75.6% respectively. However, a meta-analysis evaluating the efficacy of advanced MRI techniques (including MRP and MRS) compared with PET (including FDG and amino acid–PET)

found instead a significantly improved diagnostic performance with advanced MRI in differentiating metastatic tumor recurrence from RN after SRS.[37]

Single-Photon Emission Computed Tomography

Single-photon emission computed tomography (SPECT) is a nuclear medicine imaging technique that functions in a similar fashion to conventional nuclear medicine planar imaging, but provides three-dimensional information through the use of gamma rays. Several radiotracer agents have been used in SPECT for brain imaging, including intravenous technetium-99m, thallium-201 (^{201}Tl), and iodine-123-alpha-methyl tyrosine. Of these agents, ^{201}Tl-SPECT has been studied to the greatest extent; however, reported variability in the diagnostic sensitivity and specificity remains a limiting issue.[46,60] In addition, SPECT offers significantly lower spatial resolution compared with PET and suffers low signal/noise ratio. These factors, along with others, including a high radiation dose, have made SPECT a less popular imaging modality compared with MRP, MRS, or PET, in the differentiation of metastatic brain tumor recurrence and RN.

Other Imaging Modalities and Diagnostics

In addition to the various diagnostic techniques described earlier, several others, including measurement of water exchange,[61] gas chromatography with time-of-flight spectrometry,[62] radiomics,[63–66] and treatment response assessment maps (TRAMs),[67] have been reported. TRAMs are high-resolution maps calculated using delayed contrast T1-weighted MRI scans that are acquired immediately and 1 hour following a conventional injection of contrast agent.[67] Colorimetric heat maps of the subtracted images are generated to represent contrast clearance. Blue regions in the TRAMs represent effective clearance of contrast material from the vascular lumen, which is thought to indicate recurrent tumor. Red regions in the TRAMs represent contrast accumulation, which is thought to indicate RN, which causes contrast leakage and pooling. In their study of 150 patients, of which 77 were BMs, Zach and colleagues[67] compared presurgical TRAM predictions with histopathologic data obtained from biopsies. TRAMs were found to have a sensitivity and positive predictive value for active tumor of 100% and 89% respectively. This finding represented similar specificity and significantly improved sensitivity compared with rCBV analysis using DSC-MRI.

TREATMENT
Steroids and Bevacizumab

Corticosteroid therapy has long been a mainstay in the symptomatic treatment of RN. Steroids can rapidly improve symptoms by reducing production of inflammatory cytokines and vascular permeability, thereby resolving associated edema.[18,68] However, RN ultimately becomes refractory to steroid treatment in up to 70% of patients.[69,70] Steroids are also associated with significant adverse effects, including immunosuppression, metabolic dysfunction, insomnia, psychosis, and Cushing syndrome with extended use. Iatrogenic immunosuppression is of particular concern in the modern era of cancer immunotherapy. Steroid use may counteract the antitumor immune response stimulated by ICI therapy and should be limited in patients receiving such therapy.[71]

Considering the central role of VEGF in RN pathogenesis, bevacizumab, a monoclonal anti-VEGF antibody, is a logical alternative to steroids. Bevacizumab has been shown to be an effective option in prospective trials, including 2 randomized controlled trials and 1 single-arm phase 2 study for patients with RN.[70,72,73] These trials have shown that bevacizumab treatment results in a significant reduction in enhancing lesion volume and perilesional edema compared with placebo and dexamethasone (see **Fig. 2**). The improvement in radiographic findings was dramatic, with a reported average maximum decrease in gadolinium-enhancement volume of 25.5% to 92.8% and an average maximum decrease in fluid-attenuated inversion recovery (FLAIR) volume of 51.8% to 63% (**Table 2**). The radiographic effects of bevacizumab administration were not permanent, with regression starting roughly 1 month after bevacizumab discontinuation; however, most patients did not return to their prebevacizumab radiographic volumes.[70,72] Bevacizumab therapy resulted in significant improvement of clinical symptoms compared with both placebo and dexamethasone, and steroid dose requirements were reduced in 76% to 80% of patients.[70,72,73]

Bevacizumab was generally safe in the prospective trials. The most commonly reported adverse effect was hypertension, which occurs in up to 34.1% of patients, and is generally controllable with standard antihypertensives.[70,73] Severe adverse events (grade 3 or greater) occurred in 1.7% to 24.4% of patients. Thromboembolic or ischemic events, which are a particular concern with bevacizumab, occurred in fewer than 5% of patients.[70,73]

The published prospective studies of RN treated with bevacizumab predominantly evaluated patients with primary (nonmetastatic) tumors. Two retrospective studies of patients with RN resulting from SRS treatment of BMs have shown similar results.[74,75] The BeST trial, a prospective randomized study of corticosteroids plus bevacizumab versus corticosteroids plus placebo for RN after SRS for BM, has completed enrollment and is expected to report results later this year (NCT02490878). This study will definitively show the benefits and adverse effects of bevacizumab in this patient population. Prospective studies are also needed to determine the optimal dose of bevacizumab for treatment of RN, because anecdotal evidence suggests that dosing and frequency can be substantially reduced from the dosing used for tumor treatment, such as in glioblastoma.

Hyperbaric Oxygen Therapy

Hyperbaric oxygen therapy (HBOT) has been used in the treatment of a diverse range of medical conditions, including RN. HBOT greater than atmospheric pressure is thought to increase dissolved plasma oxygen sufficient to meet tissue oxygen demands independent of hemoglobin-binding capacity, promoting angiogenesis.[76] Evidence for HBOT in brain metastasis treated with SRS is limited. A retrospective analysis of 78 patients treated with or without HBOT before SRS showed a reduction in white matter injury and RN in the HBOT group (11% vs 20%).[77] However, although a systematic review of HBOT for RN by the Cochrane Collaboration found some benefit for head and neck and colorectal cancers, there was no benefit for neural tissue.[78] Two prospective clinical trials testing HBOT for RN in the brain (NCT00087815, NCT02714465) have been initiated, but results have not yet been reported. More data are needed for the recommendation of HBOT for RN caused by SRS.

Anticoagulant and Antiplatelet Therapy

Because vascular abnormalities are thought to be involved in the pathogenesis of RN, small, single-institution reports trialing anticoagulant or antiplatelet therapy, most commonly warfarin or heparin, have been published.[79–81] The small sample size and marginal benefit of these therapies in RN are thus far unsatisfactory, and this has not been further investigated.

Laser Interstitial Thermal Therapy

Although significant improvement has been made in the accuracy of various diagnostic modalities in differentiating BM recurrence from RN, no single modality or combination of diagnostic tests has proved to be perfect. Even the gold standard of

Table 2
Studies of bevacizumab for radiation necrosis

Study	Dose (mg/kg)	Imaging Response (Change in Volume)		Clinical Response (No. of Patients)	Reduction in Steroids (No. of Patients)
		T1 + Contrast	T2 FLAIR		
Levin et al,[72] 2011	7.5 mg/kg Q 3 wk	−63%	−59%	12/12 (100%)	4/5 (80%)
Boothe et al,[74] 2013	10 mg/kg Q 2 wk	−64%	−64%	10/11 (91%)	9/9 (100%)
Furuse et al,[73] 2016	5 mg/kg Q 2 wk	−93%	−63%	16/38 (42%)	30/38 (79%)
Glitza et al,[75] 2017	5–10 mg/kg Q 2 wk	85% of patients improved		7/7 (100%)	NR
Xu et al,[70] 2018	5 mg/kg Q 2 wk	−26%	−52%	53.4%	Steroid naive

Abbreviation: Q, every.

stereotactic biopsy with histopathologic evaluation remains imperfect, because of sampling bias in mixed lesions containing both areas of tumor recurrence and RN. For most treatment modalities, accurate assessment of the underlying pathophysiology is critical to selecting the right treatment. Reirradiation of RN worsens the disease, and management of edema only in a recurrent tumor allows further progression. There is only 1 treatment approach that is equivalently effective for RN and tumor recurrence, allowing intervention regardless of the underlying disorder: laser interstitial thermal therapy (LITT).

LITT is a minimally invasive ablative technique that has been adopted for the treatment of many disorders, including primary and metastatic intracranial tumors, RN, and epilepsy.[82] In addition to ablation of the lesion, a simultaneous stereotactic biopsy can be performed during probe placement to inform on the disorder, allowing better management of systemic therapy after treatment.[83] Several studies have examined the safety and efficacy of LITT in the treatment of recurrent metastatic brain tumors and RN following radiation therapy for metastatic brain tumors.[84–92] A critical end point is the rate of local lesion control following LITT, although there is variability in the definition across studies. The control rate of recurrent tumor, expectedly, depends on the degree of lesion ablation. Carpentier and colleagues[85] reported on local control in recurrent BM treated with LITT, finding that the median progression-free survival for totally ablated lesions (n = 9) was 15 months, compared with 6 months for partially ablated lesions (n = 6). Further evidence supporting the importance of total ablation for recurrent tumor has been shown in subsequent studies,[89,90] and a recent meta-analysis found that total ablation of recurrent tumors resulted in 3-month local control rates of 80% to 100%.[93]

Most studies of LITT have evaluated local control rates of RN and recurrent metastases together.[88,90–92] Rao and colleagues[88] found a local control rate of 75% at a median follow-up of 24 weeks, a median progression-free survival of 37 weeks, and an overall survival rate of 57% for recurrence and RN. Similar or improved control rates of greater than 80% with follow-up periods of 6 to 11 months have subsequently been reported.[91,94,95] The local control rates for RN are particularly robust, with a complete response rate of 100% reported for total ablations, and no progressive disease reported regardless of the degree of ablation.[90] Studies comparing outcomes of LITT versus the gold standard, craniotomy, for recurrent lesions (RN or tumor) after SRS found no significant differences in progression-free survival, overall survival, ability to taper off steroids, perioperative complications, or neurologic outcomes between the 2 groups.[92] LITT was associated with a significantly shorter hospital length of stay, with multiple studies reporting stays of 24 hours or less,[84,85,88] compared with a historical length of stay following craniotomy of 5 to 7 days.[96,97]

There has been little discussion about the impact of repeat SRS on tumor control following LITT for recurrent BM, likely because most studies in the literature evaluated patients with an extensive prior history of radiation who were not candidates for further treatment. However, in practice, patients develop changes concerning for recurrence versus RN even after a single SRS treatment. For such patients, repeat SRS is an option if RN can be ruled out definitively. As indicated in the review of diagnostic techniques, stereotactic biopsy remains the most accurate method to differentiate recurrence from RN. If biopsy is going to be performed, simultaneous LITT should be considered. For RN, LITT can definitively treat

A B

C D

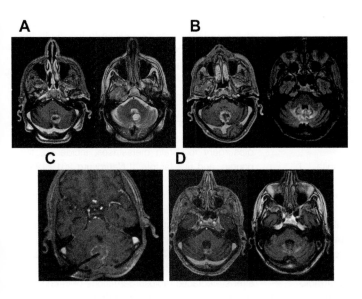

Fig. 3. Radionecrosis following stereotactic radiosurgery treated with LITT. An 80-year-old man with a history of stage IIIb lung squamous cell carcinoma after resection, systemic chemotherapy, and local radiotherapy, who presented with new-onset ataxia and nausea. He was found to have a solitary cerebellar metastasis. (*A*) T1-weighted postcontrast (*left*) and T2-weighted (*right*) MRI at the time of stereotactic radiosurgery for the cerebellar tumor. The patient was treated with a marginal dose of 18 Gy in a single fraction to the lesion without complication. Four months after treatment, the patient developed severe nausea and dysarthria. (*B*) T1-weighted postcontrast (*left*) and FLAIR (*right*) MRI showing progression of the cerebellar lesion and surrounding edema, which was suspected to be radionecrosis and the patient underwent LITT with simultaneous biopsy to characterize the lesion. The biopsy showed necrotic changes without viable tumor. (*C*) T1-weighted postcontrast MRI at completion of the LITT procedure with the fiber still in place. Treatment substantially reduced the enhancement of the lesion and surrounding edema. By postoperative day 1, the patient's nausea had almost completely resolved. (*D*) T1-weighted postcontrast (*left*) and FLAIR (*right*) MRI 3 months after LITT treatment.

the lesion without the need for prolonged steroids or bevacizumab (**Fig. 3**). More data are necessary to determine whether LITT plus repeat SRS can enhance tumor control or allow dose reduction of SRS to decrease complications.

SUMMARY

Some degree of RN occurs in approximately 10% to 25% of patients with BMs treated with SRS, with most cases occurring greater than 6 months after treatment. Dose/volume parameters such as total target volume and V12 Gy are the most important factors in predicting RN risk. Although concern has been raised over the use of ICIs with SRS, most of the data indicate that the risk of RN in these patients is not significantly increased. Several noninvasive advanced imaging modalities exist to differentiate RN from recurrent tumor with high sensitivity and specificity. However, stereotactic biopsy remains the gold standard. Treatment of RN usually involves management of edema with steroids and/or bevacizumab. To avoid prolonged use of these agents, surgical intervention can be considered. Although resection of RN can be performed to control mass-related symptoms, minimally invasive ablation with LITT is equally effective and reduces hospital length of stay and perioperative pain.

DISCLOSURE

The authors have nothing to disclose.

REFERENCES

1. Graber JJ, Cobbs CS, Olson JJ. Congress of neurological surgeons systematic review and evidence-based guidelines on the use of stereotactic radiosurgery in the treatment of adults with metastatic brain tumors. Neurosurgery 2019;84(3):E168–70.
2. Ammirati M, Cobbs CS, Linskey ME, et al. The role of retreatment in the management of recurrent/progressive brain metastases: a systematic review and evidence-based clinical practice guideline. J Neurooncol 2010;96(1):85–96.
3. Kirkpatrick JP, Soltys SG, Lo SS, et al. The radiosurgery fractionation quandary: single fraction or hypo-fractionation? Neuro Oncol 2017;19(suppl_2):ii38–49.
4. Sahgal A, Ruschin M, Ma L, et al. Stereotactic radiosurgery alone for multiple brain metastases? A review of clinical and technical issues. Neuro Oncol 2017;19(suppl_2):ii2–15.
5. Hopewell JW, van der Kogel AJ. Pathophysiological mechanisms leading to the development of late radiation-induced damage to the central nervous system. Front Radiat Ther Oncol 1999;33:265–75.
6. Miyatake S, Nonoguchi N, Furuse M, et al. Pathophysiology, diagnosis, and treatment of radiation

necrosis in the brain. Neurol Med Chir (Tokyo) 2015; 55(Suppl 1):50–9.

7. Calvo W, Hopewell JW, Reinhold HS, et al. Time- and dose-related changes in the white matter of the rat brain after single doses of X rays. Br J Radiol 1988;61(731):1043–52.

8. Li YQ, Chen P, Haimovitz-Friedman A, et al. Endothelial apoptosis initiates acute blood-brain barrier disruption after ionizing radiation. Cancer Res 2003;63(18):5950–6.

9. Yamaguchi N, Yamashima T, Yamashita J. A histological and flow cytometric study of dog brain endothelial cell injuries in delayed radiation necrosis. J Neurosurg 1991;74(4):625–32.

10. Ansari R, Gaber MW, Wang B, et al. Anti-TNFA (TNF-alpha) treatment abrogates radiation-induced changes in vascular density and tissue oxygenation. Radiat Res 2007;167(1):80–6.

11. Yoshii Y. Pathological review of late cerebral radionecrosis. Brain Tumor Pathol 2008;25(2):51–8.

12. Yoritsune E, Furuse M, Kuwabara H, et al. Inflammation as well as angiogenesis may participate in the pathophysiology of brain radiation necrosis. J Radiat Res 2014;55(4):803–11.

13. Nonoguchi N, Miyatake S, Fukumoto M, et al. The distribution of vascular endothelial growth factor-producing cells in clinical radiation necrosis of the brain: pathological consideration of their potential roles. J Neurooncol 2011;105(2):423–31.

14. Kureshi SA, Hofman FM, Schneider JH, et al. Cytokine expression in radiation-induced delayed cerebral injury. Neurosurgery 1994;35(5):822–9 [discussion: 829–30].

15. Teicher BA, Fricker SP. CXCL12 (SDF-1)/CXCR4 pathway in cancer. Clin Cancer Res 2010;16(11): 2927–31.

16. Wilson CM, Gaber MW, Sabek OM, et al. Radiation-induced astrogliosis and blood-brain barrier damage can be abrogated using anti-TNF treatment. Int J Radiat Oncol Biol Phys 2009;74(3): 934–41.

17. Chao ST, Ahluwalia MS, Barnett GH, et al. Challenges with the diagnosis and treatment of cerebral radiation necrosis. Int J Radiat Oncol Biol Phys 2013;87(3):449–57.

18. Giglio P, Gilbert MR. Cerebral radiation necrosis. Neurologist 2003;9(4):180–8.

19. New P. Radiation injury to the nervous system. Curr Opin Neurol 2001;14(6):725–34.

20. Kohutek ZA, Yamada Y, Chan TA, et al. Long-term risk of radionecrosis and imaging changes after stereotactic radiosurgery for brain metastases. J Neurooncol 2015;125(1):149–56.

21. Minniti G, Clarke E, Lanzetta G, et al. Stereotactic radiosurgery for brain metastases: analysis of outcome and risk of brain radionecrosis. Radiat Oncol 2011;6:48.

22. Ohtakara K, Hayashi S, Nakayama N, et al. Significance of target location relative to the depth from the brain surface and high-dose irradiated volume in the development of brain radionecrosis after micromultileaf collimator-based stereotactic radiosurgery for brain metastases. J Neurooncol 2012; 108(1):201–9.

23. Sneed PK, Mendez J, Vemer-van den Hoek JG, et al. Adverse radiation effect after stereotactic radiosurgery for brain metastases: incidence, time course, and risk factors. J Neurosurg 2015;123(2): 373–86.

24. Blonigen BJ, Steinmetz RD, Levin L, et al. Irradiated volume as a predictor of brain radionecrosis after linear accelerator stereotactic radiosurgery. Int J Radiat Oncol Biol Phys 2010;77(4):996–1001.

25. Schuttrumpf LH, Niyazi M, Nachbichler SB, et al. Prognostic factors for survival and radiation necrosis after stereotactic radiosurgery alone or in combination with whole brain radiation therapy for 1-3 cerebral metastases. Radiat Oncol 2014;9:105.

26. Fang P, Jiang W, Allen P, et al. Radiation necrosis with stereotactic radiosurgery combined with CTLA-4 blockade and PD-1 inhibition for treatment of intracranial disease in metastatic melanoma. J Neurooncol 2017;133(3):595–602.

27. Korytko T, Radivoyevitch T, Colussi V, et al. 12 Gy gamma knife radiosurgical volume is a predictor for radiation necrosis in non-AVM intracranial tumors. Int J Radiat Oncol Biol Phys 2006;64(2): 419–24.

28. Colaco RJ, Martin P, Kluger HM, et al. Does immunotherapy increase the rate of radiation necrosis after radiosurgical treatment of brain metastases? J Neurosurg 2016;125(1):17–23.

29. Martin AM, Cagney DN, Catalano PJ, et al. Immunotherapy and Symptomatic Radiation Necrosis in Patients With Brain Metastases Treated With Stereotactic Radiation. JAMA Oncol 2018;4(8): 1123–4.

30. Kaidar-Person O, Zagar TM, Deal A, et al. The incidence of radiation necrosis following stereotactic radiotherapy for melanoma brain metastases: the potential impact of immunotherapy. Anti Cancer Drugs 2017;28(6):669–75.

31. Patel KR, Shoukat S, Oliver DE, et al. Ipilimumab and Stereotactic Radiosurgery Versus Stereotactic Radiosurgery Alone for Newly Diagnosed Melanoma Brain Metastases. Am J Clin Oncol 2017;40(5): 444–50.

32. Diao K, Bian SX, Routman DM, et al. Combination ipilimumab and radiosurgery for brain metastases: tumor, edema, and adverse radiation effects. J Neurosurg 2018;129(6):1397–406.

33. Koenig JL, Shi S, Sborov K, et al. Adverse radiation effect and disease control in patients undergoing stereotactic radiosurgery and immune checkpoint

inhibitor therapy for brain metastases. World Neurosurg 2019;126:e1399–411.

34. Weingarten N, Kruser TJ, Bloch O. Symptomatic radiation necrosis in brain metastasis patients treated with stereotactic radiosurgery and immunotherapy. Clin Neurol Neurosurg 2019;179:14–8.

35. Chen L, Douglass J, Kleinberg L, et al. Concurrent immune checkpoint inhibitors and stereotactic radiosurgery for brain metastases in non-small cell lung cancer, melanoma, and renal cell carcinoma. Int J Radiat Oncol Biol Phys 2018;100(4):916–25.

36. Kim JM, Miller JA, Kotecha R, et al. The risk of radiation necrosis following stereotactic radiosurgery with concurrent systemic therapies. J Neurooncol 2017;133(2):357–68.

37. Suh CH, Kim HS, Jung SC, et al. Comparison of MRI and PET as potential surrogate endpoints for treatment response after stereotactic radiosurgery in patients with brain metastasis. AJR Am J Roentgenol 2018;211(6):1332–41.

38. Mitsuya K, Nakasu Y, Horiguchi S, et al. Perfusion weighted magnetic resonance imaging to distinguish the recurrence of metastatic brain tumors from radiation necrosis after stereotactic radiosurgery. J Neurooncol 2010;99(1):81–8.

39. Chuang MT, Liu YS, Tsai YS, et al. Differentiating radiation-induced necrosis from recurrent brain tumor using MR perfusion and spectroscopy: a meta-analysis. PLoS One 2016;11(1):e0141438.

40. Cicone F, Minniti G, Romano A, et al. Accuracy of F-DOPA PET and perfusion-MRI for differentiating radionecrotic from progressive brain metastases after radiosurgery. Eur J Nucl Med Mol Imaging 2015; 42(1):103–11.

41. Muto M, Frauenfelder G, Senese R, et al. Dynamic susceptibility contrast (DSC) perfusion MRI in differential diagnosis between radionecrosis and neoangiogenesis in cerebral metastases using rCBV, rCBF and K2. Radiol Med 2018;123(7):545–52.

42. Morabito R, Alafaci C, Pergolizzi S, et al. DCE and DSC perfusion MRI diagnostic accuracy in the follow-up of primary and metastatic intra-axial brain tumors treated by radiosurgery with cyberknife. Radiat Oncol 2019;14(1):65.

43. Kimura T, Sako K, Gotoh T, et al. In vivo single-voxel proton MR spectroscopy in brain lesions with ring-like enhancement. NMR Biomed 2001;14(6):339–49.

44. Kimura T, Sako K, Tohyama Y, et al. Diagnosis and treatment of progressive space-occupying radiation necrosis following stereotactic radiosurgery for brain metastasis: value of proton magnetic resonance spectroscopy. Acta Neurochir (Wein) 2003;145(7): 557–64 [discussion: 564].

45. Kimura T, Sako K, Tanaka K, et al. Evaluation of the response of metastatic brain tumors to stereotactic radiosurgery by proton magnetic resonance spectroscopy, 201TlCl single-photon emission

computerized tomography, and gadolinium-enhanced magnetic resonance imaging. J Neurosurg 2004;100(5):835–41.

46. Lai G, Mahadevan A, Hackney D, et al. Diagnostic Accuracy of PET, SPECT, and Arterial Spin-Labeling in Differentiating Tumor Recurrence from Necrosis in Cerebral Metastasis after Stereotactic Radiosurgery. AJNR Am J Neuroradiol 2015; 36(12):2250–5.

47. Chernov M, Hayashi M, Izawa M, et al. Differentiation of the radiation-induced necrosis and tumor recurrence after gamma knife radiosurgery for brain metastases: importance of multi-voxel proton MRS. Minimally Invasive Neurosurg 2005;48(4):228–34.

48. Chao ST, Suh JH, Raja S, et al. The sensitivity and specificity of FDG PET in distinguishing recurrent brain tumor from radionecrosis in patients treated with stereotactic radiosurgery. Int J Cancer 2001; 96(3):191–7.

49. Belohlavek O, Simonova G, Kantorova I, et al. Brain metastases after stereotactic radiosurgery using the Leksell gamma knife: can FDG PET help to differentiate radionecrosis from tumour progression? Eur J Nucl Med Mol Imaging 2003;30(1):96–100.

50. Horky LL, Hsiao EM, Weiss SE, et al. Dual phase FDG-PET imaging of brain metastases provides superior assessment of recurrence versus post-treatment necrosis. J Neurooncol 2011;103(1): 137–46.

51. Hatzoglou V, Yang TJ, Omuro A, et al. A prospective trial of dynamic contrast-enhanced MRI perfusion and fluorine-18 FDG PET-CT in differentiating brain tumor progression from radiation injury after cranial irradiation. Neuro Oncol. 2016;18(6):873–80.

52. Tomura N, Kokubun M, Saginoya T, et al. Differentiation between Treatment-Induced Necrosis and Recurrent Tumors in Patients with Metastatic Brain Tumors: Comparison among (11)C-Methionine-PET, FDG-PET, MR Permeability Imaging, and MRI-ADC-Preliminary Results. AJNR Am J Neuroradiol 2017;38(8):1520–7.

53. Galldiks N, Langen KJ, Pope WB. From the clinician's point of view - What is the status quo of positron emission tomography in patients with brain tumors? Neuro Oncol 2015;17(11):1434–44.

54. Langen KJ, Galldiks N, Hattingen E, et al. Advances in neuro-oncology imaging. Nat Rev Neurol 2017; 13(5):279–89.

55. Tsuyuguchi N, Sunada I, Iwai Y, et al. Methionine positron emission tomography of recurrent metastatic brain tumor and radiation necrosis after stereotactic radiosurgery: is a differential diagnosis possible? J Neurosurg 2003;98(5):1056–64.

56. Terakawa Y, Tsuyuguchi N, Iwai Y, et al. Diagnostic accuracy of 11C-methionine PET for differentiation of recurrent brain tumors from radiation necrosis after radiotherapy. J Nucl Med 2008;49(5):694–9.

57. Yomo S, Oguchi K. Prospective study of (11)C-methionine PET for distinguishing between recurrent brain metastases and radiation necrosis: limitations of diagnostic accuracy and long-term results of salvage treatment. BMC Cancer 2017;17(1):713.

58. Galldiks N, Stoffels G, Filss CP, et al. Role of O-(2-(18)F-fluoroethyl)-L-tyrosine PET for differentiation of local recurrent brain metastasis from radiation necrosis. J Nucl Med 2012;53(9):1367–74.

59. Grosu AL, Astner ST, Riedel E, et al. An interindividual comparison of O-(2-[18F]fluoroethyl)-L-tyrosine (FET)- and L-[methyl-11C]methionine (MET)-PET in patients with brain gliomas and metastases. Int J Radiat Oncol Biol Phys 2011;81(4):1049–58.

60. Serizawa T, Saeki N, Higuchi Y, et al. Diagnostic value of thallium-201 chloride single-photon emission computerized tomography in differentiating tumor recurrence from radiation injury after gamma knife surgery for metastatic brain tumors. J Neurosurg 2005;102(Suppl):266–71.

61. Mehrabian H, Detsky J, Soliman H, et al. Advanced Magnetic Resonance Imaging Techniques in Management of Brain Metastases. Front Oncol 2019;9: 440.

62. Lu AY, Turban JL, Damisah EC, et al. Novel biomarker identification using metabolomic profiling to differentiate radiation necrosis and recurrent tumor following Gamma Knife radiosurgery. J Neurosurg 2017;127(2):388–96.

63. Lohmann P, Stoffels G, Ceccon G, et al. Radiation injury vs. recurrent brain metastasis: combining textural feature radiomics analysis and standard parameters may increase (18)F-FET PET accuracy without dynamic scans. Eur Radiol 2017;27(7): 2916–27.

64. Peng L, Parekh V, Huang P, et al. Distinguishing True Progression From Radionecrosis After Stereotactic Radiation Therapy for Brain Metastases With Machine Learning and Radiomics. Int J Radiat Oncol Biol Phys 2018;102(4):1236–43.

65. Lohmann P, Kocher M, Steger J, et al. Radiomics derived from amino-acid PET and conventional MRI in patients with high-grade gliomas. Q J Nucl Med Mol Imaging 2018;62(3):272–80.

66. Lohmann P, Kocher M, Ceccon G, et al. Combined FET PET/MRI radiomics differentiates radiation injury from recurrent brain metastasis. Neuroimage Clin 2018;20:537–42.

67. Zach L, Guez D, Last D, et al. Delayed contrast extravasation MRI: a new paradigm in neuro-oncology. Neuro Oncol 2015;17(3):457–65.

68. Vellayappan B, Tan CL, Yong C, et al. Diagnosis and Management of Radiation Necrosis in Patients With Brain Metastases. Front Oncol 2018;8:395.

69. Zhuo X, Huang X, Yan M, et al. Comparison between high-dose and low-dose intravenous methylprednisolone therapy in patients with brain necrosis after radiotherapy for nasopharyngeal carcinoma. Radiother Oncol 2019;137:16–23.

70. Xu Y, Rong X, Hu W, et al. Bevacizumab Monotherapy Reduces Radiation-induced Brain Necrosis in Nasopharyngeal Carcinoma Patients: A Randomized Controlled Trial. Int J Radiat Oncol Biol Phys 2018;101(5):1087–95.

71. Ramakrishna R, Formenti S. Radiosurgery and Immunotherapy in the Treatment of Brain Metastases. World Neurosurg 2019;130:615–22.

72. Levin VA, Bidaut L, Hou P, et al. Randomized double-blind placebo-controlled trial of bevacizumab therapy for radiation necrosis of the central nervous system. Int J Radiat Oncol Biol Phys 2011; 79(5):1487–95.

73. Furuse M, Nonoguchi N, Kuroiwa T, et al. A prospective, multicentre, single-arm clinical trial of bevacizumab for patients with surgically untreatable, symptomatic brain radiation necrosis(dagger). Neurooncol Pract 2016;3(4):272–80.

74. Boothe D, Young R, Yamada Y, et al. Bevacizumab as a treatment for radiation necrosis of brain metastases post stereotactic radiosurgery. Neuro Oncol 2013;15(9):1257–63.

75. Glitza IC, Guha-Thakurta N, D'Souza NM, et al. Bevacizumab as an effective treatment for radiation necrosis after radiotherapy for melanoma brain metastases. Melanoma Res 2017;27(6): 580–4.

76. Tibbles PM, Edelsberg JS. Hyperbaric-oxygen therapy. N Engl J Med 1996;334(25):1642–8.

77. Ohguri T, Imada H, Kohshi K, et al. Effect of prophylactic hyperbaric oxygen treatment for radiation-induced brain injury after stereotactic radiosurgery of brain metastases. Int J Radiat Oncol Biol Phys 2007;67(1):248–55.

78. Bennett MH, Feldmeier J, Hampson NB, et al. Hyperbaric oxygen therapy for late radiation tissue injury. Cochrane Database Syst Rev 2016;(4): CD005005.

79. Glantz MJ, Burger PC, Friedman AH, et al. Treatment of radiation-induced nervous system injury with heparin and warfarin. Neurology 1994;44(11): 2020–7.

80. Rizzoli HV, Pagnanelli DM. Treatment of delayed radiation necrosis of the brain. A clinical observation. J Neurosurg 1984;60(3):589–94.

81. Happold C, Ernemann U, Roth P, et al. Anticoagulation for radiation-induced neurotoxicity revisited. J Neurooncol 2008;90(3):357–62.

82. Rennert RC, Khan U, Bartek J, et al. Laser Ablation of Abnormal Neurological Tissue Using Robotic Neuroblate System (LAANTERN): Procedural Safety and Hospitalization. Neurosurgery 2020;86(4): 538–47.

83. Shah AH, Semonche A, Eichberg DG, et al. The role of laser interstitial thermal therapy in surgical neuro-

oncology: series of 100 consecutive patients. Neurosurgery 2020;87(2):266–75.

84. Carpentier A, McNichols RJ, Stafford RJ, et al. Real-time magnetic resonance-guided laser thermal therapy for focal metastatic brain tumors. Neurosurgery 2008;63(1 Suppl 1):ONS21–8 [discussion: ONS28-29].

85. Carpentier A, McNichols RJ, Stafford RJ, et al. Laser thermal therapy: real-time MRI-guided and computer-controlled procedures for metastatic brain tumors. Lasers Surg Med 2011;43(10):943–50.

86. Rahmathulla G, Recinos PF, Valerio JE, et al. Laser interstitial thermal therapy for focal cerebral radiation necrosis: a case report and literature review. Stereotact Funct Neurosurg 2012;90(3):192–200.

87. Torres-Reveron J, Tomasiewicz HC, Shetty A, et al. Stereotactic laser induced thermotherapy (LITT): a novel treatment for brain lesions regrowing after radiosurgery. J Neurooncol 2013;113(3):495–503.

88. Rao MS, Hargreaves EL, Khan AJ, et al. Magnetic resonance-guided laser ablation improves local control for postradiosurgery recurrence and/or radiation necrosis. Neurosurgery 2014;74(6):658–67 [discussion: 667].

89. Ali MA, Carroll KT, Rennert RC, et al. Stereotactic laser ablation as treatment for brain metastases that recur after stereotactic radiosurgery: a multiinstitutional experience. Neurosurg Focus 2016; 41(4):E11.

90. Ahluwalia M, Barnett GH, Deng D, et al. Laser ablation after stereotactic radiosurgery: a multicenter prospective study in patients with metastatic brain tumors and radiation necrosis. J Neurosurg 2018; 130(3):804–11.

91. Bastos DCA, Rao G, Oliva ICG, et al. Predictors of Local Control of Brain Metastasis Treated With Laser Interstitial Thermal Therapy. Neurosurgery 2020; 87(1):112–22.

92. Hong CS, Deng D, Vera A, et al. Laser-interstitial thermal therapy compared to craniotomy for treatment of radiation necrosis or recurrent tumor in brain metastases failing radiosurgery. J Neurooncol 2019; 142(2):309–17.

93. Alattar AA, Bartek J Jr, Chiang VL, et al. Stereotactic Laser Ablation as Treatment of Brain Metastases Recurring after Stereotactic Radiosurgery: A Systematic Literature Review. World Neurosurg 2019; 128:134–42.

94. Chaunzwa TL, Deng D, Leuthardt EC, et al. Laser Thermal Ablation for Metastases Failing Radiosurgery: A Multicentered Retrospective Study. Neurosurgery 2018;82(1):56–63.

95. Hernandez RN, Carminucci A, Patel P, et al. Magnetic Resonance-Guided Laser-Induced Thermal Therapy for the Treatment of Progressive Enhancing Inflammatory Reactions Following Stereotactic Radiosurgery, or PEIRs, for Metastatic Brain Disease. Neurosurgery 2019;85(1):84–90.

96. Sawaya R, Hammoud M, Schoppa D, et al. Neurosurgical outcomes in a modern series of 400 craniotomies for treatment of parenchymal tumors. Neurosurgery 1998;42(5):1044–55 [discussion: 1055–6].

97. Long DM, Gordon T, Bowman H, et al. Outcome and cost of craniotomy performed to treat tumors in regional academic referral centers. Neurosurgery 2003;52(5):1056–63 [discussion: 1063–5].

Antiepileptic Drugs in the Management of Cerebral Metastases

Meredith A. Monsour, BS[a], Patrick D. Kelly, MD[b], Lola B. Chambless, MD[b],*

KEYWORDS

• AED • Anticonvulsant • Antiepileptic • Seizure • Metastasis

KEY POINTS

- Between 15% and 25% of patients with brain metastases experience a seizure at some point in the disease course.
- Patients who have not had a seizure or seizurelike episode should not be routinely placed on seizure prophylaxis preoperatively.
- Nonoperative patients do not require seizure prophylaxis in the absence of prior seizure history.
- Existing literature does not support the routine use of postoperative seizure prophylaxis, although the practice is common among neurosurgeons.
- Timing of antiepileptic drug cessation should be guided by patient-specific factors, including risk of recurrence, life expectancy, and adverse reactions to antiepileptic agents.

INTRODUCTION

Approximately 10% to 40% of adult patients with cancer develop brain metastases.[1–3] Although seizures are less common among those with metastatic lesions compared with primary brain tumors, the incidence remains as high as 15% to 25%.[4–6] Seizures can be effectively treated or prevented with any number of antiepileptic drugs (AEDs), but these agents have associated risks and side effects. The decision to treat a patient with AEDs must be made carefully, balancing the risks of seizure with potential adverse effects of therapy.

The ill effects of seizures for patients with metastatic brain tumors are numerous. Epilepsy is considered to be the most important risk factor for long-term disability in patients with brain tumors.[7] Postoperative seizures in particular are associated with considerable morbidity, longer length of hospital stay, and higher rates of readmission.[8–12] Concerns about seizure-associated morbidity often prompt physicians to seek to aggressively treat or prevent epilepsy.

However, AEDs are associated with adverse effects that can result in substantial disability, morbidity, and mortality. The incidence and severity of adverse effects of anticonvulsants may be 20% to 40% worse in patients with brain tumors compared with the general population.[13] More broadly, AEDs may profoundly affect a patient's quality of life, and are associated with perceived increase in cognitive deficits, social dysfunction, and adverse events such as fatigue, nausea, and weight changes.[7] A careful analysis of the risks and benefits must therefore be heavily weighed before initiating treatment, particularly prophylactically.

Funding: P.D. Kelly is supported by a training grant from the National Cancer Institute of the National Institutes of Health under award number T32CA106183.
[a] Vanderbilt University School of Medicine, 2209 Garland Avenue, Nashville, TN 37240-0002, USA;
[b] Department of Neurological Surgery, Vanderbilt University Medical Center, T-4224 Medical Center North, Nashville, TN 37232-2380, USA
* Corresponding author.
E-mail address: Lola.chambless@vumc.org

Neurosurg Clin N Am 31 (2020) 589–601
https://doi.org/10.1016/j.nec.2020.06.008
1042-3680/20/© 2020 Elsevier Inc. All rights reserved.

Although several systematic reviews and meta-analyses on the issue have suggested no benefit to prophylactic therapy,[14–17] a recent survey study found that greater than 63% of surgeons administer seizure prophylaxis after brain tumor resection in patients without history of antecedent seizure.[18] Given the significant discrepancy between evidence and practice as well as the lack of consensus on treatment decisions, this article provides a concise summary of current evidence and clinical recommendations regarding the use of AEDs among patients with brain metastases.

INDICATIONS FOR TREATMENT

Antiepileptic therapy may be administered in the preoperative, intraoperative, and postoperative periods, with the goal of either primary or secondary prevention. Primary prevention is synonymous with traditional prophylaxis. Secondary prevention refers to AED therapy designed to mitigate the risk of additional seizures in patients who have already experienced one. This article considers the indications for treatment within each phase of care and for both types of prevention. Summaries of guidelines and studies on the issue of AED prophylaxis are provided in **Tables 1** and **2**, respectively.

Primary Prevention

Preoperative prophylaxis
The American Academy of Neurology (AAN) published guidelines on AED prophylaxis in patients with newly diagnosed brain tumors in 2000; these guidelines recommend against AED prophylaxis in patients who have not had a seizure.[13] Similarly, a systematic review and clinical practice guideline published by the Congress of Neurological Surgeons (CNS) in 2010 did not recommend prophylactic anticonvulsant use for patients with CNS metastases who had not had a seizure (level 3 American Association of Neurological Surgeons/CNS recommendation, see **Table 1**).[15]

In 2019, the CNS published updated guidelines in prophylactic AED therapy for patients with brain metastases.[19] These guidelines also suggested against AED prophylaxis in the absence of a seizure history, a recommendation that has subsequently been endorsed by both the American Society of Clinical Oncology (ASCO) and the Society for Neuro-Oncology (SNO).[20]

Many of the studies included in these evidence-based reviews compared patients not receiving any prophylactic AED therapy with those who received prophylaxis preoperatively, postoperatively, or both.[21–23] No studies directly addressed the independent effect of preoperative prophylaxis on rates of postoperative seizures.

Intraoperative prophylaxis
Intraoperative AED use has not been specifically assessed in the literature, although many studies of postoperative prophylaxis included an

---

Table 1
Synopsis of published guidelines and practice parameters

Organization	Year	Recommendations
AAN[13]	2000	• "In patients with newly diagnosed brain tumors, anticonvulsant medications are not effective in preventing first seizures. Because of their lack of efficacy and their potential side effects, prophylactic anticonvulsants should not be used routinely in patients with newly diagnosed brain tumors" • "In patients with brain tumors who have not had a seizure, tapering and discontinuing anticonvulsants after the first postoperative week is appropriate, particularly in those patients who are medically stable and who are experiencing anticonvulsant-related side effects"
CNS[15]	2010	• "For adults with brain metastases who have not experienced a seizure due to their metastatic brain disease, routine prophylactic use of anticonvulsants is not recommended"
CNS[19]	2019	• "Prophylactic AEDs are not recommended for patients with brain metastases who did not undergo surgical resection and are otherwise seizure-free." • "Routine postcraniotomy AED use for seizure-free patients with brain metastases is not recommended"

Abbreviations: AAN, American Academy of Neurology; CNS: Congress of Neurological Surgeons.

Table 2
Details of study design for retrospective reviews and randomized-controlled trials evaluating the use of prophylactic antiepileptic drugs among patients with central nervous system metastases

Reference	Study Design	Total (N)	Patients with Cerebral Metastases (N)	Time Frame of AED Administration	AED Used	Duration of Therapy	Adverse Effects Reported	Key Findings
North et al,[65] 1983	RCT	140 AED; 141 control	6 AED; 7 control	Treatment started in the recovery room	Phenytoin	12 mo	12 patients in AED group withdrawn because of adverse drug reaction, unspecified	Significant reduction in frequency of epilepsy was observed in the AED group up to the 10th postoperative week
Lee et al,[66] 1989	RCT	189 AED; 185 control	3 AED; 2 control	Intraoperative	Phenytoin	3 postoperative days	None reported	Results suggest incidence of early postoperative seizure may be lower in AED group (not statistically significant)
Franceschetti et al,[27] 1990	RCT	106 AED total, 63 without antecedent seizure; 22 control	13 (no. in each cohort unclear)	Unclear	Phenobarbital or phenytoin	Duration not specified, but serum concentrations tested every 6 mo (minimum follow-up of 6 mo)	None reported/ unable to access full text of article	Results suggest some effectiveness of short-term preventive AED administration to prevent early postoperative seizure among patients without seizure history (not statistically significant)

(continued on next page)

Table 2
(continued)

Reference	Study Design	Total (N)	Patients with Cerebral Metastases (N)	Time Frame of AED Administration	AED Used	Duration of Therapy	Adverse Effects Reported	Key Findings
Glantz et al,[22] 1996	RCT	74	31 AED; 28 control	Randomization 15 d after diagnosis; unclear when in perioperative period AED was started	Valproic acid	Minimum follow-up of 7 mo	2 patients in AED group and 1 in control group developed rashes	AED prophylaxis with valproic acid is not effective at preventing first seizure
Forsyth et al,[23] 2003	RCT	100	26 AED; 34 control	Randomization 1 mo after diagnosis; unclear when in perioperative period AED was started	Phenytoin; phenobarbital if patient could not tolerate phenytoin	Throughout study; mean follow-up of 5.44 mo	Nausea (9%), rash (7%), sore gums (2%), myelosuppression (2%), increased LDH level (2%)	Incidence of seizure and seizure-free survival did not differ significantly (in total and when only analyzing patients with metastatic brain tumor), although study was underpowered

Study	Design	N	N	Timing	AED	Duration	Adverse events	Outcome
Wu et al,[28] 2013	RCT	62 AED; 61 control	39 AED; 38 control	Intraoperative	Phenytoin	Tapered on POD 8	12 events in 7 patients among metastasis group; 8 events in 4 patients in the glioma group. Rash (4 events), thrombocytopenia (2), decrease LOC (1), confusion (2), increased LFTs (4), nausea (1) vomiting (1), dry skin (1), ataxia (1), photophobia (1), aphasia (2)	No statistically significant difference in early or late seizure frequency between AED and control groups, although study was stopped early. Extremely low seizure rate in control arm casts doubt about usefulness of perioperative AED prophylaxis
Ansari et al,[29] 2014	Retrospective review	134 AED; 68 control	53 AED; 33 control	Postoperative	Phenytoin, levetiracetam, carbamazepine, phenobarbital, topiramate, and valproate	Unspecified	Not reported	The odds of seizure were 1.62 times higher in the AED group than in the control group. This finding was not statistically significant
Lockney et al,[21] 2017	Retrospective review	162 AED; 234 control (no. of patients without antecedent seizure)	51 AED; 54 control	Treatment initiated preoperatively or postoperatively	Levetiracetam, phenytoin, carbamazepine, lacosamide, lamotrigine, clonazepam, lorazepam, topiramate, or diazepam	Variable; many continued through duration of follow-up	Reported adverse events included supratherapeutic AED levels, nystagmus, gait difficulty, somnolence, irritability, insomnia, nausea/vomiting, and visual disturbance	Prophylactic AEDs did not significantly reduce number of postoperative seizures

(continued on next page)

Table 2
(continued)

Reference	Study Design	Total (N)	Patients with Cerebral Metastases (N)	Time Frame of AED Administration	AED Used	Duration of Therapy	Adverse Effects Reported	Key Findings
Kamenova et al,[30] 2019	Two-center retrospective matched cohort study	109 AED; 207 control	14 AED; 41 control	Intraoperative	Levetiracetam	At discretion of treating surgeon; usually 14–30 d postoperatively	None reported	No significant difference in postoperative seizure rate between AED and control groups

Abbreviations: LDH, lactate dehydrogenase; LFTs, liver function tests; LOC, level of consciousness; POD, postoperative day.

intraoperative dose as part of the treatment regimen (see **Table 2**). Intraoperative treatment is of particular concern for patients undergoing awake craniotomy (primarily for resection of gliomas) but, even in this setting, practice is varied.[24,25] One retrospective review found no association between type of AED and timing of administration for intraoperative seizure and rates of failed awake craniotomy.[25]

Postoperative prophylaxis

Postoperative seizure prophylaxis has been extensively studied but remains a contentious issue. Postcraniotomy seizure rates for patients with no prior history of seizure range between 7% and 18% in the literature.[8,26] The 2000 AAN guidelines suggest that postoperative prophylaxis be left to the surgeon's discretion.[13] Many surgeons are in favor of the use of prophylactic AEDs for patients undergoing any supratentorial craniotomy (irrespective of indication) to prevent early postoperative seizures. Although the evidence for this practice is weak and the baseline risk of seizure is low, high value is placed on avoiding early postoperative seizures because of their potentially severe neurologic consequences.[8–10]

In contrast, the CNS currently offers a level 3 recommendation against the use of postoperative seizure prophylaxis among patients with no prior history of seizure.[19] This guideline is based on 3 studies published in 1990, 2013, and 2014.

The 1990 study published by Franceschetti and colleagues[27] prospectively randomized 63 patients to receive AED treatment (phenytoin or second-line phenobarbital) or routine care after undergoing operation for supratentorial tumor resection. Thirteen patients (10.2%) across groups had cerebral metastases. Seven percent of the AED cohort experienced early postoperative seizures (within 1 week of surgery) compared with 18% of the non-AED cohort (P = .64). Late seizures (>1 week after surgery) occurred in 12% of the AED cohort compared with 21% of the non-AED cohort (P = .64).

The 2013 study by Wu and colleagues[28] prospectively randomized 123 patients with brain tumors to either phenytoin or no AED for 7 days postoperatively. Thirty-nine patients in the AED group (62.9%) and 38 patients in the control group (62.3%) had cerebral metastases. Across disorders, 24% of the phenytoin cohort had seizures within 30 days of surgery compared with 18% of the non-AED cohort (P = .51).

The 2014 study by Ansari and colleagues[29] retrospectively reviewed AED usage and seizure frequency among 202 patients with no antecedent seizure who underwent brain tumor resection.

Fifty-three patients in the AED group (39.6%) and 33 patients in the control group (48.5%) had cerebral metastases. Overall, the study found no difference in postoperative seizure risk (up to 321 days after surgery) between those who received AED prophylaxis and those who did not. The fact that brain metastases were not the sole disorder evaluated in any of the included studies is an important limitation given the heterogeneity in seizure risk and AED responsiveness among different histologies.

In the interval since the literature search was conducted for the 2019 CNS guidelines, Kamenova and colleagues[30] compared prophylactic postoperative AED treatment against no treatment among matched cohorts of patients undergoing brain tumor resection at 2 institutions. Fourteen patients in the AED group (12.8%) and 41 patients in the control group (19.3%) had metastases. Importantly, this study used levetiracetam, a newer agent with fewer side effects that is favored among neurosurgeons.[18] The investigators found no statistically significant difference in the occurrence of postoperative seizures between the two groups, further supporting recommendations against the use of prophylactic postoperative AEDs (n = 10 in the levetiracetam group, n = 21 in the control group; P = .69).

Nonsurgical patients

The 2019 CNS guidelines posed the question of whether AED prophylaxis decreases the risk of seizures in nonsurgical patients with brain metastases. Based on a thorough literature review, the CNS proposed a level 3 recommendation against the use of prophylactic AEDs in this patient population.[19] Two independent RCTs, by Forsyth and colleagues[23] (2003) and Glantz and colleagues[22] (1996), were used to formulate this recommendation. The study by Forsyth and colleagues[23] randomized 100 patients (60 of whom had cerebral metastases) to receive either 3 months of AED (phenytoin or phenobarbital) or no AED. The incidence of seizure did not differ significantly in total or in subgroup analysis of patients with metastasis. Glantz and colleagues[22] randomized 74 patients to receive valproic acid or placebo (59 of whom had cerebral metastases). The study found no statistically significant difference in seizure incidence within 12 months.

Radiosurgery patients

Stereotactic radiosurgery (SRS) is increasingly used in the management of brain metastases. Compared with whole-brain radiation therapy (WBRT), SRS carries a lower risk of seizure, ranging from 5% to 13%.[31–35] No clear guidelines for AED administration in this population currently exist, leading to heterogeneity in provider practice. Many clinicians take a conservative approach; a recent survey of 500 radiation oncologists found that 79% of respondents stated that they rarely or never prescribe anticonvulsants, and less than 10% usually or always recommend AED usage. Among those who prescribed AEDs during or after SRS, the recommended duration of therapy was less than 1 week, 1 to 2 weeks, and greater than 2 weeks among 35%, 25%, and 41% of respondents, respectively.[36] Some providers may recommend AEDs to select patients based on perceived seizure risk; for instance, there is a suspected higher seizure risk in patients with lesions in eloquent cortex.[31,33,37] Nevertheless, there is no evidence at this time to support the use of prophylactic AEDs before SRS.

Secondary Prevention

There is professional consensus that any patient with a brain tumor who presents with a first seizure should be started on an AED given the high likelihood that seizures will recur in those with structural disorders of the brain.[31,38] When these patients go on to receive surgical treatment, they are at a greater risk of postoperative seizure than those who have never seized.[39] For this reason, preoperative AED therapy should be continued into the postoperative period, as well.[27]

CHOICE OF THERAPY
Selection of Agent

Once an indication for AED treatment is established, determining a safe and effective medication regimen for patients requires knowledge of potential adverse effects and drug-drug interactions of each agent. Drug interactions are of particular importance within the brain metastasis population given that many of these patients are receiving concurrent, potent systemic chemotherapeutic agents.

Older agents such as carbamazepine, phenytoin, phenobarbital, and valproic acid are the most well-studied AEDs among patients with brain tumors. However, current physician practice seems to be incongruent with the agents assessed in the brain tumor literature. Among the estimated 63% of surgeons who administer seizure prophylaxis after tumor resection in patients without history of antecedent seizure, 85% use the drug levetiracetam.[18] This preference has been attributed to the efficacy of levetiracetam for treating both partial and generalized epilepsy, its comparatively favorable side effect profile, and the fact that routine monitoring of serum concentration is not necessary.[40]

Preference for levetiracetam is likely also driven by physician desire to avoid enzyme-inducing AEDs that may interfere with chemotherapeutic treatment.[41] **Table 3** lists major interactions between common AEDs and US Food and Drug Administration (FDA)–approved chemotherapeutic agents for lung, breast, colon, renal, and head and neck cancer. Strong inducers of the cytochrome P450 3A4 enzyme (eg, carbamazepine, phenobarbital, and phenytoin) have many interactions and decrease the serum concentration of several chemotherapeutic agents.[42,43] Furthermore, phenytoin, carbamazepine, and phenobarbital significantly decrease the serum concentration of dexamethasone, which is given almost ubiquitously to patients with brain tumor in order to reduce symptomatic cerebral edema.[44–46]

Nonhepatically cleared drugs such as lamotrigine, levetiracetam, topiramate, and gabapentin have far fewer drug-drug interactions, but not all of these agents have been assessed for prevention of seizures specifically in patients with brain tumors.[16] Only recently have reviews and meta-analyses evaluated the efficacy of levetiracetam, suggesting that this agent may be superior to older agents such as phenytoin and valproic acid.[47–49] Lacosamide is a newer agent that was shown to be effective in treating brain tumor–related epilepsy (BTRE) in 2 multicenter, observational, retrospective studies, and has few adverse effects.[50–53]

Because of the limited and heterogeneous evidence for particular AED agents in this population, selection of an agent is primarily guided by physicians' experiences and judgment.[38] The benefits of newer agents (primarily levetiracetam) in terms of safety, compatibility with other treatments, and lack of need for blood level monitoring support its use for seizures caused by brain tumors.[54,55] At the current time, there is reasonable evidence to support levetiracetam's use as a first-line agent, particularly as postcraniotomy prophylaxis among patients without prior history of seizure.

Number of Agents

Regardless of agent used, monotherapy is preferable because of improved compliance, diminished toxicity or risk of drug interactions, and decreased costs. Further, patients with BTRE who receive AED monotherapy have significantly better view of their health and perceive less adverse effects relative to those on polytherapy.[7] Fortunately, more than 50% of adults with tumor-related epilepsy respond to monotherapy.[56] If seizures are poorly controlled on 1 agent, serum levels should be verified to be therapeutic and then the drug dose may be increased as

Table 3
Common antiepileptic drugs and their major interactions with Food and Drug Administration–approved chemotherapeutic drugs for lung, breast, colon, melanoma, renal cell, head and neck, and skin (melanoma) cancer

Antiepileptic Agent	Chemotherapeutic Agents with Major Interaction		
Carbamazepine	Abemaciclib	Entrectinib	Osimertinib mesylate
	Afatinib dimaleate	Erlotinib	Paclitaxel
	Alpelisib	Etoposide	Formulation
	Axitinib	Everolimus	Palbociclib
	Brigatinib	Exemestane	Regorafenib
	Cabozantinib-S-malate	Gefitinib	Ribociclib
	Ceritinib	Irinotecan	Sorafenib tosylate
	Cobimetinib	Ixabepilone	Tamoxifen
	Crizotinib	Lapatinib	Temsirolimus
	Dabrafenib mesylate	Lorlatinib	Toremifene
	Docetaxel	Neratinib maleate	Vemurafenib
	Doxorubicin	Olaparib	
Clonazepam	Dabrafenib mesylate	—	—
Felbamate	Dabrafenib mesylate	—	—
Gabapentin	—	—	—
Lamotrigine	—	—	—
Levetiracetam	—	—	—
Oxcarbazepine	—	—	—
Phenobarbital	Afatinib dimaleate	Osimertinib mesylate	Ribociclib
	Brigatinib	Paclitaxel	Tamoxifen
	Ceritinib	Formulation	Toremifene
	Crizotinib	Abemaciclib	Vinblastine
	Dabrafenib mesylate	Alpelisib	Axitinib
	Docetaxel	Exemestane	Cabozantinib-S-maleate
	Doxorubicin	Irinotecan	Pazopanib
	Entrectinib	Ixabepilone	Sorafenib Tosylate
	Erlotinib	Lapatinib ditosylate	Sunitinib malate
	Etoposide	Neratinib maleate	Temsirolimus
	Everolimus	Olaparib	Cobimetinib
	Gefitinib	Palbociclib	Vemurafenib
	Lorlatinib	Regorafenib	
Phenytoin	5-Fluorouracil	Docetaxel	Osimertinib mesylate
	Abemaciclib	Doxorubicin	Paclitaxel
	Afatinib dimaleate	Entrectinib	Palbociclib
	Alpelisib	Erlotinib	Pazopanib
	Axitinib	Etoposide	Regorafenib
	Brigatinib	Everolimus	Ribociclib
	Cabozantinib-S-malate	Exemestane	Sorafenib tosylate
	Capecitabine	Gefitinib	Sunitinib malate
	Ceritinib	Irinotecan	Tamoxifen
	Cobimetinib	Ixabepilone	Temsirolimus
	Crizotinib	Lapatinib ditosylate	Topotecan
	Dabrafenib mesylate	Lorlatinib	Toremifene
	Dabrafenib mesylate	Neratinib maleate	Vemurafenib
	Dexamethasone	Olaparib	Vinblastine
Tiagabine	Dabrafenib mesylate	—	—
Valproic acid	—	—	—
Zonisamide	Dabrafenib mesylate	—	—

tolerated. Failing this, a trial of an alternative monotherapy or adjuvant therapy with another agent can then be pursued.

Adverse Effects of Antiepileptic Drugs

A 2008 Cochrane Review found that, compared with placebo or observational controls, phenytoin, phenobarbital, and divalproex sodium had higher rates of adverse events (relative risk, 6.10; 95% confidence interval, 1.10–34.63) and did not decrease the rate of seizures among patients with brain tumors.[17] The adverse effect profiles of specific AEDs are continuously refined, and the literature is advancing rapidly in understanding individual factors that may predispose patients to experience them.[57] Although a thorough description of each agent's potential adverse effects is outside the scope of this article, common reactions across agents include somnolence, rash, weight change, cognitive dysfunction, and teratogenicity.

As previously stated, adverse drug events and interactions with chemotherapeutic agents are less common with newer AEDs such as levetiracetam, making them preferable for the treatment of BTRE.[54,58,59] A systematic review of 21 studies suggested that the most common adverse effect associated with levetiracetam was somnolence, and this was typically mild.[55] However, prospective studies of patients treated with levetiracetam show a 7-fold increased risk for the development of neuropsychiatric adverse events such as agitation, depression, anxiety, emotional lability, and psychotic symptoms, regardless of tumor site.[54] Patients with frontal lobe tumors who were treated with levetiracetam are more severely affected, suggesting a synergistic effect between tumor location and agent.[54,60] Accurate monitoring of neuropsychiatric side effects is paramount, because decreased compliance because of these side effects may lead to worse seizure control.[54,57,61]

DURATION OF THERAPY

Duration of therapy is inconsistently documented in studies of AED use in patients with brain tumors, with many describing protracted treatment courses lasting through many months of follow-up (see **Table 2**). Although there is no standard duration among these studies, there is no evidence to suggest that prophylactic AEDs should be continued on a long-term basis.

The few studies showing a benefit to postoperative prophylaxis have primarily reported efficacy and safety up to only 1 week after surgery, suggesting that long-term therapy offers no benefit.[40]

Furthermore, increased duration of therapy, regardless of the AED used, is associated with patient perception of worsened cognition and social functioning, worse side effects, and greater distress.[7]

The AAN guidelines suggest that tapering and discontinuing anticonvulsants after the first postoperative week is appropriate, particularly in patients who are stable and are experiencing AED-related adverse effects.[13] A 1996 AAN practice parameter on discontinuing AED therapy in the general epilepsy population suggested that adults with a seizure-free interval of 2 to 5 years, a single seizure type, normal neurologic examination/intelligence quotient, and a normal electroencephalogram have at least a 61% chance of seizure freedom with AED discontinuation.[62] Because there are no rigorous studies on discontinuing AED treatment among patients with brain tumors, these criteria as well as the likelihood of tumor recurrence and prognosis for long-term survival should be considered.[38,63,64]

NEUROLOGY CONSULTATION

There is no practice guideline suggesting whether or when a neurologist should be consulted to manage or comanage AED therapy. In light of the growing number of novel AED agents, consideration for neurology referral is appropriate when a patient has contraindications to or side effects from AEDs traditionally prescribed by neurosurgeons. Multidrug treatment regimens may also be best monitored by neurologists, particularly when blood level monitoring, titration schedules, or nonstandard tapering of therapy are necessary.

LIMITATIONS AND FUTURE AREAS OF INVESTIGATION

Existing research on antiepileptic therapy for brain metastases is plagued by several methodological issues. Studies have included heterogeneous agents, various regimen schedules, small sample sizes, and inconsistent inclusion criteria, all predisposing to substantial bias.[55] The problem is confounded by low outcome event frequency, leading to underpowered results and early study termination.[23,28] In addition, there is a paucity of studies evaluating newer AEDs despite their popularity among practicing neurosurgeons.

CONCLUDING REMARKS

Seizures represent a common and debilitating complication of CNS metastases. The use of prophylactic AEDs in the preoperative period remains controversial, but the preponderance of evidence suggests that it is not helpful in preventing seizure and instead poses a substantial risk of adverse events. Studies of postoperative seizure prophylaxis have not shown substantial benefit, but this practice remains widespread. Careful analysis of the risk of seizure based on patient-specific factors, such as tumor location and primary tumor histology, should guide the physician's decision on the initiation and cessation of prophylactic AED therapy.

DISCLOSURE

The authors have no conflicts to disclose.

REFERENCES

1. Gavrilovic IT, Posner JB. Brain metastases: epidemiology and pathophysiology. J Neurooncol 2005; 75(1):5–14.
2. Patchell RA. The management of brain metastases. Cancer Treat Rev 2003;29(6):533–40.
3. Bradley KA, Mehta MP. Management of brain metastases. Seminars in Oncology 2004;31(5):693-701. doi:10.1053/j.seminoncol.2004.07.012.
4. Oberndorfer S, Schmal T, Lahrmann H, et al. The frequency of seizures in patients with primary brain tumors or cerebral metastases. An evaluation from the Ludwig Boltzmann Institute of Neuro-Oncology and the Department of Neurology, Kaiser Franz Josef Hospital, Vienna. Wien Klin Wochenschr 2002; 114(21–22):911–6 [in German].
5. Lote K, Stenwig AE, Skullerud K, et al. Prevalence and prognostic significance of epilepsy in patients with gliomas. Eur J Cancer 1998;34(1):98–102.
6. Chan V, Sahgal A, Egeto P, et al. Incidence of seizure in adult patients with intracranial metastatic disease. J Neurooncol 2017;131(3):619–24.
7. Maschio M, Sperati F, Dinapoli L, et al. Weight of epilepsy in brain tumor patients. J Neurooncol 2014; 118(2):385–93.
8. Dewan MC, White-Dzuro GA, Brinson PR, et al. Perioperative seizure in patients with glioma is associated with longer hospitalization, higher readmission, and decreased overall survival. J Neurosurg 2016;125(4):1033–41.
9. Klimek M, Dammers R. Antiepileptic drug therapy in the perioperative course of neurosurgical patients. Curr Opin Anaesthesiol 2010;23(5):564–7.
10. Kuijlen JM, Teernstra OP, Kessels AG, et al. Effectiveness of antiepileptic prophylaxis used with supratentorial craniotomies: a meta-analysis. Seizure 1996;5(4):291–8.
11. Marcus LP, McCutcheon BA, Noorbakhsh A, et al. Incidence and predictors of 30-day readmission for patients discharged home after craniotomy for malignant supratentorial tumors in California (1995-2010). J Neurosurg 2014;120(5):1201–11.
12. Dasenbrock HH, Yan SC, Smith TR, et al. Readmission After Craniotomy for Tumor: A National Surgical Quality Improvement Program Analysis. Neurosurgery 2017;80(4):551–62.
13. Glantz MJ, Cole BF, Forsyth PA, et al. Practice parameter: anticonvulsant prophylaxis in patients with newly diagnosed brain tumors. Report of the Quality Standards Subcommittee of the American Academy of Neurology. Neurology 2000;54(10): 1886–93.
14. Chandra V, Rock AK, Opalak C, et al. A systematic review of perioperative seizure prophylaxis during brain tumor resection: the case for a multicenter randomized clinical trial. Neurosurg Focus 2017;43(5): E18.
15. Mikkelsen T, Paleologos NA, Robinson PD, et al. The role of prophylactic anticonvulsants in the management of brain metastases: a systematic review and evidence-based clinical practice guideline. J Neurooncol 2010;96(1):97–102.
16. Sirven JI, Wingerchuk DM, Drazkowski JF, et al. Seizure prophylaxis in patients with brain tumors: a meta-analysis. Mayo Clin Proc 2004;79(12): 1489–94.
17. Tremont-Lukats IW, Ratilal BO, Armstrong T, et al. Antiepileptic drugs for preventing seizures in people with brain tumors. Cochrane Database Syst Rev 2008;(2):CD004424.
18. Dewan MC, Thompson RC, Kalkanis SN, et al. Prophylactic antiepileptic drug administration following brain tumor resection: results of a recent AANS/CNS Section on Tumors survey. J Neurosurg 2016; 126(6):1772–8.
19. Chen CC, Rennert RC, Olson JJ. Congress of neurological surgeons systematic review and evidence-based guidelines on the role of prophylactic anticonvulsants in the treatment of adults with metastatic brain tumors. Neurosurgery 2019; 84(3):E195–7.
20. Chang SM, Messersmith H, Ahluwalia M, et al. Anticonvulsant prophylaxis and steroid use in adults with metastatic brain tumors: summary of SNO and ASCO endorsement of the Congress of Neurological Surgeons guidelines. Neuro Oncol 2019;21(4): 424–7.
21. Lockney DT, Vaziri S, Walch F, et al. Prophylactic Antiepileptic Drug Use in Patients with Brain Tumors Undergoing Craniotomy. World Neurosurg 2017;98: 28–33.
22. Glantz MJ, Cole BF, Friedberg MH, et al. A randomized, blinded, placebo-controlled trial of divalproex sodium prophylaxis in adults with newly diagnosed brain tumors. Neurology 1996;46(4): 985–91.

23. Forsyth PA, Weaver S, Fulton D, et al. Prophylactic anticonvulsants in patients with brain tumour. Can J Neurol Sci 2003;30(2):106–12.

24. Spena G, Schucht P, Seidel K, et al. Brain tumors in eloquent areas: A European multicenter survey of intraoperative mapping techniques, intraoperative seizures occurrence, and antiepileptic drug prophylaxis. Neurosurg Rev 2017;40(2): 287–98.

25. Nossek E, Matot I, Shahar T, et al. Failed awake craniotomy: a retrospective analysis in 424 patients undergoing craniotomy for brain tumor. J Neurosurg 2013;118(2):243–9.

26. Dewan MC, White-Dzuro GA, Brinson PR, et al. The Influence of Perioperative Seizure Prophylaxis on Seizure Rate and Hospital Quality Metrics Following Glioma Resection. Neurosurgery 2017;80(4): 563–70.

27. Franceschetti S, Binelli S, Casazza M, et al. Influence of surgery and antiepileptic drugs on seizures symptomatic of cerebral tumours. Acta Neurochir (Wien) 1990;103(1–2):47–51.

28. Wu AS, Trinh VT, Suki D, et al. A prospective randomized trial of perioperative seizure prophylaxis in patients with intraparenchymal brain tumors. J Neurosurg 2013;118(4):873–83.

29. Ansari SF, Bohnstedt BN, Perkins SM, et al. Efficacy of postoperative seizure prophylaxis in intra-axial brain tumor resections. J Neurooncol 2014;118(1): 117–22.

30. Kamenova M, Stein M, Ram Z, et al. Prophylactic antiepileptic treatment with levetiracetam for patients undergoing supratentorial brain tumor surgery: a two-center matched cohort study. Neurosurgical review 2019. doi:10.1007/s10143-019-01111-6

31. Julie DAR, Ahmed Z, Karceski SC, et al. An overview of anti-epileptic therapy management of patients with malignant tumors of the brain undergoing radiation therapy. Seizure 2019;70:30–7.

32. Aoyama H, Shirato H, Tago M, et al. Stereotactic Radiosurgery Plus Whole-Brain Radiation Therapy vs Stereotactic Radiosurgery Alone for Treatment of Brain Metastases: A Randomized Controlled Trial. JAMA 2006;295(21):2483–91.

33. Brian JW, Dima S, Benjamin DF, et al. Stereotactic radiosurgery for metastatic brain tumors: a comprehensive review of complications. J Neurosurg 2009; 111(3):439–48.

34. Minniti G, Clarke E, Lanzetta G, et al. Stereotactic radiosurgery for brain metastases: analysis of outcome and risk of brain radionecrosis. Radiat Oncol 2011;6(1):48.

35. Chitapanarux I, Goss B, Vongtama R, et al. Prospective study of stereotactic radiosurgery without whole brain radiotherapy in patients with four or less brain metastases: incidence of intracranial progression and salvage radiotherapy. J Neurooncol 2003; 61(2):143–9.

36. Arvold ND, Pinnell NE, Mahadevan A, et al. Steroid and anticonvulsant prophylaxis for stereotactic radiosurgery: Large variation in physician recommendations. Pract Radiat Oncol 2016;6(4): e89–96.

37. Gelblum DY, Lee H, Bilsky M, et al. Radiographic findings and morbidity in patients treated with stereotactic radiosurgery. Int J Radiat Oncol Biol Phys 1998;42(2):391–5.

38. Perucca E. Optimizing antiepileptic drug treatment in tumoral epilepsy. Epilepsia 2013;54(Suppl 9): 97–104.

39. Milligan TA, Hurwitz S, Bromfield EB. Efficacy and tolerability of levetiracetam versus phenytoin after supratentorial neurosurgery. Neurology 2008;71(9): 665–9.

40. Iuchi T, Kuwabara K, Matsumoto M, et al. Levetiracetam versus phenytoin for seizure prophylaxis during and early after craniotomy for brain tumours: a phase II prospective, randomised study. J Neurol Neurosurg Psychiatry 2015;86(10):1158–62.

41. Rossetti AO, Stupp R. Epilepsy in brain tumor patients. Curr Opin Neurol 2010;23(6):603–9.

42. Restrepo JG, Garcia-Martin E, Martinez C, et al. Polymorphic drug metabolism in anaesthesia. Curr Drug Metab 2009;10(3):236–46.

43. Nation RL, Evans AM, Milne RW. Pharmacokinetic drug interactions with phenytoin (Part I). Clin Pharmacokinet 1990;18(1):37–60.

44. Lawson LA, Blouin RA, Smith RB, et al. Phenytoindexamethasone interaction: a previously unreported observation. Surg Neurol 1981;16(1):23–4.

45. Ma RC, Chan WB, So WY, et al. Carbamazepine and false positive dexamethasone suppression tests for Cushing's syndrome. BMJ 2005;330(7486):299–300.

46. Waxman DJ, Azaroff L. Phenobarbital induction of cytochrome P-450 gene expression. Biochem J 1992;281(Pt 3):577–92.

47. Weston J, Greenhalgh J, Marson AG. Antiepileptic drugs as prophylaxis for post-craniotomy seizures. Cochrane Database Syst Rev 2015;(3):CD007286.

48. Pourzitaki C, Tsaousi G, Apostolidou E, et al. Efficacy and safety of prophylactic levetiracetam in supratentorial brain tumour surgery: a systematic review and meta-analysis. Br J Clin Pharmacol 2016; 82(1):315–25.

49. Lee C-H, Koo H-W, Han SR, et al. Phenytoin versus levetiracetam as prophylaxis for postcraniotomy seizure in patients with no history of seizures: systematic review and meta-analysis. J Neurosurg 2018;1(aop):1–8.

50. Villanueva V, Saiz-Diaz R, Toledo M, et al. NEOPLASM study: Real-life use of lacosamide in patients with brain tumor-related epilepsy. Epilepsy Behav 2016;65:25–32.

51. Sepulveda-Sanchez JM, Conde-Moreno A, Baron M, et al. Efficacy and tolerability of lacosamide for secondary epileptic seizures in patients with brain tumor: A multicenter, observational retrospective study. Oncol Lett 2017;13(6):4093–100.

52. Sepulveda-Sanchez JM, Conde-Moreno A, Baron M, et al. Erratum: Efficacy and tolerability of lacosamide for secondary epileptic seizures in patients with brain tumor: A multicenter, observational retrospective study. Oncol Lett 2017;14(4):4410.

53. Toledo M, Molins A, Quintana M, et al. Outcome of cancer-related seizures in patients treated with lacosamide. Acta Neurol Scand 2018;137(1):67–75.

54. Bedetti C, Romoli M, Maschio M, et al. Neuropsychiatric adverse events of antiepileptic drugs in brain tumour-related epilepsy: an Italian multicentre prospective observational study. Eur J Neurol 2017; 24(10):1283–9.

55. Nasr ZG, Paravattil B, Wilby KJ. Levetiracetam for seizure prevention in brain tumor patients: a systematic review. J Neurooncol 2016;129(1):1–13.

56. van Breemen MS, Rijsman RM, Taphoorn MJ, et al. Efficacy of anti-epileptic drugs in patients with gliomas and seizures. J Neurol 2009;256(9):1519–26.

57. Perucca P, Gilliam FG. Adverse effects of antiepileptic drugs. Lancet Neurol 2012;11(9):792–802.

58. Huberfeld G, Vecht CJ. Seizures and gliomas–towards a single therapeutic approach. Nat Rev Neurol 2016;12(4):204–16.

59. Laghari AA, Ahmed SI, Qadeer N, et al. Choice of therapeutic anti-seizure medication in patients with brain tumour. J Pak Med Assoc 2019;69(3):442–4.

60. Belcastro V, Pisani LR, Bellocchi S, et al. Brain tumor location influences the onset of acute psychiatric adverse events of levetiracetam therapy: an observational study. J Neurol 2017;264(5):921–7.

61. Feyissa AM. Antiepileptic drug-related neuropsychiatric adverse events in brain tumor-related epilepsy: levetiracetam front and center. Eur J Neurol 2017; 24(12):1435–6.

62. Practice Parameter: A guideline for discontinuing antiepileptic drugs in seizure-free patients–Summary Statement. Neurology 1996;47(2):600–2. https://doi.org/10.1212/wnl.47.2.600.

63. Chassoux F, Landre E. Prevention and management of postoperative seizures in neuro-oncology. Neuro Chir 2017;63(3):197–203.

64. Fröscher W, Kirschstein T, Rösche J. Antiepileptikabehandlung bei Hirntumor-bedingten epileptischen Anfällen [Anticonvulsant therapy for brain tumour-related epilepsy]. Fortschr Neurol Psychiatr 2014; 84(12):678–90.   https://doi.org/10.1055/s-0034-1385475.

65. North JB, Penhall RK, Hanieh A, et al. Phenytoin and postoperative epilepsy. A double-blind study. J Neurosurg 1983;58(5):672–7. https://doi.org/10.3171/jns.1983.58.5.0672.

66. Lee ST, Lui TN, Chang CN, et al. Prophylactic anticonvulsants for prevention of immediate and early postcraniotomy seizures. Surg Neurol 1989;31(5): 361–4.   https://doi.org/10.1016/0090-3019(89) 90067-0.

Chemotherapy for the Management of Cerebral Metastases

Chase H. Foster, MD, MS[a], Pooja Dave, BS[b], Jonathan H. Sherman, MD[c],*

KEYWORDS

- Cerebral metastasis • Brain • Tumor • Chemotherapy • Neurosurgery

KEY POINTS

- Chemotherapy has historically played a minor role as an adjuvant therapy in cerebral metastasis (CM) largely because of poor penetration through the blood-brain barrier (BBB).
- Focused ultrasound and the "molecular Trojan horses" for the delivery of chemotherapeutic agents are two novel methods of improving BBB penetration.
- There is sufficient evidence to suggest that inhibition of CM angiogenesis with bevacizumab is an efficacious adjuvant agent.
- There are some high-level data to support the use of signal transduction inhibition with tyrosine kinase inhibitors, primarily in breast cancer with CM.
- Checkpoint inhibitors have thus far shown only modest benefit in melanoma and non–small cell lung cancer with CM, but several clinical trials are ongoing.

INTRODUCTION

The multidisciplinary approach of modern neuro-oncologic care has increased 1-year survival after diagnosis of cerebral metastasis (CM) by 19% in patients with favorable prognostic characteristics.[1] Yet survival rates following CM diagnosis across all primaries remain low, especially in patients with unfavorable characterisitcs.[1–3] Although the exact effect size of chemotherapy for CM is currently unknown because of a paucity of high-level data, chemotherapy has been shown in some studies and with certain primaries to prolong survival when included in a multimodal treatment strategem.[3–5] This review focuses on published data on novel agents.

HISTORY OF CHEMOTHERAPY FOR CEREBRAL METASTASIS

Understanding past treatment failures helps to contextualize current treatment strategies. The blood-brain barrier (BBB) is a widely known obstacle to CM chemotherapy.[6–9] The endothelial tight junctions and specific transport proteins in the BBB selectively allow molecules of a specific charge, lipophilicity, size, and binding affinity into the brain.[10] Moreover, efflux pumps in the so-called "blood-tumor barrier" (BTB), such as permeability glycoprotein 1 (P-GP) and breast cancer resistance protein (BCRP), have been found to actively reduce the intracranial concentration of a variety of chemotherapeutic agents.[6,11–15] Even agents that readily cross the BBB and are commonly used in the treatment of

[a] Department of Neurological Surgery, George Washington University Hospital, 2150 Pennsylvania Avenue, Northwest, Suite 7-420, Washington, DC 20037, USA; [b] The GW School of Medicine & Health Sciences, 2150 Pennsylvania Avenue, Northwest, Suite 7-420, Washington, DC 20037, USA; [c] West Virginia University, Eastern Division, 800 North Tennessee Avenue, Suite 104, Martinsburg, WV 25401, USA
* Corresponding author.
E-mail address: jsherman0620@gmail.com

Neurosurg Clin N Am 31 (2020) 603–611
https://doi.org/10.1016/j.nec.2020.06.009
1042-3680/20/© 2020 Elsevier Inc. All rights reserved.

CM, such as alkylating agents (eg, temozolamide), topoisomerase inhibitors (eg, irinotecan, topotecan), procarbazine, and carboplatin,[10,16] have demonstrated only limited effect on overall survival (OS) in at least one randomized clinical trial.[17]

Taken together, the pathologic milieu of CM alerted researchers to the unique obstacles that they faced in treating this unique form of cancer.[18,19] This underscored the need for the development of new and esoteric methods to increase the effectiveness of systemic chemotherapy to improve patients' quality of life.

NOVEL DELIVERY SYSTEMS
Biochemical Disruption

Researchers have known since the early 1970s that giving mannitol caused shrinkage of brain cells and concurrent "loosening" of tight junctions, increasing the permeability of the central nervous system (CNS).[20,21] However, major drawbacks to this approach are its nonspecificity and duration of effect, which can cause highly morbid clinical consequences, such as seizures secondary to brain edema and altered physiology.[14,21] In the 1980s, Raymond and colleagues[22] used vasoactive compounds (eg, bradykinin) to enhance large molecular movement across the BTB. This approach faces the same shortcomings. Although a variety of other vasoactive agents have been investigated for their potential in enhancing chemotherapy delivery across the BBB (eg, interleukin-2, necrosis factor-α,[23] alkylglycerols), none have shown tenable success because of limited effectiveness, significant side effects,[24] and a still-incompletely understood role in CM as opposed to primary CNS tumors.[16]

Focused Ultrasound

Physical disruption of the BBB has emerged as a recent and promising solution to these issues.[25] A form of thermotherapy, the acoustic waves emitted during focused ultrasound transiently increases BBB permeability through a variety of mechanisms[24] as detected by concurrent MRI.[13,25–27] Several studies[13,28,29] and at least one clinical trial[30] have recapitulated this finding. The technique is valued for its practicality, ubiquity, inexpensiveness, and noninvasiveness. It allows for the passage of molecules up to 2000 kDa,[31,32] and has not been reported to have known deleterious effects in animal studies.[24] Its use as an adjunct in other chemotherapeutic regimens to augment drug delivery further underscores its importance in the neurosurgical oncologist's armamentarium.[13,28,33–37]

Trojan Horse Strategies

Transcytosis commandeers the endogenous mechanisms by which native molecules with specific ligands bind to receptors on the endothelial cells of the BBB to pass therapeutic agents into the CNS.[16,38,39] Colloquially referred to as "molecular Trojan horses,"[10,40] these methods include but are not limited to: tagged conjugated-insulin and hormonal signalers,[41] the use of engineered recombinant fusion proteins attached to effector moieties,[10] and the compartmentalization of chemotherapy into liposomes that bind to tumor- or BBB-specific receptors.[42] Several groups have used nanoparticles and microparticles[43] to transport conjugated chemotherapy predominantly in murine models.[42,44–46] More recent animal data have shown that the transport of these novel nanovehicles across the BBB is further enhanced when deployed in combination with the aforementioned focused ultrasound techniques.[13,28,35] However, the efficacy of nanoparticle-based carrier systems has yet to be realized according to some authors.[15]

NOVEL AGENTS

Newer agents, such as tyrosine kinase inhibitors (TKIs), non-TKIs, and checkpoint inhibitors, have been described as targeted therapies,[47] a reference to their molecular tropism (**Table 1**). Research into such agents has accelerated dramatically in recent years, incensed by promising early results from several low-level data[19,47–51] as well as randomized clinical trials.[52–54]

Angiogenesis Inhibition

Research has shown that the BBB might become compromised once a CM grows to a size larger than 1 to 2 mm because new tumor-associated vessels lack normal BBB characteristics.[12,55] Bevacizumab, a recombinant monoclonal antibody (MAb) against vascular endothelial growth factor (VEGF), has been shown to act as a chemosensitizer and improve response rates to chemotherapy by reducing tumor neovascularization and improving drug penetrance.[6,47,56] For this reason, it was included in the first Food and Drug Administration–approved first-line systemic treatment regimen for non–small cell lung cancer (NSCLC) along with platinum-based chemotherapy.[48]

Several randomized studies, including those published by Johnson and colleagues[57] and Sandler and colleagues[58] in the early 2000s and more recently recapitulated by the retrospective analysis by Tang and colleagues,[48] have shown

Table 1
Novel chemotherapeutic agents for CM

Molecular Target	Drugs	Mechanism of Action	Miscellaneous
VEGF	1. Bevacizumab, cabozantinib 2. Lenvatinib	1. Binds circulating VEGF 2. TKI against VEGFR-2 receptors and c-MET[15]	a. High doses can lead to thromboembolism b. Bevacizumab with sunitinib can cause micro-angiopathic hemolytic anemia[96]
Multiple kinases of antiangiogenesis	Sunitinib, sorafenib, pazopanib, vandetanib	Blocks VEGF, platelet-derived growth factor, and C-kit to create antiangiogenesis and antitumor effects[97]	a. Sunitinib has a higher response rate than sorafenib[12] b. When given in combination with WBRT there is a pseudoprogression of the tumor before it improves[12]
HEGFR (EGFR/HER-2)	1. Erlotinib, gefitinib 2. Lapatinib 3. Afatinib	1. Blocks the EGFR tyrosine kinase domain 2. Effect on EGFR and HER-2 receptors 3. Blocker of ErbB family of epidermal growth factor receptors	a. Erlotinib has higher CSF concentrations in the brain than gefitinib[6] b. Giving erlotinib with WBRT might sensitize cells to radiation[6]
BRAF	Dabrafenib, vemurafenib	Inhibitors of type I BRAF V600E kinase in the mitogen-activated protein kinase pathway[98]	96% of participants in 1 pilot study experienced at least 1 adverse event[78]
ALK	1. Crizotinib 2.Ceritinib 3.Alectinib	1. Inhibits ALK/c-MET 2. Inhibits ALK/IGF-1 3. New generation	a. Crizotinib reaches very low CSF concentrations b. Alectinib may be useful in crizotinib-resistant NSCLC metastases[6]
CKD 4/6	Abemaciclib, palbociclib, ribociclib	Blocks downstream mitogenic signals in cell growth and division, disinhibiting native antiproliferative cell machinery[99]	
PI3K	Alpelisib, buparlisib, dactolisib	Reduces microglia-mediated CNS import of tumor cells and disrupts inherent CM PI3K signaling[84]	Buparlisib reaches significant CSF concentrations with 90% bioavailability[84]
CTLA-4	Ipilimumab	Disinhibits T-cell antitumor activity by blocking inhibitory signals from B7[89]	Greater risk of toxicity when used in combination with nivolumab[89]
PD-1	Pembrolizumab, nivolumab	Blocks PD-L1-mediated suppression of effector T cells to prevent quiescence[89]	a. Pembrolizumab is highly PD-1 selective, and indicated for EGFR-/ALK-metastatic NSCLC[74,89] b. Radiation necrosis and immunotherapy may be linked[51,100]

Abbreviations: ALK, anaplastic lymphoma kinase; CDK, cyclin-dependent kinase; CSF, cerebrospinal fluid; CTLA-4, cytotoxic T-lymphocyte-associated protein 4; EGFR, epidermal growth factor receptor; HEGFR, human epidermal growth factor receptor; HER-2, human epidermal growth factor receptor-2; PD-1, program cell death protein-1; PD-L1, programmed death ligand 1; PI3K, phosphoinositide-3 kinase; VEGF, vascular endothelial growth factor; WBRT, whole-brain radiation therapy.

statistically significant increases in OS rates when bevacizumab is used with targeted therapies compared with chemotherapy alone.[59,60] Phase II data have also suggested bevacizumab's potentiating effect when used with pembrolizumab, a MAb against program cell death protein-1 (PD-1), presumably secondary to improved permeation of the latter.[48]

Two inhibitors of vascular endothelial growth factor receptor 2 (VEGFR-2), cabozantinib and lenvatinib, have also been investigated for their therapeutic potential in breast cancer with CM (BCCM) according to a comprehensive review by Shah and colleagues.[15] Cabozantinib, an inhibitor of the VEGFR-2 and radiotherapy resistance-inducing c-MET tyrosine kinases,[47] has been studied in several phase II trials investigating its effect in CM when used with conventional agents.[50] Lenvatinib is being similarly studied in hormone-positive BCCM, but results are not yet available.

Tumor angiogenesis can also be inhibited by systemic administration of sorafenib, sunitinib, pazopanib, and vandetanib via inhibition of a variety of mechanisms (see **Table 1**).[6,61] These aptly named multikinase inhibitors have unfortunately been shown to have poor CNS concentration in at least two separate animal studies,[6,62,63] likely by mechanisms similar to active TKI efflux from tumor cells by P-GP and BCRP.[14,64] As noted by Gabay and colleagues,[61] whereas several phase II trials have aimed to establish the safety and efficacy of these agents in patients with NSCLC and renal cell carcinoma, data on its effectiveness are largely limited to case reports and series.

Signal Transduction Inhibition

A large number of signal transduction inhibitors have been described and investigated for their effect on OS in patients with CM (see **Table 1**). The development of agents against epidermal growth factor receptor (EGFR) and human epidermal growth factor receptor 2 (HER-2) perhaps heralded the arrival of these targeted therapies. Numerous studies have demonstrated that NSCLC responds to TKIs directed against EGFR mutations, such as the first-generation agents erlotinib and gefitinib.[48,49,65] In their phase II study, Wu and colleagues[49] reported an increase in progression-free survival (PFS) of nearly 11 months between EGFR mutated and EGFR wild-type groups treated with erlotinib.

Similarly, retrospective data reported by Heon and colleagues[66] demonstrated a 15% decrease in "CNS progression" in NSCLC when these drugs were used instead of conventional chemotherapy. However, resistance to EGFR-directed targeted therapy occurs at an estimated rate of 30%,[67] resulting in only a transient response.[65] Second-generation TKIs against EGFR, HER-2, and other signal transduction mediators, such as afatinib and neratinib, have been designed to rectify these shortcomings, but with little published clinical success.[6]

Lapatinib is an inhibitor of EGFR and HER-2, and is often deployed alongside trastuzumab (a targeted MAb against HER-2) in the treatment of metastatic breast cancer.[61] Data from several phase II trials[68–70] have demonstrated lapatinib to have a modest but appreciable effect on reducing CNS tumor volume.[50] Furthermore, the use of lapatinib in combination with capecitabine reduced the rate of CM progression by 4% compared with conventional chemotherapy alone in one study of 399 women.[71] Bachelot and colleagues[72] further reported an objective CNS response as measured by volumetric CM reduction in 65% of their cohort of previously untreated BCCM. Recent reviews of the major phase III trials on this topic (CLEOPATRA, EMILIA, and TH3RESA) and resultant modern chemotherapy regimens concur that lapatinib has a specific role in the management of this subgroup of CM.[73]

Dabrafenib and vemurafenib are examples of type 1 BRAF V600E kinase inhibitors (see **Table 1**).[61,74] The former has been seen to reduce CM tumor volume in a small cohort of patients with untreated asymptomatic lesions.[75] However, small sample sizes and the negligible effect on PFS despite proven activity seen in the phase II trials[76,77] and pilot study[78] that followed seem to have stymied ongoing research. Nevertheless, some authors posit that these agents may still be useful in inducing CM regression in subsets of patients with BRAF-positive metastatic melanoma with CM (MMCM) when used in combination with other treatments.[74]

Crizotinib is an inhibitor of anaplastic lymphoma kinase (ALK), a rare mutation in aggressive NSCLC subtypes.[79] Despite low cerebrospinal fluid concentrations,[80] crizotinib has shown some effect in early phase II studies. However, the newer generation agents ceritinib and alectinib improved on this effect, and are thought to represent the future of ALK–positive NSCLC CM treatment,[65,74] especially in cases resistant or refractory to crizotinib first-line therapy.[6,81] These early data prompted the phase III clinical trial ALEX (NCT02075840) comparing these agents' efficacy head-to-head in treating NSCLC with CM.[65,77] The results, published in 2017, lauded the superior efficacy and lower toxicity of alectinib compared with crizotinib, with a statistically significant event-free PFS rate of 68.4% versus 48.7%, respectively.[82]

Therapies targeted against cyclin-dependent kinases 4 and 6 (CDK4/6) and phosphoinositide 3-kinase (PI3K) are currently limited to metastatic breast cancer. Several phase II and even some phase III clinical trials have investigated the safety and efficacy of CDK4/6 inhibitors when used as first-line therapies and in conjunction with antihormonal systemic chemotherapies, including the MONARCH and monarcHER2 (NCT02675231) series of trials (abemaciclib); the PATINA (NCT02947685) and PALINA (NCT02692755) trials (palbociclib); and the MONALEESA-3, TEEL, and PALOMA-2 (NCT01740427) and PALOMA-3 (NCT01942135) trials (ribociclib).[15] Although meta-analysis of the resultant data has confirmed improvement in PFS for each of these agents,[83] BCCM was an exclusion criterion in many of these studies and only included with strict requisites in others.[15] Others have not yet published their results, but expanded access to these trials may rectify the issue.

The PI3K inhibitors alpelisib, buparlisib, and dactolisib share the same promise but also the same challenges. PI3K and its ability to promote CM during CNS colonization has previously been shown through laboratory research.[84] The phase III SOLAR-1 trial (alpelisib, NCT02437318), the phase III BELLE-2 (NCT01610284) and BELLE-3 trials (NCT01633060) and phase II/III BELLE-4 series of trials (NCT01572727), the phase Ib B-YOND trial (NCT02058381), and phase II STAR Cape trial (all buparlisib, NCT02000882), and at least one phase I trial investigating dactolisib have randomized some BCCM patients to receive a combination of PI3K inhibitors and trastuzumab, capecitabine, or other hormone therapy.[15] Although some results from these studies are pending, others have found statistically but not pragmatically significant change in PFS rates,[85–87] suggesting further research is needed on these targeted therapies and patients with BCCM, especially that majority with symptomatic CM.

Data from controlled clinical trials on BCCM and mammalian target of rapamycin (mTOR) inhibitors (see **Table 1**) are even more sparse. Early data suggest its inclusion in a multidrug chemotherapeutic regimen may be reasonable (note that the BELLE-3 trial was premised on patients who had failed or progressed on mTOR therapy[87]), but studies inclusive of CM are needed for validation.[47] At least one recently published phase I trial has investigated a combination of bevacizumab with everolimus in the treatment of a small pediatric cohort of five patients with recurrent brain tumors.[88] Another trial is investigating its effect in BCCM when used with an aromatase inhibitor, the aforementioned palbociclib, or the PI3K inhibitors taselisib and pictilisib.[15]

Checkpoint Inhibition

Immunotherapy or so-called "checkpoint inhibition" operates on the premise that native immune cells can be programmed against CM via activation or inhibition of immune receptor molecules, thereby preventing immune tolerance to cancer tumor markers[89] and allowing cytotoxic immune cells to prevent tumor quiescence (see **Table 1** for common drugs in this category).[9] Research into these checkpoint inhibitors has thus far been mostly limited to retrospective studies on MM and NSCLC.[19]

A phase III trial by Hodi and colleagues[90] in 2010 demonstrated a modest increase in OS of 4 months when ipilimumab was administered to patients with previously treated MM. However, MMCM patients were excluded. Two years later, a prospective phase II trial of 72 patients with melanoma and CM found that ipilimumab as monotherapy had activity in the asymptomatic CM subgroup of their cohort.[91] Additional studies have queried various combinations of ipilimumab, pembrolizumab, and nivolumab with other adjuvant treatment options, including radiotherapy.[51]

The phase II clinical trial CheckMate 204 demonstrated an intracranial clinical benefit rate of 57% for patients with MMCM treated with four doses of nivolumab and ipilimumab every 3 weeks.[92] The similarly designed ABC trial reported a 6-month intracranial PFS rate of 53% and OS rate of 78% in maximally treated patients with this combination.[52] This combination was associated with a significant adverse event rate in both studies: 55% overall and 97% in the combination treatment arm, respectively. The most common grade 3 or 4 adverse events were rash, diarrhea, transaminitis, hepatitis, and increased lipase.[52,92]

Chemotherapeutic strategies targeting PD-1 alone with pembrolizumab have been applied to melanoma and NSCLC. One phase II trial reported intracranial response rates of 33% and 22% in NSCLC and MMCM, respectively, for patients treated with pembrolizumab.[93] Prospective and randomized clinical data are lacking. Retrospective studies, however, have been performed with cautiously promising results.[48,94]

Ongoing clinical trials notwithstanding, a clinically significant improvement in PFS or OS in patients with CM has only been seen in scattered case reports.[19] One systematic review of MMCM studies available in 2016 found that although checkpoint inhibitors have a measurable response in at least this cancer type, the median OS in retrospective studies and clinical trials was just 4.3 and 7 months, respectively.[90,95]

SUMMARY

The use of chemotherapy in the treatment of CM has traditionally been limited by such obstacles as the BBB and BTB. Recent research from several retrospective and prospective reviews and a small number of phase III clinical trials suggests that novel means of instilling systemic next-generation chemotherapeutic agents can produce a modest survival benefit in patients with CM. However, these results are cautiously reported, because statistical significance has not yet translated to meaningful patient benefit across tumor subtypes. Future research looks to maximize efficacy of these chemotherapeutics via techniques that bypass the aforementioned barriers while minimizing adverse effects of these drugs.

DISCLOSURE

The authors have nothing to disclose.

REFERENCES

1. Nieder C, Spanne O, Mehta MP, et al. Presentation, patterns of care, and survival in patients with brain metastases: what has changed in the last 20 years? Cancer 2011;117(11):2505–12.

2. Fox BD, Cheung VJ, Patel AJ, et al. Epidemiology of metastatic brain tumors. Neurosurg Clin N Am 2011;22(1):1–6, v.

3. Tabouret E, Chinot O, Metellus P, et al. Recent trends in epidemiology of brain metastases: an overview. Anticancer Res 2012;32(11):4655–62.

4. Melisko ME, Moore DH, Sneed PK, et al. Brain metastases in breast cancer: clinical and pathologic characteristics associated with improvements in survival. J Neurooncol 2008;88(3):359–65.

5. McKee MJ, Keith K, Deal AM, et al. A multidisciplinary breast cancer brain metastases clinic: the University of North Carolina experience. The oncologist 2016;21(1):16–20.

6. Bohn J-P, Pall G, Stockhammer G, et al. Targeted therapies for the treatment of brain metastases in solid tumors. Target Oncol 2016;11(3):263–75.

7. Pitz MW, Desai A, Grossman SA, et al. Tissue concentration of systemically administered antineoplastic agents in human brain tumors. J Neurooncol 2011;104(3):629–38.

8. Walbert T, Gilbert MR. The role of chemotherapy in the treatment of patients with brain metastases from solid tumors. Int J Clin Oncol 2009;14(4):299–306.

9. Lin X, DeAngelis LM. Treatment of brain metastases. J Clin Oncol 2015;33(30):3475–84.

10. Weidle UH, Niewöhner J, Tiefenthaler G. The blood-brain barrier challenge for the treatment of brain cancer, secondary brain metastases, and neurological diseases. Cancer Genomics Proteomics 2015;12(4):167–77.

11. Abbott NJ, Rönnbäck L, Hansson E. Astrocyte-endothelial interactions at the blood-brain barrier. Nat Rev Neurosci 2006;7(1):41–53.

12. Grimm SA. Treatment of brain metastases: chemotherapy. Curr Oncol Rep 2012;14(1):85–90.

13. Arvanitis CD, Askoxylakis V, Guo Y, et al. Mechanisms of enhanced drug delivery in brain metastases with focused ultrasound-induced blood-tumor barrier disruption. Proc Natl Acad Sci U S A 2018;115(37):E8717–26.

14. Kemper EM, Boogerd W, Thuis I, et al. Modulation of the blood-brain barrier in oncology: therapeutic opportunities for the treatment of brain tumours? Cancer Treat Rev 2004;30(5):415–23.

15. Shah N, Mohammad AS, Saralkar P, et al. Investigational chemotherapy and novel pharmacokinetic mechanisms for the treatment of breast cancer brain metastases. Pharmacol Res 2018;132:47–68.

16. Peereboom DM. Chemotherapy in brain metastases. Neurosurgery 2005;57(5 Suppl):S54.

17. Pesce GA, Klingbiel D, Ribi K, et al. Outcome, quality of life and cognitive function of patients with brain metastases from non-small cell lung cancer treated with whole brain radiotherapy combined with gefitinib or temozolomide. A randomised phase II trial of the Swiss Group for Clinical Cancer Research (SAKK 70/03). Eur J Cancer 2012;48(3):377–84.

18. Kim S-J, Kim J-S, Park ES, et al. Astrocytes upregulate survival genes in tumor cells and induce protection from chemotherapy. Neoplasia 2011;13(3):286–98.

19. Tan AC, Heimberger AB, Menzies AM, et al. Immune checkpoint inhibitors for brain metastases. Curr Oncol Rep 2017;19(6):38.

20. Rapoport SI. Effect of concentrated solutions on blood-brain barrier. Am J Physiol 1970;219(1):270–4.

21. Kroll RA, Neuwelt EA. Outwitting the blood-brain barrier for therapeutic purposes: osmotic opening and other means. Neurosurgery 1998;42(5):1083–99 [discussion: 1099–100].

22. Raymond JJ, Robertson DM, Dinsdale HB. Pharmacological modification of bradykinin induced breakdown of the blood-brain barrier. Can J Neurol Sci 1986;13(3):214–20.

23. Connell JJ, Chatain G, Cornelissen B, et al. Selective permeabilization of the blood-brain barrier at sites of metastasis. J Natl Cancer Inst 2013;105(21):1634–43.

24. Hendricks BK, Cohen-Gadol AA, Miller JC. Novel delivery methods bypassing the blood-brain and blood-tumor barriers. Neurosurg Focus 2015;38(3):E10.

25. McDannold N, Arvanitis CD, Vykhodtseva N, et al. Temporary disruption of the blood-brain barrier by use of ultrasound and microbubbles: safety and efficacy evaluation in rhesus macaques. Cancer Res 2012;72(14):3652–63.

26. Aryal M, Arvanitis CD, Alexander PM, et al. Ultrasound-mediated blood-brain barrier disruption for targeted drug delivery in the central nervous system. Adv Drug Deliv Rev 2014;72:94–109.

27. Hynynen K, McDannold N, Vykhodtseva N, et al. Noninvasive MR imaging-guided focal opening of the blood-brain barrier in rabbits. Radiology 2001; 220(3):640–6.

28. Yang FY, Wang HE, Lin GL, et al. Evaluation of the increase in permeability of the blood-brain barrier during tumor progression after pulsed focused ultrasound. Int J Nanomed 2012;7:723–30.

29. Sheikov N, McDannold N, Vykhodtseva N, et al. Cellular mechanisms of the blood-brain barrier opening induced by ultrasound in presence of microbubbles. Ultrasound Med Biol 2004;30(7): 979–89.

30. Carpentier A, Canney M, Vignot A, et al. Clinical trial of blood-brain barrier disruption by pulsed ultrasound. Sci Transl Med 2016;8(343):343re342.

31. Chen H, Konofagou EE. The size of blood-brain barrier opening induced by focused ultrasound is dictated by the acoustic pressure. J Cereb Blood Flow Metab 2014;34(7):1197–204.

32. Choi JJ, Wang S, Tung YS, et al. Molecules of various pharmacologically-relevant sizes can cross the ultrasound-induced blood-brain barrier opening in vivo. Ultrasound Med Biol 2010;36(1): 58–67.

33. Park EJ, Zhang YZ, Vykhodtseva N, et al. Ultrasound-mediated blood-brain/blood-tumor barrier disruption improves outcomes with trastuzumab in a breast cancer brain metastasis model. J Control Release 2012;163(3):277–84

34. Kobus T, Zervantonakis IK, Zhang Y, et al. Growth inhibition in a brain metastasis model by antibody delivery using focused ultrasound-mediated blood-brain barrier disruption. J Control Release 2016;238:281–8.

35. Baghirov H, Snipstad S, Sulheim E, et al. Ultrasound-mediated delivery and distribution of polymeric nanoparticles in the normal brain parenchyma of a metastatic brain tumour model. PLoS One 2018;13(1):e0191102.

36. Askoxylakis V, Arvanitis CD, Wong CSF, et al. Emerging strategies for delivering antiangiogenic therapies to primary and metastatic brain tumors. Adv Drug Deliv Rev 2017;119:159–74.

37. Nossek E, Matot I, Shahar T, et al. Failed awake craniotomy: a retrospective analysis in 424 patients undergoing craniotomy for brain tumor. J Neurosurg 2013;118(2):243–9.

38. Lajoie JM, Shusta EV. Targeting receptor-mediated transport for delivery of biologics across the blood-brain barrier. Annu Rev Pharmacol Toxicol 2015;55: 613–31.

39. Morad G, Carman CV, Hagedorn EJ, et al. Tumor-derived extracellular vesicles breach the intact blood-brain barrier via transcytosis. ACS Nano 2019;13(12):13853–65.

40. Pardridge WM. Re-engineering biopharmaceuticals for delivery to brain with molecular Trojan horses. Bioconjug Chem 2008;19(7): 1327–38.

41. Rautioa J, Chikhale PJ. Drug delivery systems for brain tumor therapy. Curr Pharm Des 2004; 10(12):1341–53.

42. Sun C, Ding Y, Zhou L, et al. Noninvasive nanoparticle strategies for brain tumor targeting. Nanomedicine 2017;13(8):2605–21.

43. Shahani K, Swaminathan SK, Freeman D, et al. Injectable sustained release microparticles of curcumin: a new concept for cancer chemoprevention. Cancer Res 2010;70(11):4443–52.

44. Silva GA. Nanotechnology approaches to crossing the blood-brain barrier and drug delivery to the CNS. BMC Neurosci 2008;9(Suppl 3):S4.

45. Schroeder U, Schroeder H, Sabel BA. Body distribution of 3H-labelled dalargin bound to poly(butyl cyanoacrylate) nanoparticles after i.v. injections to mice. Life Sci 2000;66(6):495–502.

46. Alyautdin RN, Petrov VE, Langer K, et al. Delivery of loperamide across the blood-brain barrier with polysorbate 80-coated polybutylcyanoacrylate nanoparticles. Pharm Res 1997;14(3): 325–8.

47. Hardesty DA, Nakaji P. The current and future treatment of brain metastases. Front Surg 2016;3:30.

48. Tang N, Guo J, Zhang Q, et al. Greater efficacy of chemotherapy plus bevacizumab compared to chemo- and targeted therapy alone on non-small cell lung cancer patients with brain metastasis. Oncotarget 2016;7(3):3635–44.

49. Wu YL, Zhou C, Cheng Y, et al. Erlotinib as second-line treatment in patients with advanced non-small-cell lung cancer and asymptomatic brain metastases: a phase II study (CTONG-0803). Ann Oncol 2013;24(4):993–9.

50. Duchnowska R, Loibl S, Jassem J. Tyrosine kinase inhibitors for brain metastases in HER2-positive breast cancer. Cancer Treat Rev 2018;67:71–7.

51. Diao K, Bian SX, Routman DM, et al. Combination ipilimumab and radiosurgery for brain metastases: tumor, edema, and adverse radiation effects. J Neurosurg 2018;129(6):1397–406.

52. Long GV, Atkinson V, Lo S, et al. Combination nivolumab and ipilimumab or nivolumab alone in melanoma brain metastases: a multicentre randomised phase 2 study. Lancet Oncol 2018;19(5):672–81.

53. Wu J, Neale N, Huang Y, et al. Comparison of adjuvant radiation therapy alone and chemotherapy alone in surgically resected low-grade gliomas: survival analyses of 2253 cases from the National Cancer Data Base. World Neurosurg 2018;112: e812–22.

54. Di Giacomo AM, Ascierto PA, Queirolo P, et al. Three-year follow-up of advanced melanoma patients who received ipilimumab plus fotemustine in the Italian Network for Tumor Biotherapy (NI-BIT)-M1 phase II study. Ann Oncol 2015;26(4): 798–803.

55. Eichler AF, Chung E, Kodack DP, et al. The biology of brain metastases-translation to new therapies. Nat Rev Clin Oncol 2011;8(6):344–56.

56. Lu YS, Chen TW, Lin CH, et al. Bevacizumab preconditioning followed by etoposide and cisplatin is highly effective in treating brain metastases of breast cancer progressing from whole-brain radiotherapy. Clin Cancer Res 2015;21(8):1851–8.

57. Johnson DH, Fehrenbacher L, Novotny WF, et al. Randomized phase II trial comparing bevacizumab plus carboplatin and paclitaxel with carboplatin and paclitaxel alone in previously untreated locally advanced or metastatic non-small-cell lung cancer. J Clin Oncol 2004;22(11):2184–91.

58. Sandler A, Gray R, Perry MC, et al. Paclitaxel-carboplatin alone or with bevacizumab for non-small-cell lung cancer. N Engl J Med 2006;355(24): 2542–50.

59. Besse B, Le Moulec S, Mazieres J, et al. Bevacizumab in Patients with Nonsquamous Non-Small Cell Lung Cancer and Asymptomatic, Untreated Brain Metastases (BRAIN): a nonrandomized, phase II study. Clin Cancer Res 2015;21(8):1896–903.

60. Labidi SI, Bachelot T, Ray-Coquard I, et al. Bevacizumab and paclitaxel for breast cancer patients with central nervous system metastases: a case series. Clin Breast Cancer 2009;9(2):118–21.

61. Gabay MP, Wirth SM, Stachnik JM, et al. Oral targeted therapies and central nervous system (CNS) metastases. CNS Drugs 2015;29(11): 935–52.

62. Kim A, McCully C, Cruz R, et al. The plasma and cerebrospinal fluid pharmacokinetics of sorafenib after intravenous administration in non-human primates. Invest New Drugs 2012;30(2):524–8.

63. Dudek AZ, Raza A, Chi M, et al. Brain metastases from renal cell carcinoma in the era of tyrosine kinase inhibitors. Clin Genitourin Cancer 2013; 11(2):155–60.

64. Minocha M, Khurana V, Qin B, et al. Enhanced brain accumulation of pazopanib by modulating P-gp and Bcrp1 mediated efflux with canertinib or erlotinib. Int J Pharm 2012;436(1–2):127–34.

65. Dempke WC, Edvardsen K, Lu S, et al. Brain metastases in NSCLC: are TKIs changing the treatment strategy? Anticancer Res 2015;35(11): 5797–806.

66. Heon S, Yeap BY, Lindeman NI, et al. The impact of initial gefitinib or erlotinib versus chemotherapy on central nervous system progression in advanced non-small cell lung cancer with EGFR mutations. Clin Cancer Res 2012;18(16): 4406–14.

67. Benedettini E, Sholl LM, Peyton M, et al. Met activation in non-small cell lung cancer is associated with de novo resistance to EGFR inhibitors and the development of brain metastasis. Am J Pathol 2010;177(1):415–23.

68. Gluck S, Castrellon A. Lapatinib plus capecitabine resolved human epidermal growth factor receptor 2-positive brain metastases. Am J Ther 2009; 16(6):585–90.

69. Lin NU, Carey LA, Liu MC, et al. Phase II trial of lapatinib for brain metastases in patients with human epidermal growth factor receptor 2-positive breast cancer. J Clin Oncol 2008;26(12):1993–9.

70. Lin NU, Dieras V, Paul D, et al. Multicenter phase II study of lapatinib in patients with brain metastases from HER2-positive breast cancer. Clin Cancer Res 2009;15(4):1452–9.

71. Cameron D, Casey M, Press M, et al. A phase III randomized comparison of lapatinib plus capecitabine versus capecitabine alone in women with advanced breast cancer that has progressed on trastuzumab: updated efficacy and biomarker analyses. Breast Cancer Res Treat 2008;112(3): 533–43.

72. Bachelot T, Romieu G, Campone M, et al. Lapatinib plus capecitabine in patients with previously untreated brain metastases from HER2-positive metastatic breast cancer (LANDSCAPE): a single-group phase 2 study. Lancet Oncol 2013; 14(1):64–71.

73. Larionov AA. Current therapies for human epidermal growth factor receptor 2-positive metastatic breast cancer patients. Front Oncol 2018;8:89.

74. Rick JW, Shahin M, Chandra A, et al. Systemic therapy for brain metastases. Crit Rev Oncol Hematol 2019;142:44–50.

75. Falchook GS, Long GV, Kurzrock R, et al. Dabrafenib in patients with melanoma, untreated brain metastases, and other solid tumours: a phase 1 dose-escalation trial. Lancet 2012;379(9829): 1893–901.

76. Davies MA, Saiag P, Robert C, et al. Dabrafenib plus trametinib in patients with BRAF(V600)-mutant melanoma brain metastases (COMBI-MB): a multicentre, multicohort, open-label, phase 2 trial. Lancet Oncol 2017;18(7):863–73.

77. Long GV, Trefzer U, Davies MA, et al. Dabrafenib in patients with Val600Glu or Val600Lys BRAF-mutant melanoma metastatic to the brain (BREAK-MB): a

multicentre, open-label, phase 2 trial. Lancet Oncol 2012;13(11):1087–95.

78. Dummer R, Goldinger SM, Turtschi CP, et al. Vemurafenib in patients with BRAF(V600) mutation-positive melanoma with symptomatic brain metastases: final results of an open-label pilot study. Eur J Cancer 2014;50(3):611–21.

79. Kwak EL, Bang YJ, Camidge DR, et al. Anaplastic lymphoma kinase inhibition in non-small-cell lung cancer. N Engl J Med 2010;363(18):1693–703.

80. Costa DB, Kobayashi S, Pandya SS, et al. CSF concentration of the anaplastic lymphoma kinase inhibitor crizotinib. J Clin Oncol 2011;29(15):e443–5.

81. McKeage K. Alectinib: a review of its use in advanced ALK-rearranged non-small cell lung cancer. Drugs 2015;75(1):75–82.

82. Peters S, Camidge DR, Shaw AT, et al. Alectinib versus crizotinib in untreated ALK-positive non-small-cell lung cancer. N Engl J Med 2017;377(9):829–38.

83. Rossi V, Berchialla P, Giannarelli D, et al. Should all patients with HR-positive HER2-negative metastatic breast cancer receive CDK 4/6 inhibitor as first-line based therapy? A network meta-analysis of data from the PALOMA 2, MONALEESA 2, MONALEESA 7, MONARCH 3, FALCON, SWOG and FACT trials. Cancers (Basel) 2019;11(11).

84. Blazquez R, Wlochowitz D, Wolff A, et al. PI3K: a master regulator of brain metastasis-promoting macrophages/microglia. Glia 2018;66(11):2438–55.

85. Andre F, Ciruelos E, Rubovszky G, et al. Alpelisib for PIK3CA-mutated, hormone receptor-positive advanced breast cancer. N Engl J Med 2019;380(20):1929–40.

86. Baselga J, Im SA, Iwata H, et al. Buparlisib plus fulvestrant versus placebo plus fulvestrant in postmenopausal, hormone receptor-positive, HER2-negative, advanced breast cancer (BELLE-2): a randomised, double-blind, placebo-controlled, phase 3 trial. Lancet Oncol 2017;18(7):904–16.

87. Di Leo A, Johnston S, Lee KS, et al. Buparlisib plus fulvestrant in postmenopausal women with hormone-receptor-positive, HER2-negative, advanced breast cancer progressing on or after mTOR inhibition (BELLE-3): a randomised, double-blind, placebo-controlled, phase 3 trial. Lancet Oncol 2018;19(1):87–100.

88. Santana VM, Sahr N, Tatevossian RG, et al. A phase 1 trial of everolimus and bevacizumab in children with recurrent solid tumors. Cancer 2020;126(8):1749–57.

89. Lauko A, Thapa B, Venur VA, et al. Management of brain metastases in the new era of checkpoint inhibition. Curr Neurol Neurosci Rep 2018;18(10):70.

90. Hodi FS, O'Day SJ, McDermott DF, et al. Improved survival with ipilimumab in patients with metastatic melanoma. N Engl J Med 2010;363(8):711–23.

91. Margolin K, Ernstoff MS, Hamid O, et al. Ipilimumab in patients with melanoma and brain metastases: an open-label, phase 2 trial. Lancet Oncol 2012;13(5):459–65.

92. Tawbi HA, Forsyth PA, Algazi A, et al. Combined nivolumab and ipilimumab in melanoma metastatic to the brain. N Engl J Med 2018;379(8):722–30.

93. Goldberg SB, Gettinger SN, Mahajan A, et al. Pembrolizumab for patients with melanoma or non-small-cell lung cancer and untreated brain metastases: early analysis of a non-randomised, open-label, phase 2 trial. Lancet Oncol 2016;17(7):976–83.

94. Kirchberger MC, Hauschild A, Schuler G, et al. Combined low-dose ipilimumab and pembrolizumab after sequential ipilimumab and pembrolizumab failure in advanced melanoma. Eur J Cancer 2016;65:182–4.

95. Spagnolo F, Picasso V, Lambertini M, et al. Survival of patients with metastatic melanoma and brain metastases in the era of MAP-kinase inhibitors and immunologic checkpoint blockade antibodies: a systematic review. Cancer Treat Rev 2016;45:38–45.

96. Kazazi-Hyseni F, Beijnen JH, Schellens JHM. Bevacizumab. Oncologist 2010;15(8):819–25.

97. Carrato Mena A, Grande Pulido E, Guillén-Ponce C. Understanding the molecular-based mechanism of action of the tyrosine kinase inhibitor: sunitinib. Anti Cancer Drugs 2010;21 Suppl 1(1):S3–11.

98. Rahman MA, Salajegheh A, Smith RA, et al. BRAF inhibitors: from the laboratory to clinical trials. Crit Rev Oncol Hematol 2014;90(3):220–32.

99. Knudsen ES, Witkiewicz AK. The strange case of CDK4/6 inhibitors: mechanisms, resistance, and combination Strategies. Trends Cancer 2017;3(1):39–55.

100. Colaco RJ, Martin P, Kluger HM, et al. Does immunotherapy increase the rate of radiation necrosis after radiosurgical treatment of brain metastases? J Neurosurg 2016;125(1):17–23.

Leptomeningeal Carcinomatosis
Molecular Landscape, Current Management, and Emerging Therapies

Hriday P. Bhambhvani, BS[a], Adrian J. Rodrigues, BS[a],
Maxine C. Umeh-Garcia, PhD, MSc[c], Melanie Hayden Gephart, MD, MAS[a,b,*]

KEYWORDS

- Cellular • Disease • Metastasis • Cell • Pathophysiology • Translational • Brain

KEY POINTS

- Despite advances in the cellular and genetic characterization of primary cancers, the underlying molecular alterations that enable leptomeningeal spread are poorly understood. However, recent work has begun to elucidate several factors that may play a role in leptomeningeal carcinomatosis (LMC) pathogenesis.
- Liquid biopsy of cerebrospinal fluid (CSF) is a promising tool in both the genetic characterization and diagnosis of LMC. CSF-derived circulating tumor DNA more accurately represents the genomic landscape of leptomeningeal metastasis compared with circulating tumor DNA derived from blood plasma.
- There exists a high degree of genetic divergence between a primary tumor and its leptomeningeal metastasis, suggesting the existence of premetastatic, subclonal populations of cancer cells within the primary tumor that are predisposed to leptomeningeal colonization.
- Thus far, studies of immunotherapy and novel experimental methods to treat LMC have been limited, with low-grade evidence of treatment efficacy. Further research with rigorous, randomized controlled studies is necessary.

INTRODUCTION

Leptomeningeal carcinomatosis (LMC), also known as leptomeningeal metastasis or leptomeningeal disease, is the metastatic spread of cancer to the pia mater, arachnoid, and subarachnoid space.[1] LMC occurs in 5% to 15% of patients with cancer, has limited therapeutic options, and has an average survival time of 2 to 6 months.[1–6] LMC most commonly arises as a result of metastasis from primary cancers originating outside the central nervous system (CNS), but LMC can also arise from primary CNS tumors, including astrocytomas, medulloblastomas, and ependymomas.[7] The incidence of LMC continues to steadily increase across primary tumor types, likely because of more sensitive detection methods and improved efficacy of therapeutics able to control systemic disease.[1,8] Currently, whole brain or cranial-spinal radiation and intrathecal (IT) or systemic chemotherapy have offered limited survival benefit with substantial risks of treatment-related toxicity.[5,9] Thus, the need for a more comprehensive characterization of disease pathogenesis in order to identify novel therapeutic

[a] Department of Neurosurgery, Stanford University Medical Center, 300 Pasteur Drive, Palo Alto, CA, 94305 USA; [b] Department of Neurosurgery, Brain Tumor Center, Stanford University School of Medicine, 300 Pasteur Drive, Palo Alto, CA 94305, USA
* Corresponding author.
E-mail address: mghayden@stanford.edu

Neurosurg Clin N Am 31 (2020) 613–625
https://doi.org/10.1016/j.nec.2020.06.010
1042-3680/20/© 2020 Elsevier Inc. All rights reserved.

targets has become increasingly urgent. Although recent scientific advances have increased the understanding of how malignant cells seed and thrive within the leptomeninges, more studies are still required. In this review, the authors summarize their current understanding of the molecular landscape of LMC, outline clinical management of these patients, and highlight emerging therapeutic options.

EPIDEMIOLOGY

Nearly every primary tumor type has been reported to metastasize to the leptomeninges. Approximately 5% to 8% of solid tumors and 5% to 15% of hematologic malignancies metastasize to the leptomeninges. The most common cancers that give rise to LMC are lung (9%–25%), breast (5%–8%), melanoma (6%–18%), acute lymphoblastic leukemia (1%–10%), and non-Hodgkin lymphoma (5%-10%).[4–6,10–15] The incidence of LMC also varies based on the molecular and/or histologic subtypes of the primary cancer, as seen in breast and lung groups. For example, in a study of 118 patients with breast LMC, 35% of patients had breast tumors that exhibited lobular histology.[16] Considering that only 10% of all primary breast cancers are invasive lobular carcinoma, there is a clear overrepresentation of this histologic subgroup in LMC.[17] In addition, the triple-negative molecular subtype of breast cancer (TNBC) comprises roughly 40% of breast LMC cases, although TNBC accounts for only 10% of all diagnosed breast cancers.[16,18] TNBC patients are at 4 times higher risk of developing LMC compared with patients with hormone receptor positive and HER2[+] breast cancer.[19] With respect to lung cancer, patients with non–small cell lung cancer (NSCLC), specifically those with epidermal growth factor receptor (EGFR)-mutant disease, are more than 3 times as likely to develop LMC as compared with those with EGFR-wild-type tumors.[20,21] Given difficulties in diagnosis and rapid mortality, these rates are likely underestimates of the true incidence of LMC.[1] In fact, 1 postmortem analysis of patients with cancer that exhibited neurologic symptoms revealed that 18% had evidence of leptomeningeal infiltration.[20]

The median interval between diagnosis of systemic disease and LMC diagnosis is 1.2 to 2 years for solid tumors, and 11 months for hematologic malignancies.[7,9,22,23] If left untreated, LMC is typically fatal within 4 to 6 weeks.[5] Because treatments for systemic cancers improve, the incidence of LMC is likely to continue to increase, and because survival from LMC is poor, treatment advances are critically needed.

PATHOPHYSIOLOGY AND MOLECULAR LANDSCAPE
Pathophysiology

The anatomic route taken by malignant cells to seed the leptomeninges may include spread from the brain parenchyma,[6,24] choroid plexus, blood,[6,7] or cerebrospinal fluid (CSF) after surgical resection[25,26] (**Fig. 1**). The blood-brain barrier (BBB) frequently blocks otherwise effective systemic therapies, creating a pharmacologically protected space for tumor cells to proliferate once they seed the leptomeninges. Once LMC develops, tumor growth can lead to cranial nerve dysfunction, inflammation, and hydrocephalus. Circulation of the blood and/or CSF frequently leads to the spread of metastatic cells resulting in multifocal CNS disease.[5,6] The diffuse nature of LMC combined with the relative inaccessibility of the brain to treatment contributes to the severe morbidity and rapid mortality observed in patients with LMC.

Similar to the metastatic microenvironment in other areas of the body, the leptomeningeal membranes possess a rich ecosystem of vasculature, fibroblasts, infiltrating immune cells, and extracellular matrix.[27] As such, metastatic disease progression at this site is likely a combination of cell intrinsic (eg, gene expression, metabolism, glycosylation) and cell extrinsic (eg, brain microenvironment) factors. Despite advances in the cellular and genetic characterization of primary cancers, the underlying molecular alterations that enable leptomeningeal spread remain poorly understood. Malignant metastatic cells from different primary sites likely have shared properties that allow survival in the leptomeninges.[5] Such properties may include anoikis and immune system evasion as cancer cells travel through the blood and CSF, tissue invasion through epithelial cells in the choroid plexus and parenchyma, and angiogenesis required for thriving within the leptomeninges.[28] In 1 study, analysis of lung cancer primary tumors and matched leptomeningeal metastases using next-generation sequencing revealed a high degree of genetic divergence and clonal heterogeneity between the paired samples.[29] A variety of potential sources may underlie this genetic divergence, such as mutations acquired during metastasis formation or in response to pressures from the leptomeningeal microenvironment. However, it is also possible that some of the genetic divergence observed is due to clonal evolution of a subset of cells in the primary tumor predisposed to metastasize to the leptomeninges. In line with this, studies have shown that the leptomeninges upregulate stromal derived factor-1 alpha and vascular

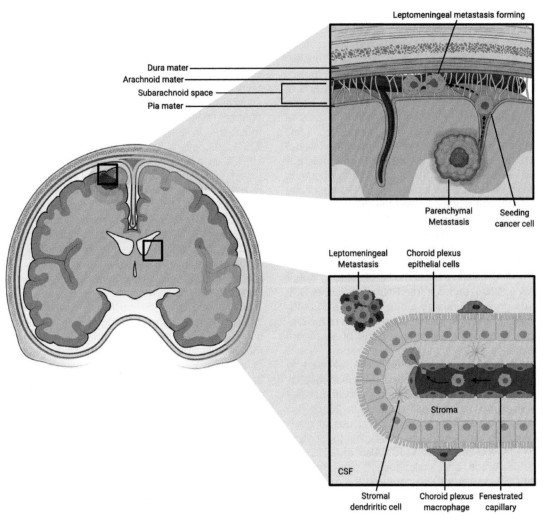

Fig. 1. Potential routes of spread to the leptomeninges.

endothelial growth factor, which hone tumor cells to the CNS and increase blood supply to metastatic tumors, respectively, suggesting that the leptomeninges may inadvertently support LMC progression.[30–32]

Immune interactions may also play an important role in metastatic tumor cell implantation and outgrowth in the leptomeninges. For example, Boire and colleagues[33] found that complement protein C3 was necessary for tumor growth within the leptomeninges in 2 breast and 2 lung cancer models of LMC. The study revealed that the interaction between C3a (a cleavage product of C3) produced by cancer cells and its associated receptor C3aR resulted in reduced integrity of the choroid plexus epithelium and a breach in the blood-CSF barrier, which allowed growth factors and mitogens to enter the CSF, enabling tumorigenesis.[33] These findings were corroborated by

Smalley and colleagues,[34] who found increased expression of C3 (as well as increased expression of C2, C6, C5, C9, C8α, C8β, and C8γ) in the CSF of patients with melanoma LMC. It will be important to determine if these findings (eg, expression of C3) can be generalized across other primary cancer types in human patients. Notably, we are only just beginning to understand the molecular mechanisms that underlie the formation, outgrowth, and support of leptomeningeal metastases, a dynamic process that gives rise to a diverse group of metastatic cells.

Novel Scientific Techniques to Characterize Leptomeningeal Carcinomatosis

In recent years, exponential advances have been seen in the understanding of biology and pathology at single-cell resolution, and technological advances to suggest cell-free nucleic acid tests may act as surrogates for solid tissue biopsy. These technologies, including single-cell RNA sequencing (scRNA-seq) and expression profiling of circulating cell-free tumor-associated nucleic acids, are well positioned to investigate the molecular landscapes of highly heterogeneous and/or physically inaccessible human cancers.[35] These techniques have recently been applied to several CNS cancers; however, applications to LMC have been limited.[36] The relative inaccessibility of LMC tissue, paucity of cells in CSF, and rapid patient mortality contribute to the scarcity of human specimens available for study. LMC tumors are generally not biopsied given the diffuse nature of the disease and lack of durable treatments. However, recent efforts that pair a liquid biopsy approach with next-generation sequencing technologies have enabled the analysis of CSF-derived circulating tumor cells, circulating tumor DNA (ctDNA), and cell-free RNA. Analysis of CSF holds great potential to aid in diagnosis of LMC, genetic and epigenetic characterization of the disease, and identifying mechanisms of treatment resistance.

ctDNA refers to extracellular DNA released by cancer cells through a variety of proposed mechanisms, such as active secretion and/or passive release upon cancer cell death.[37] In 2015, Pan and colleagues[38] reported the first use of next-generation sequencing technologies to analyze CSF-derived ctDNA in LMC. Also in 2015, De Mattos-Arruda and colleagues[39] demonstrated that CSF-derived ctDNA captured the mutational landscape of a variety of CNS tumors, including LMC, with improved sensitivity as compared with plasma-derived ctDNA. In line with this, a study by Li and colleagues[40] of 26 patients with EGFR-mutant NSCLC LMC revealed that CSF ctDNA more accurately recapitulated the genomic landscape of leptomeningeal metastasis than plasma ctDNA. In this study, driver genes were detected in 100% of CSF ctDNA samples compared with 73.1% of ctDNA derived from plasma. Among patients with anaplastic lymphoma kinase (ALK)-rearranged NSCLC, similar results have been reported with driver genes detected in 81.8% of CSF ctDNA samples versus 45.5% in plasma ctDNA samples.[41] Importantly, analysis of CSF-derived ctDNA, even very small amounts, has proven reliable and reproducible, with multiple studies characterizing the genetic landscape of LMC. A comprehensive summary of ctDNA studies in LMCs from lung, breast, and melanoma is summarized in **Table 1**.[38,40–54]

Most ctDNA studies have focused on patients with primary lung cancer-derived LMC, whereby driver mutations are more common and directly linked to therapy (eg, EGFR, ALK). However, CSF ctDNA may also prove useful for the diagnosis of LMC from other primary cancer types. For example, in a small study of breast LMC, analysis of CSF ctDNA was more sensitive than cytologic testing of CSF in 2 of 3 patients, and equally sensitive in the third patient.[39] Specifically, the investigators tested for POLE, ARID5B, and PCDH1 mutations in patient 1; PTEN, MRPS33, and ESR1 in patient 2; and AKT3, CDC73, and HERC2 in patient 3. At present, the only other report of liquid biopsy in breast LMC is a case report of a patient with both parenchymal brain metastasis and LMC from HER2+ breast cancer.[50] CSF-derived ctDNA analysis revealed mutations in TP53 and PIK3CA, as well as amplification of ERBB2 and cMYC. Given the low sensitivity of cytology and MRI for LMC diagnosis, assessment of CSF ctDNA holds the potential to significantly improve LMC diagnosis.

scRNA-seq, like CSF ctDNA, is well suited to investigate rare and heterogeneous biological samples, as is the case with LMC. Although many studies have investigated the transcriptional diversity of primary brain tumors using scRNA-seq, there is only 1 report of scRNA-seq in CSF samples and no peer-reviewed reports of its use in LMC.[55] The authors' group and others are currently refining techniques necessary for the application of scRNA-seq to LMC. Their initial analysis has identified altered cancer-specific genes that demonstrated pathologic effects in vitro (Li et al., in revision, 2020). These data, and future studies of scRNA-seq of LMC, will allow further investigation of the transcriptional heterogeneity both within and between LMC patient samples and will help identify molecular pathways that underlie mechanisms of treatment resistance.

Animal Models of Leptomeningeal Carcinomatosis

Rodent models of LMC are most commonly established through injection of cancer cells directly into the cisterna magna, or into the subarachnoid space of the spinal cord.[33,56,57] The authors' laboratory has recently demonstrated that injection of cancer cells into the internal carotid artery of mice, a technique previously described as a method to recapitulate brain metastasis in mice, also leads to the formation of LMC (Chernikova et al., under review). Using this technique, the authors model TNBC LMC and show improvements in survival following treatment with the chemotherapeutic Cyclophosphamide, or a novel, brain penetrant chemotherapeutic QBS10072S. Using a mouse model of lung LMC to investigate

Table 1
Studies involving cerebrospinal fluid-derived circulating tumor DNA in leptomeningeal carcinomatosis

Study	Primary Site	Detection Method	Mutation Genes
Pan et al,[38] 2015	Lung	NGS	578 gene panel
De Mattos-Arruda et al,[39] 2015	Breast	ddPCR	POLE, ARID5B, PCDH1, PTEN, MRPS33, ESR1, AKT3, CDC73, HERC2
Li et al,[40] 2018	Lung	NGS	N/A
Song et al,[42] 2019	Lung	NGS	1021 gene panel
Ge et al,[43] 2019	Lung	NGS	10–59 gene panel
Huang et al,[44] 2019	Lung	ddPCR	EGFR
Ma et al,[45] 2019	Lung	NGS	N/A
Aldea et al,[46] 2020	Lung	NGS	Sentosa NSCLC panel
van Bussel et al,[47] 2020	Lung	ddPCR	EGFR
Ma et al,[48] 2020	Lung	NGS	Cancer HotSpot panel v2
Li et al,[49] 2018	Lung	ddPCR NGS NGS	EGFR, TP53 Whole-exome sequencing MSK-IMPACT
Siravegna et al,[50] 2017	Breast	ddPCR NGS	ERBB2, MYC, TP53, PIK3CA Whole-exome sequencing
Pentsova et al,[51] 2016	Lung, melanoma	NGS	MSK-IMPACT
Li et al,[52] 2016	Melanoma	ddPCR NGS	BRAF Whole-exome sequencing
Ballester et al,[53] 2018	Melanoma	ddPCR NGS	BRAF Cancer HotSpot panel v2
Momtaz et al,[54] 2016	Melanoma	ddPCR	BRAF

Abbreviations: ddPCR, digital droplet polymerase chain reaction; N/A, not applicable; NGS, next-generation sequencing.

mechanisms of resistance to Gefitinib, Nanjo and colleagues[58] found that copy number gain of the MET oncogene, and its subsequent activation, is implicated in the development of drug resistance. In a similarly themed study seeking to elucidate mechanisms of ALK-tyrosine kinase inhibitors (TKI) resistance in lung LMC, Arai and colleagues[59] found that decreased expression of microRNA-449a led to overexpression of amphiregulin (a ligand of EGFR) and subsequent EGFR activation, regulating the development of resistance to the ALK-TKI Alectinib. AZD3759, a BBB-penetrant EGFR inhibitor, has demonstrated tumor regression in a mouse model of lung LMC,[56] with clinical trials currently underway [NCT02228369]. Not only have animal models deepened the understanding of LMC formation and progression but they have also enabled preclinical testing of promising therapies.

CURRENT TREATMENT AND IMAGING

The National Comprehensive Cancer Network (NCCN) has published comprehensive guidelines to stratify patients with CNS cancer and identify those who should receive aggressive therapy. Patients with high Karnofsky performance scale scores (ie, low functional impairment), no fixed neurologic deficits, and limited systemic disease are expected to receive the most benefit from multimodal intervention.[60] LMC has traditionally been treated with whole-brain radiation therapy (WBRT), CNS penetrant systemic therapy, and palliation. Because most systemic chemotherapies have limited ability to cross the BBB, they are often paired with radiation to slow neurologic decline, stabilize quality of life, and slightly prolong survival.[4] For example, in patients with breast cancer who received LMC treatment, median time to neurologic progression was only 49 days, with 56% of patients dying with simultaneous progression of LMC and their primary breast cancer.[61,62] Even with aggressive intervention, survival time is only increased, on average, by 4 to 12 weeks.[9] Ideally, LMC treatment would involve the entire neuroaxis, because disseminated tumor cells may migrate with CSF flow circulating from the choroid plexus to the base of the sacral subarachnoid space.[5] Such a therapy could involve a combination of radiation to the leptomeningeal metastases, IT chemotherapy for CNS-specific disease control, and systemic chemotherapy for extra-CNS disease control.

Radiation

Although radiation has failed to prolong overall survival (OS) in LMC patients, it can result in dramatic symptom relief and improved quality of life for patients with symptomatic disease.[63,64] In particular, LMC arising from breast and hematologic malignancies is more radiosensitive, and these patients are predicted to benefit most from WBRT.[5,65,66] Irradiation-induced tumor shrinkage can reduce hydrocephalus, which not only improves IT chemotherapy by facilitating CSF flow but also relieves elevated intracranial pressure-related symptoms.[7,67] Typically, patients undergo WBRT of 30 Gy in 10 fractions[5,7]; however, an attenuated course of 20 Gy in 4-Gy fractions can be administered to patients who are unlikely to tolerate higher doses of radiation or longer courses of treatment.[68] Unfortunately, in addition to the routine toxicities associated with radiation, some evidence suggests that the risk of leukoencephalopathy (brain white-matter neurotoxicity) is increased when LMC irradiation is combined with intravenous or IT methotrexate.[69–71] Total eradication of LMC tumor cells would require irradiating the entire neuroaxis, including the spine; however, this treatment choice is rarely an option for solid tumor malignancies because of bone marrow suppression caused by irradiation and systemic chemotherapies would not prevent reseeding from the systemic disease and lacks durable efficacy.[7]

Systemic Chemotherapy

Systemic chemotherapy has the obvious advantage of simultaneously treating extra-CNS disease and LMC; numerous studies have identified this treatment strategy as providing a survival benefit, although modest.[3,72,73] However, it still remains a challenge for systemic chemotherapies to reach therapeutic concentrations in the CSF.[5] Moreover, the BBB, although damaged by LMC, remains a selective filter often preventing the 1:1 CSF:plasma ratio concentration needed for chemotherapeutics. The chemotherapy drug Thiotepa, which is a DNA alkylating agent, is best able to cross the BBB, with a ratio of 1:1, but it is most commonly used as an IT agent in the treatment of breast cancer LMC.[74,75] Temozolomide (TMZ), a widely used chemotherapeutic for primary brain cancers, has less BBB penetration (CSF:plasma ratio of 0.20) and is not commonly used for LMC treatment. A phase 2 randomized clinical trial examining systemic TMZ treatment in LMC patients with solid tumors (breast and NSCLC) was terminated prematurely because of poor accrual; median time to progression was 28 days (95% confidence interval 14–42 days), and clinical benefit was observed in only 3 of 19 patients.[76] High-dose Methotrexate has shown efficacy in patients with LMC originating from solid tumors.[77,78] Similarly, Capecitabine has been reported to offer clinical benefit to patients with breast cancer LMC.[79–82] To treat EGFR-mutated NSCLC LMC, the TKI Erlotinib is "pulsed" intermittently at high doses to deliver therapeutic concentrations to the CSF.[83] For LMC arising from nonsolid tumors, high-dose Cytarabine has been effective against CNS leukemias.[84,85] Ultimately, the chemotherapeutic agent chosen will depend on the primary cancer of the patient and their ability to safely tolerate the toxicities associated with high-dose cytotoxic therapeutics.

Intrathecal Chemotherapy

In theory, IT chemotherapy delivers cytotoxic agents directly to the site of ventricular disease and to tumor cells present throughout the CSF. Bypassing the BBB also allows a lower dose of chemotherapy to be delivered, lowering the likelihood of systemic toxicity. The most commonly used IT chemotherapies are Methotrexate, Cytarabine (and its long-acting liposomal formulation), Trastuzumab, and Thiotepa. Regardless of the specific agent, most IT chemotherapy involves a high-dose induction phase, an intermediate-dose consolidation phase, and a low-dose maintenance phase.[86] Patients with LMC can receive IT chemotherapy through either a lumbar puncture or a ventricular reservoir. Each method has associated risks, with reservoir placements carrying the risks of catheter misplacement, tip occlusion, and infection.[87] IT chemotherapy carries procedural risks not associated with systemic chemotherapy or radiation therapy, including CNS infection, CSF leak, and cerebral herniation.[5] Aseptic and chemical meningitis has been observed in up to 43% of LMC patients who receive IT chemotherapy, and septic meningitis has been seen in 8% to 24% of patients.[87–89] These complications often require treatment with hydration, corticosteroids and antibiotics, and cessation of therapy.[90] In addition, CSF flow, required for IT chemotherapy, may be disrupted by obstruction of the ventricles or venous outflow, in which case the IT medication is rapidly degraded.

The only randomized clinical trial to study IT chemotherapy against standard-of-care therapy was conducted by Boogerd and colleagues.[91] Of 35 patients with breast cancer LMC, 17 were randomized to receive IT chemotherapy, systemic chemotherapy, and radiotherapy, whereas the other 18 received only systemic chemotherapy and radiotherapy. No difference in patient survival or neurologic response was noted between groups, and the trial was terminated prematurely because of decreasing accrual. Similarly, a large retrospective study of 104 LMC patients who received systemic therapy and radiation ± IT chemotherapy did not show a survival benefit.[92] This finding is in contrast to 2 previous studies that showed IT chemotherapy prolonged patient survival. The first study examined breast cancer LMC patients, whereas the second study examined lung cancer LMC patients. Patients from both studies underwent similar treatment regimen, with all patients receiving IT Methotrexate and some patients additionally receiving IT Cytarabine and Thiotepa. Median survival was 7.5 months for the breast LMC study,[62] and 5 months for lung LMC.[67] Both survival times are longer than the average survival time of all patients with LMD, suggesting that IT chemotherapy may provide clinical benefit. Because of conflicting results of the studies, at this time there is inadequate evidence to determine whether IT chemotherapy improves patient prognosis, but further studies are currently underway.

Imaging

Although the gold standard of LMC diagnosis remains CSF cytology, the diagnosis is often made in modern practice with the use of MRI; even patients with clear LMC on MRI may have negative cytology. T1-weighted gadolinium-enhanced MRI (gdMRI) is the imaging modality of choice, which is reported to have a specificity and sensitivity of roughly 75%.[93] In a study of 14 patients with cytologically confirmed leptomeningeal metastasis, T1-weighted gdMRI was able to detect foci of abnormal enhancement in twice as many patients as compared with contrast-enhanced CT.[94] The classical appearance of LMC on gdMRI is serpentine, nodular, or plaquelike contrast enhancement within the CSF or along the leptomeninges, subependyma, cranial, and spinal nerves, as well as communicating hydrocephalus.[5,95] Typical imaging findings of LMC are depicted in **Fig. 2**. In a subset of patients without clear disease on contrast-weighted imaging, LMC can be associated with fluid-attenuated inversion recovery or T2-weighted imaging,[95] and these sequences should be included in patients whose symptoms are consistent with LMC.

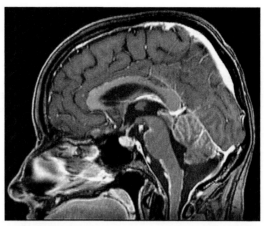

Fig. 2. Typical leptomeningeal enhancement on MRI.

EMERGING THERAPIES
Immunotherapy

Immunotherapeutic agents acting to inhibit checkpoint proteins, such as PD-1 or CTLA-4, have been shown to promote an antitumor immune response with remarkable clinical activity in a wide array of malignancies, ranging from bladder cancer to Hodgkin lymphoma.[96] Although many studies have examined the efficacy of immunotherapy in systemic disease, there are few studies examining such treatments in intracranial malignancies, and even fewer studies specifically in LMC. **Table 2** summarizes studies exploring the effectiveness of immunotherapy in LMC.[97–105] Notable studies are highlighted in later discussion.

In a study of patients with melanoma LMC, the median survival of 10 patients treated with Ipilimumab, a monoclonal antibody against CTLA-4, was 15.8 weeks.[98] In comparison, the median survival of patients receiving any treatment was 16.9 weeks, demonstrating no improvement with Ipilimumab. A study of 42 patients with melanoma LMC treated with IT interleukin-2 (IL-2) found median OS among these patients to be 9.1 months with greater than 16% surviving more than 24 months.[99] This improvement is notable over a median survival of roughly 2 to 6 months among patients with any form of treatment.[1] This finding was corroborated by another study of patients with melanoma LMC, in which patients who received IT administration of IL-2 had remarkably increased survival time (7.8 months) compared with patients who did not (1.6 months).[100]

With regard to lung cancer, 1 study of 19 patients with NSCLC LMC treated with immune checkpoint inhibitors found mean progression-free survival among these patients to be 2 months,

Table 2
Summary of studies involving immunotherapy in leptomeningeal carcinomatosis

Study	Primary Site	Type of Study	Therapy	Outcome
Bot et al[97]	Melanoma	Case report	WBRT + Ipilimumab	1.5-y OS
Geukes foppen et al[98]	Melanoma	Nonrandomized, retrospective cohort	Multiple treatment arms consisting of RT ± BRAF inhibitor ± MEK inhibitor ± Ipilimumab	Median OS of 15.8 wk among patients receiving ipilimumab
Glitza et al[99]	Melanoma	Nonrandomized, retrospective cohort	IT IL-2 ± RT ± systemic therapy before IL-2 administration	Median OS of 9.1 mo
Ferguson et al[100]	Melanoma	Nonrandomized, retrospective cohort	IT IL-2	Median OS of 7.8 mo
Hendriks et al[101]	Lung	Nonrandomized, retrospective cohort	Pembrolizumab or Nivolumab	Median progression-free survival of 2.0 mo
Bover et al[102]	Lung	Case report	Nivolumab	4-y OS
Gion et al,[103]	Lung	Case report	Nivolumab	7 mo of progression-free survival
Dudnik et al[104]	Lung	Case series (2 patients)	Nivolumab	One patient surviving 7 mo, other not reported
Brastianos et al[105]	15 Breast, 2 lung, 1 gastric	Prospective cohort	Pembrolizumab	3-mo OS rate of 44%

a 6-month OS rate of 36.8%, and a median survival of 5.1 months.[101] Although this is not particularly impressive compared with other treatment methods, the investigators noted that a subset of patients, particularly those classified as having good prognosis per NCCN guidelines, exhibited prolonged survival. Consistent with this, multiple case reports have documented sustained pathologic complete response among some patients with NCCN-defined favorable prognosis lung LMC.[102,103,106] In a cohort of 18 LMC patients (15 of whom had primary breast cancer), Pembrolizumab, a monoclonal antibody against PD-1, demonstrated limited efficacy with a 3-month OS rate of 44%.[105] It is likely that the relatively lackluster response to immunotherapy among patients with LMC may be due in part to limited delivery of systemic drugs to the CNS. Pembrolizumab, Nivolumab, and Ipilimumab each have a molecular weight of ≥145 kDa, making penetration of the BBB and blood-CSF barrier challenging.[107] Nevertheless, further study of these agents in a more rigorous, prospective fashion is warranted.

Experimental Therapies

Focused ultrasound (FUS) has emerged in the last 2 decades as a method to invoke focal and transient permeability of the BBB.[108] In an initial study of the efficacy of FUS, Kinoshita and colleagues[109] were able to greatly enhance delivery of Trastuzumab to the CNS in a rodent model of breast cancer brain metastasis. Although some clinical trials of FUS have been initiated as a result of promising preclinical data, the technique remains largely experimental. Because LMC is considered a disease of diffuse tumor cell growth throughout the leptomeninges, it would reason that increased permeability across regions of the BBB would increase therapeutic response and enhance clinical benefit; however, to date there are no reports of FUS use in LMC patients.[110,111] A recent study examined, for the first time, the efficacy of ultrasound-mediated delivery of Trastuzumab in a mouse model of breast LMC.[112] The study found a statistically significant decrease in tumor volume in the Trastuzumab + FUS group compared with the Trastuzumab-alone group; however, no significant increase in survival was observed, which the investigators surmised was due to systemic disease progression. More investigation is needed to characterize the safety, feasibility, and efficacy of this novel treatment paradigm.

Enthusiasm has grown for the use of chimeric antigen receptor (CAR) T cells in cancer immunotherapy, including in the treatment of CNS tumors. CAR T cells, which can be expanded rapidly ex vivo, are genetically modified T cells engineered to target a single surface antigen on cancer cells.[113] In a mouse model of breast cancer brain metastasis and LMC, Priceman and colleagues[114] found that intraventricular delivery of HER2-CAR T cells demonstrated a potent antitumor effect and conferred a marked increase in survival compared with intraventricular delivery of mock T cells lacking a CAR. Immunotherapy involving tumor-infiltrating lymphocytes (TILs) has also shown success primarily among patients with metastatic melanoma. TILs are extracted from the host's tumor, expanded ex vivo, and reimplanted.[115] Clinical trials for TIL therapy are underway, and in a case report of a patient with melanoma LMC, IT administration of TILs halted LMC progression, although the patient ultimately died 5 months after the initiation of therapy because of systemic disease progression.[116,117]

Recently, promising results of a phase 2 clinical study on the efficacy of ANG1005, a novel taxane derivative with increased BBB permeability, in breast cancer LMC were reported.[118] Among 28 patients, 79% exhibited intracranial disease control and median survival times of 8 months. As a follow-up to these promising results, a randomized phase 3 study, comparing the use of ANG1005 to a physician's best choice control, is currently underway [NCT03613181].

The results from these aforementioned studies highlight that many experimental therapies for the treatment of LMC are currently on the horizon. Studies using FUS, CAR T cells, TILs, and BBB-penetrating compounds like ANG1005 may hold promise for clinical benefit; however, to date, these studies remain preliminary and inconclusive. Further investigation is required to determine which emerging experimental therapies, if any, will provide significant improvements to LMC treatment.

SUMMARY

LMC is a rapidly fatal consequence of systemic cancer spread. Current therapeutic options are predominantly palliative and do not significantly prolong patient survival. It is likely that the dismal response to current treatments among patients with LMC may be due to a variety of factors, such as limited delivery of therapeutic drugs to the CNS due to the BBB, the inherently aggressive biology of the subset of tumors cells predisposed to metastasize to the leptomeninges, shared intrinsic properties of LMC tumor cells that drive therapy resistance, and the LMC microenvironment, including normal leptomeningeal cells and infiltrating immune cells. Most of these factors have yet to be studied because of the diffuse nature of LMC tumors, rapid morbidity/mortality of patients, and lack of patient samples for basic research. Contemporary experimental techniques, including analysis of CSF ctDNA, scRNA-seq, and animal models, have provided a means for deeper understanding of the biology underlying formation, outgrowth, and maintenance of leptomeningeal metastasis. Continued efforts to understand the basic pathophysiology of LMC will also be necessary to guide the development of more efficacious treatments.

DISCLOSURE

The authors have no conflicts of interest to report. This research did not receive any specific grant from funding agencies in the public, commercial, or not-for-profit sectors. M.H. Gephart's salary is supported in part by NIH grant K08 NS901527.

REFERENCES

1. Nayar G, Ejikeme T, Chongsathidkiet P, et al. Leptomeningeal disease: current diagnostic and therapeutic strategies. Oncotarget 2017;8(42): 73312–28.
2. Thomas KH, Ramirez RA. Leptomeningeal disease and the evolving role of molecular targeted therapy and immunotherapy. Ochsner J 2017;17(4): 362–78.
3. Herrlinger U, Förschler H, Küker W, et al. Leptomeningeal metastasis: survival and prognostic factors in 155 patients. J Neurol Sci 2004;223(2):167–78.
4. Beauchesne P. Intrathecal chemotherapy for treatment of leptomeningeal dissemination of metastatic tumours. Lancet Oncol 2010;11(9):871–9.
5. Groves MD. Leptomeningeal disease. Neurosurg Clin N Am 2011;22(1):67–78, vii.
6. Le Rhun E, Taillibert S, Chamberlain MC. Carcinomatous meningitis: leptomeningeal metastases in solid tumors. Surg Neurol Int 2013;4(Suppl 4): S265–88.
7. Wang N, Bertalan MS, Brastianos PK. Leptomeningeal metastasis from systemic cancer: review and update on management. Cancer 2018;124(1): 21–35.

8. Leal T, Chang JE, Mehta M, et al. Leptomeningeal metastasis: challenges in diagnosis and treatment. Curr Cancer Ther Rev 2011;7(4):319–27.

9. Balm M, Hammack J. Leptomeningeal carcinomatosis: presenting features and prognostic factors. Arch Neurol 1996;53(7):626–32.

10. Amer MH, Al-Sarraf M, Baker LH, et al. Malignant melanoma and central nervous system metastases: incidence, diagnosis, treatment and survival. Cancer 1978;42(2):660–8.

11. Rosen ST, Aisner J, Makuch RW, et al. Carcinomatous leptomeningitis in small cell lung cancer: a clinicopathologic review of the National Cancer Institute experience. Medicine 1982;61(1):45–53.

12. Yap HY, Yap BS, Tashima CK, et al. Meningeal carcinomatosis in breast cancer. Cancer 1978;42(1):283–6.

13. DeAngelis LM, Posner JB. Neurologic complications of cancer (Contemporary neurology series). New York: Oxford University Press; 2009.

14. Tsukada Y, Fouad A, Pickren JW, et al. Central nervous system metastasis from breast carcinoma. Autopsy study. Cancer 1983;52(12):2349–54.

15. Aroney RS, Dalley DN, Chan WK, et al. Meningeal carcinomatosis in small cell carcinoma of the lung. Am J Med 1981;71(1):26–32.

16. Niwińska A, Rudnicka H, Murawska M. Breast cancer leptomeningeal metastasis: propensity of breast cancer subtypes for leptomeninges and the analysis of factors influencing survival. Med Oncol 2013;30(1):408.

17. Arpino G, Bardou VJ, Clark GM, et al. Infiltrating lobular carcinoma of the breast: tumor characteristics and clinical outcome. Breast Cancer Res 2004;6(3):R149–56.

18. Brewster AM, Chavez-macgregor M, Brown P. Epidemiology, biology, and treatment of triple-negative breast cancer in women of African ancestry. Lancet Oncol 2014;15(13):e625–34.

19. Yust-Katz S, Garciarena P, Liu D, et al. Breast cancer and leptomeningeal disease (LMD): hormone receptor status influences time to development of LMD and survival from LMD diagnosis. J Neurooncol 2013;114:229–35.

20. Glass JP, Melamed M, Chernik NL, et al. Malignant cells in cerebrospinal fluid (CSF): the meaning of a positive CSF cytology. Neurology 1979;29(10):1369–75.

21. Li YS, Jiang BY, Yang JJ, et al. Leptomeningeal metastases in patients with NSCLC with EGFR mutations. J Thorac Oncol 2016;11(11):1962–9.

22. Clarke JL, Perez HR, Jacks LM, et al. Leptomeningeal metastases in the MRI era. Neurology 2010;74(18):1449–54.

23. Waki F, Ando M, Takashima A, et al. Prognostic factors and clinical outcomes in patients with leptomeningeal metastasis from solid tumors. J Neurooncol 2009;93(2):205–12.

24. Boyle R, Thomas M, Adams JH. Diffuse involvement of the leptomeninges by tumour—a clinical and pathological study of 63 cases. Postgrad Med J 1980;56(653):149–58.

25. Suki D, Abouassi H, Patel AJ, et al. Comparative risk of leptomeningeal disease after resection or stereotactic radiosurgery for solid tumor metastasis to the posterior fossa. J Neurosurg 2008;108(2):248–57.

26. Suki D, Hatiboglu MA, Patel AJ, et al. Comparative risk of leptomeningeal dissemination of cancer after surgery or stereotactic radiosurgery for a single supratentorial solid tumor metastasis. Neurosurgery 2009;64(4):664–74.

27. Spector R, Robert snodgrass S, Johanson CE. A balanced view of the cerebrospinal fluid composition and functions: focus on adult humans. Exp Neurol 2015;273:57–68.

28. Chiang AC, Massagué J. Molecular basis of metastasis. N Engl J Med 2008;359(26):2814–23.

29. Fan Y, Zhu X, Xu Y, et al. Cell-cycle and DNA-damage response pathway is involved in leptomeningeal metastasis of non-small cell lung cancer. Clin Cancer Res 2018;24(1):209–16.

30. Groves MD, Hess KR, Puduvalli VK, et al. Biomarkers of disease: cerebrospinal fluid vascular endothelial growth factor (VEGF) and stromal cell derived factor (SDF)-1 levels in patients with neoplastic meningitis (NM) due to breast cancer, lung cancer and melanoma. J Neurooncol 2009;94(2):229–34.

31. Herrlinger U, Wiendl H, Renninger M, et al. Vascular endothelial growth factor (VEGF) in leptomeningeal metastasis: diagnostic and prognostic value. Br J Cancer 2004;91(2):219–24.

32. Reijneveld JC, Brandsma D, Boogerd W, et al. CSF levels of angiogenesis-related proteins in patients with leptomeningeal metastases. Neurology 2005;65(7):1120–2.

33. Boire A, Zou Y, Shieh J, et al. Complement component 3 adapts the cerebrospinal fluid for leptomeningeal metastasis. Cell 2017;168(6):1101–13.e13.

34. Smalley I, Law V, Wyatt C, et al. Proteomic analysis of CSF from patients with leptomeningeal melanoma metastases identifies signatures associated with disease progression and therapeutic resistance. Clin Cancer Res 2020. https://doi.org/10.1158/1078-0432.CCR-19-2840.

35. Tellez-gabriel M, Ory B, Lamoureux F, et al. Tumour heterogeneity: the key advantages of single-cell analysis. Int J Mol Sci 2016;17(12):2142.

36. Lawson DA, Kessenbrock K, Davis RT, et al. Tumour heterogeneity and metastasis at single-cell resolution. Nat Cell Biol 2018;20(12):1349–60.

37. Wan JCM, Massie C, Garcia-Corbacho J, et al. Liquid biopsies come of age: towards implementation of circulating tumour DNA. Nat Rev Cancer 2017;17(4):223–38.

38. Pan W, Gu W, Nagpal S, et al. Brain tumor mutations detected in cerebral spinal fluid. Clin Chem 2015;61(3):514–22.

39. De Mattos-Arruda L, Mayor R, Ng CKY, et al. Cerebrospinal fluid-derived circulating tumour DNA better represents the genomic alterations of brain tumours than plasma. Nat Commun 2015;6:8839.

40. Li YS, Jiang BY, Yang JJ, et al. Unique genetic profiles from cerebrospinal fluid cell-free DNA in leptomeningeal metastases of EGFR-mutant non-small-cell lung cancer: a new medium of liquid biopsy. Ann Oncol 2018;29(4):945–52.

41. Zheng MM, Li YS, Jiang BY, et al. Clinical utility of cerebrospinal fluid cell-free DNA as liquid biopsy for leptomeningeal metastases in ALK-rearranged NSCLC. J Thorac Oncol 2019;14(5):924–32.

42. Song Y, Liu P, Huang Y, et al. Osimertinib quantitative and gene variation analyses in cerebrospinal fluid and plasma of a non-small cell lung cancer patient with leptomeningeal metastases. Curr Cancer Drug Targets 2019;19(8):666–73.

43. Ge M, Zhan Q, Zhang Z, et al. Different next-generation sequencing pipelines based detection of tumor DNA in cerebrospinal fluid of lung adenocarcinoma cancer patients with leptomeningeal metastases. BMC Cancer 2019;19(1):143.

44. Huang R, Xu X, Li D, et al. Digital PCR-based detection of EGFR mutations in paired plasma and CSF samples of lung adenocarcinoma patients with central nervous system metastases. Target Oncol 2019;14(3):343–50.

45. Ma C, Huang C, Tang D, et al. Afatinib for advanced non-small cell lung cancer in a case with an uncommon epidermal growth factor receptor mutation (G719A) identified in the cerebrospinal fluid. Front Oncol 2019;9:628.

46. Aldea M, Hendriks L, Mezquita L, et al. Circulating tumor DNA analysis for patients with oncogene-addicted NSCLC with isolated central nervous system progression. J Thorac Oncol 2020;15(3):383–91.

47. van Bussel MTJ, Pluim D, Milojkovic Kerklaan B, et al. Circulating epithelial tumor cell analysis in CSF in patients with leptomeningeal metastases. Neurology 2020;94(5):e521–8.

48. Ma C, Yang X, Xing W, et al. Detection of circulating tumor DNA from non-small cell lung cancer brain metastasis in cerebrospinal fluid samples. Thorac Cancer 2020;11(3):588–93.

49. Li Y, Liu B, Connolly ID, et al. Recurrently mutated genes differ between leptomeningeal and solid lung cancer brain metastases. J Thorac Oncol 2018;13(7):1022–7.

50. Siravegna G, Geuna E, Mussolin B, et al. Genotyping tumour DNA in cerebrospinal fluid and plasma of a HER2-positive breast cancer patient with brain metastases. ESMO Open 2017;2(4):e000253.

51. Pentsova EI, Shah RH, Tang J, et al. Evaluating cancer of the central nervous system through next-generation sequencing of cerebrospinal fluid. J Clin Oncol 2016;34(20):2404–15.

52. Li Y, Pan W, Connolly ID, et al. Tumor DNA in cerebral spinal fluid reflects clinical course in a patient with melanoma leptomeningeal brain metastases. J Neurooncol 2016;128(1):93–100.

53. Ballester LY, Glitza Oliva IC, Douse DY, et al. Evaluating circulating tumor DNA from the cerebrospinal fluid of patients with melanoma and leptomeningeal disease. J Neuropathol Exp Neurol 2018;77(7):628–35.

54. Momtaz P, Pentsova E, Abdel-Wahab O, et al. Quantification of tumor-derived cell free DNA (cfDNA) by digital PCR (DigPCR) in cerebrospinal fluid of patients with BRAFV600 mutated malignancies. Oncotarget 2016;7(51):85430–6.

55. Farhadian SF, Mehta SS, Zografou C, et al. Single-cell RNA sequencing reveals microglia-like cells in cerebrospinal fluid during virologically suppressed HIV. JCI Insight 2018;3(18):e121718.

56. Yang Z, Guo Q, Wang Y, et al. AZD3759, a BBB-penetrating EGFR inhibitor for the treatment of EGFR mutant NSCLC with CNS metastases. Sci Transl Med 2016;8(368):368ra172.

57. Janczewski KH, Chalk CL, Pyles RB, et al. A simple, reproducible technique for establishing leptomeningeal tumors in nude rats. J Neurosci Methods 1998;85(1):45–9.

58. Nanjo S, Arai S, Wang W, et al. MET copy number gain is associated with gefitinib resistance in leptomeningeal carcinomatosis of EGFR-mutant lung cancer. Mol Cancer Ther 2017;16(3):506–15.

59. Arai S, Takeuchi S, Fukuda K, et al. Osimertinib overcomes alectinib resistance caused by amphiregulin in a leptomeningeal carcinomatosis model of ALK-rearranged lung cancer. J Thorac Oncol 2020;15(5):752–65.

60. Grossman SA, Spence A. NCCN clinical practice guidelines for carcinomatous/lymphomatous meningitis. Oncology 1999;13(11A):144–52.

61. Jaeckle KA, Phuphanich S, Bent MJ, et al. Intrathecal treatment of neoplastic meningitis due to breast cancer with a slow-release formulation of cytarabine. Br J Cancer 2001;84(2):157–63.

62. Chamberlain MC, Kormanik PR. Carcinomatous meningitis secondary to breast cancer: predictors of response to combined modality therapy. J Neurooncol 1997;35(1):55–64.

63. Morris PG, Reiner AS, Szenberg OR, et al. Leptomeningeal metastasis from non-small cell lung

cancer: survival and the impact of whole brain radiotherapy. J Thorac Oncol 2012;7(2):382–5.

64. Gani C, Müller AC, Eckert F, et al. Outcome after whole brain radiotherapy alone in intracranial leptomeningeal carcinomatosis from solid tumors. Strahlenther Onkol 2012;188(2):148–53.

65. Gunther JR, Rahman AR, Dong W, et al. Craniospinal irradiation prior to stem cell transplant for hematologic malignancies with CNS involvement: effectiveness and toxicity after photon or proton treatment. Pract Radiat Oncol 2017;7(6):e401–8.

66. Walker GV, Shihadeh F, Kantarjian H, et al. Comprehensive craniospinal radiation for controlling central nervous system leukemia. Int J Radiat Oncol Biol Phys 2014;90(5):1119–25.

67. Chamberlain MC, Kormanik P. Carcinoma meningitis secondary to non–small cell lung cancer: combined modality therapy. Arch Neurol 1998;55(4): 506–12.

68. Souchon R, Feyer P, Thomssen C, et al. Clinical recommendations of DEGRO and AGO on preferred standard palliative radiotherapy of bone and cerebral metastases, metastatic spinal cord compression, and leptomeningeal carcinomatosis in breast cancer. Breast Care (Basel) 2010;5(6): 401–7.

69. Chang EL, Maor MH. Standard and novel radiotherapeutic approaches to neoplastic meningitis. Curr Oncol Rep 2003;5(1):24–8.

70. Soussain C, Ricard D, Fike JR, et al. CNS complications of radiotherapy and chemotherapy. Lancet 2009;374(9701):1639–51.

71. Pan Z, Yang G, He H, et al. Concurrent radiotherapy and intrathecal methotrexate for treating leptomeningeal metastasis from solid tumors with adverse prognostic factors: a prospective and single-arm study. Int J Cancer 2016;139(8): 1864–72.

72. Oechsle K, Lange-Brock V, Kruell A, et al. Prognostic factors and treatment options in patients with leptomeningeal metastases of different primary tumors: a retrospective analysis. J Cancer Res Clin Oncol 2010;136(11):1729–35.

73. Rudnicka H, Niwinska A, Murawska M. Breast cancer leptomeningeal metastasis–the role of multimodality treatment. J Neurooncol 2007;84(1):57–62.

74. Mack F, Baumert BG, Schäfer N, et al. Therapy of leptomeningeal metastasis in solid tumors. Cancer Treat Rev 2016;43:83–91.

75. Le Rhun E, Taillibert S, Zairi F, et al. A retrospective case series of 103 consecutive patients with leptomeningeal metastasis and breast cancer. J Neurooncol 2013;113(1):83–92.

76. Segura PP, Gil M, Balañá C, et al. Phase II trial of temozolomide for leptomeningeal metastases in patients with solid tumors. J Neurooncol 2012; 109(1):137–42.

77. Glantz MJ, Cole BF, Recht L, et al. High-dose intravenous methotrexate for patients with nonleukemic leptomeningeal cancer: is intrathecal chemotherapy necessary? J Clin Oncol 1998;16(4): 1561–7.

78. Lassman AB, Abrey LE, Shah GD, et al. Systemic high-dose intravenous methotrexate for central nervous system metastases. J Neurooncol 2006;78(3): 255–60.

79. Ekenel M, Hormigo AM, Peak S, et al. Capecitabine therapy of central nervous system metastases from breast cancer. J Neurooncol 2007;85(2):223–7.

80. Giglio P, Tremont-Lukats IW, Groves MD. Response of neoplastic meningitis from solid tumors to oral capecitabine. J Neurooncol 2003;65(2):167–72.

81. Paydas S, Bicakci K, Yavuz S. Dramatic response with capecitabine after cranial radiation to the brain parenchymal and leptomeningeal metastases from lung cancer. Eur J Intern Med 2009;20(1):96–9.

82. Rogers LR, Remer SE, Tejwani S. Durable response of breast cancer leptomeningeal metastasis to capecitabine monotherapy. Neuro Oncol 2004;6(1):63–4.

83. How J, Mann J, Laczniak AN, et al. Pulsatile erlotinib in EGFR-positive non-small-cell lung cancer patients with leptomeningeal and brain metastases: review of the literature. Clin Lung Cancer 2017;18(4):354–63.

84. Frick J, Ritch PS, Hansen RM, et al. Successful treatment of meningeal leukemia using systemic high-dose cytosine arabinoside. J Clin Oncol 1984;2(5):365–8.

85. Morra E, Lazzarino M, Brusamolino E, et al. The role of systemic high-dose cytarabine in the treatment of central nervous system leukemia. Clinical results in 46 patients. Cancer 1993;72(2):439–45.

86. Chamberlain MC. Neoplastic meningitis. Neurologist 2006;12(4):179–87.

87. Chamberlain MC, Kormanik PA, Barba D. Complications associated with intraventricular chemotherapy in patients with leptomeningeal metastases. J Neurosurg 1997;87(5):694–9.

88. Chamberlain MC. Neoplastic meningitis. Oncologist 2008;13(9):967–77.

89. Chamberlain MC. Leptomeningeal metastasis. Semin Neurol 2010;30(3):236–44.

90. Szvalb AD, Raad II, Weinberg JS, et al. Ommaya reservoir-related infections: clinical manifestations and treatment outcomes. J Infect 2014;68(3): 216–24.

91. Boogerd W, van den Bent MJ, Koehler PJ, et al. The relevance of intraventricular chemotherapy for leptomeningeal metastasis in breast cancer: a randomised study. Eur J Cancer 2004;40(18): 2726–33.

92. Bokstein F, Lossos A, Siegal T. Leptomeningeal metastases from solid tumors: a comparison of

two prospective series treated with and without intra-cerebrospinal fluid chemotherapy. Cancer 1998;82(9):1756–63.

93. An YJ, Cho HR, Kim TM, et al. An NMR metabolomics approach for the diagnosis of leptomeningeal carcinomatosis in lung adenocarcinoma cancer patients. Int J Cancer 2015;136(1):162–71.

94. Chamberlain MC, Sandy AD, Press GA. Leptomeningeal metastasis: a comparison of gadolinium-enhanced MR and contrast-enhanced CT of the brain. Neurology 1990;40(3 Pt 1):435–8.

95. Hatzoglou V, Karimi S, Diamond EL, et al. Nonenhancing leptomeningeal metastases: imaging characteristics and potential causative factors. Neurohospitalist 2016;6(1):24–8.

96. Darvin P, Toor SM, Sasidharan Nair V, et al. Immune checkpoint inhibitors: recent progress and potential biomarkers. Exp Mol Med 2018;50(12):1–11.

97. Bot I, Blank CU, Brandsma D. Clinical and radiological response of leptomeningeal melanoma after whole brain radiotherapy and ipilimumab. J Neurol 2012;259(9):1976–8.

98. Geukes foppen MH, Brandsma D, Blank CU, et al. Targeted treatment and immunotherapy in leptomeningeal metastases from melanoma. Ann Oncol 2016;27(6):1138–42.

99. Glitza IC, Rohlfs M, Guha-Thakurta N, et al. Retrospective review of metastatic melanoma patients with leptomeningeal disease treated with intrathecal interleukin-2. ESMO Open 2018;3(1): e000283.

100. Ferguson SD, Bindal S, Bassett RL Jr, et al. Predictors of survival in metastatic melanoma patients with leptomeningeal disease (LMD). J Neurooncol 2019;142(3):499–509.

101. Hendriks LEL, Bootsma G, Mourlanette J, et al. Survival of patients with non-small cell lung cancer having leptomeningeal metastases treated with immune checkpoint inhibitors. Eur J Cancer 2019; 116:182–9.

102. Bover M, Yarza R, Docampo LI. Four-year lasting sustained complete response after nivolumab in a patient with non-small-cell lung cancer and confirmed leptomeningeal carcinomatosis: changing the paradigm. Clin Lung Cancer 2020;21(1):e1–5.

103. Gion M, Remon J, Caramella C, et al. Symptomatic leptomeningeal metastasis improvement with nivolumab in advanced non-small cell lung cancer patient. Lung Cancer 2017;108:72–4.

104. Dudnik E, Yust-Katz S, Nechushtan H, et al. Intracranial response to nivolumab in NSCLC patients with untreated or progressing CNS metastases. Lung Cancer 2016;98:114–7.

105. Brastianos PK, Prakadan S, Alvarez-Breckenridge C, et al. Phase II study of pembrolizumab in leptomeningeal carcinomatosis. J Clin Oncol 2018;36:2007.

106. Nabors LB, Portnow J, Ammirati M, et al. NCCN guidelines insights: central nervous system cancers, version 1.2017. J Natl Compr Canc Netw 2017;15(11):1331–45.

107. Cohen JV, Kluger HM. Systemic immunotherapy for the treatment of brain metastases. Front Oncol 2016;6:49.

108. Azad TD, Pan J, Connolly ID, et al. Therapeutic strategies to improve drug delivery across the blood-brain barrier. Neurosurg Focus 2015;38(3):E9.

109. Kinoshita M, Mcdannold N, Jolesz FA, et al. Noninvasive localized delivery of herceptin to the mouse brain by MRI-guided focused ultrasound-induced blood-brain barrier disruption. Proc Natl Acad Sci U S A 2006;103(31):11719–23.

110. Carpentier A, Canney M, Vignot A, et al. Clinical trial of blood-brain barrier disruption by pulsed ultrasound. Sci Transl Med 2016;8(343):343re2.

111. Mainprize T, Lipsman N, Huang Y, et al. Blood-brain barrier opening in primary brain tumors with non-invasive MR-guided focused ultrasound: a clinical safety and feasibility study. Sci Rep 2019; 9(1):321.

112. O'reilly MA, Chinnery T, Yee ML, et al. Preliminary investigation of focused ultrasound-facilitated drug delivery for the treatment of leptomeningeal metastases. Sci Rep 2018;8(1):9013.

113. Miliotou AN, Papadopoulou LC. CAR T-cell therapy: a new era in cancer immunotherapy. Curr Pharm Biotechnol 2018;19(1):5–18.

114. Priceman SJ, Tilakawardane D, Jeang B, et al. Regional delivery of chimeric antigen receptor-engineered T cells effectively targets HER2 breast cancer metastasis to the brain. Clin Cancer Res 2018;24(1):95–105.

115. Rohaan MW, Van den berg JH, Kvistborg P, et al. Adoptive transfer of tumor-infiltrating lymphocytes in melanoma: a viable treatment option. J Immunother Cancer 2018;6(1):102.

116. Glitza IC, Haymaker C, Bernatchez C, et al. Intrathecal administration of tumor-infiltrating lymphocytes is well tolerated in a patient with leptomeningeal disease from metastatic melanoma: a case report. Cancer Immunol Res 2015; 3(11):1201–6.

117. Nguyen LT, Saibil SD, Sotov V, et al. Phase II clinical trial of adoptive cell therapy for patients with metastatic melanoma with autologous tumor-infiltrating lymphocytes and low-dose interleukin-2. Cancer Immunol Immunother 2019;68(5): 773–85.

118. Kumthekar P, Tang SC, Brenner AJ, et al. ANG1005, a brain penetrating peptide-drug conjugate, shows activity in patients with breast cancer with leptomeningeal carcinomatosis and recurrent brain metastases. Clin Cancer Res 2020;26(12): 2789–99.

Immune Therapy for Central Nervous System Metastasis

Malia B. McAvoy, BS, MS[a], Bryan D. Choi, MD, PhD[b],
Pamela S. Jones, MD, MS, MPH[c],*

KEYWORDS

- Immunotherapy • Brain metastasis • Checkpoint inhibitors • Abscopal effect

KEY POINTS

- There has been growth in the clinical use of immunotherapy for central nervous system metastases.
- Immune checkpoint inhibitors have shown efficacy in patients with melanoma, renal cell carcinoma, and lung cancer brain metastases.
- Future research into the molecular determinates that lead to greater response to immune therapy is critical to expanding the potential of these therapies.

INTRODUCTION

Brain metastases cause devastating neurologic complications leading to substantial morbidity and mortality. Current treatment of brain metastases involves a multidisciplinary approach consisting of radiation, surgery and systemic chemotherapies. These treatments have been largely palliative, failing to improve survival for most patients. Until recently, a limited number of new systemic treatments have been developed for these patients.

The few advances that have decreased mortality involve targeted therapies for patients with specific mutations. Routine screening for mutations in *EGFR*, *BRAF*, *MET*, *KRAS*, and *HER2*, rearrangements in *ALK*, *ROS1*, *RET*, *NTRK*, and *NRG1*, as well as amplifications in *HER2* and *MET*, allow identification of cellular vulnerabilities that may be exploited with specific therapies inhibiting the kinase of interest. For instance, alectinib, a selective inhibitor of anaplastic lymphoma kinase (ALK) has been shown to decrease central nervous system (CNS) progression and death among patients with ALK-positive non–small cell lung cancer

(NSCLC).[1] However, targeting specific molecular subgroups may only be relevant for a limited number of patients.

Another approach to targeting metastases more broadly involves identification of specific processes by which these tumors evolve, especially with regard to their tumor microenvironments (TMEs). The recent study of interactions between cancer cells and noncancerous cells including endothelial cells, pericytes, fibroblasts, and immune cells in metastasis has led to the identification of more targets that drive metastatic growth.[2] Moreover, the concurrent development of monoclonal antibodies disrupting these interactions, such as anti–cytotoxic T lymphocyte–associated antigen-4 (CTLA-4), anti–programmed cell death protein 1 (PD-1), and anti–programmed death-ligand 1 (PD-L1), has led to numerous US Food and Drug Administration (FDA) and European Medicines Agency approvals for treatment of metastatic melanoma, lung cancer, urothelial cancer, head and neck squamous cell carcinoma, renal cell cancer, and Hodgkin disease.[3]

Until 2010, patients with brain metastases were generally excluded from these immunotherapy

---

[a] University of Washington Medical Center, Department of Neurological Surgery, Box 356470, 1959 NE Pacific Street, Seattle, WA 98195-6470, USA; [b] Department of Neurosurgery, Massachusetts General Hospital, Harvard Medical School, 15 Parkman Street, WAC 3, Boston, MA 02114, USA; [c] Department of Neurosurgery, Massachusetts General Hospital, Harvard Medical School, 15 Parkman Street, WAC 745, Boston, MA 02114, USA
* Corresponding author.
E-mail address: psjones@mgh.harvard.edu

Neurosurg Clin N Am 31 (2020) 627–639
https://doi.org/10.1016/j.nec.2020.06.014
1042-3680/20/© 2020 Elsevier Inc. All rights reserved.

clinical trials because of the presumption that the blood-brain barrier (BBB) would prevent the therapeutic agents from reaching the brain.[4,5] The belief that the BBB is disrupted during brain metastasis has been disproved in side-by-side comparisons of drugs with and without chemical modifications allowing for BBB permeability showing only brain-permeable drugs treated brain metastasis.[6] Nevertheless, a few small molecule immune inhibitors, such as erlotinib, afatinib and lapatinib, have shown some ability to cross the BBB,[7,8] and T cells activated by systemic immunotherapies are able to pass through this barrier and mount an antitumor response within the brain.[9,10] Altogether, this work has inspired further research into immune cell interactions with metastatic brain tumors and paved the way to several clinical trials applying immune checkpoint inhibitors to patients harboring brain metastases.

SYSTEMIC IMMUNOTHERAPIES

The immune surveillance hypothesis suggests that the immune system is a key player in suppressing tumor growth. The first experimental evidence supporting this hypothesis emerged in 2001 showing the co-operation of lymphocytes and interferon-gamma in inhibiting the development of both spontaneous and carcinogen-induced tumors in genetically engineered mice lacking a functional immune system.[11] Antitumor responses by the immune system may be counteracted through regulatory mechanisms that act to mitigate T-cell responses, such as via upregulation of CTLA-4 or PD-1 receptors or through tumor-mediated immune suppression.

Validation of the immune surveillance hypothesis led to the rapid development of immune-based anticancer therapies. One strategy has been to target the receptors through which tumor cells interact with immune cells. Homeostasis of the immune system is mediated through the interplay of costimulatory (agonistic) and coinhibitory (antagonistic) signals delivered by surface receptors belonging to the immunoglobulin or tumor necrosis factor families.[12] Enhancement of antitumor immune response may be generated through development of monoclonal antibodies against these receptors, inhibiting their functions. This strategy has been referred to as immune checkpoint inhibition (CPI). Another immunotherapy is called adoptive cell therapy (ACT) with autologous tumor-infiltrating lymphocytes (TILs), in which naturally existing tumor-reactive T cells are isolated from the patient's tissue and reinfused after in vitro activation and expansion. Response rates among patients with metastatic melanoma of up to 50%, including complete tumor regression in 10% to 20% of patients, have been reported from several institutions.[13–16] One disadvantage of TIL therapy is that many cancer types can escape the T cell–mediated immune responses through downregulation or loss of their major histocompatibility complex (MHC) expression.[17] To circumvent the need for MHC expression, T cells have been engineered using viral particles to express receptors on their cell surfaces called chimeric antigen receptors (CARs). These receptors allow T cells to recognize antigens on tumor cells and mount an immune response against the tumor.

Checkpoint Inhibition

Treatment with monoclonal antibodies targeting CTLA-4 and/or PD-1 have shown significant clinical efficacy across a wide range of tumors (**Table 1**).[18] CTLA-4 lies on the surface of T cells and binds to cluster of differentiation (CD) 80/CD86 on antigen-presenting cells within the lymph node to dampen early T-cell activation.[19] Successful blockade of CTLA-4 inhibits regulatory T cell–associated immune suppression and promotes CD4+ and CD8+ T-cell effector function.[20,21] Treatment with anti–CTLA-4 monoclonal antibody, ipilimumab, led to improved survival among patients with unresectable stage III/IV melanoma. Subsequently, ipilimumab became the first CPI approved by the FDA in 2011.

The PD-1 receptor is located on the surface of activated T cells as well as B cells and myeloid cells. Binding of PD-1 to either PD-L1, expressed in a wide variety of cells, or PD-L2, expressed by dendritic cells and monocytes, occurs within target organs, leading to inhibition of the effector phase of T-cell activation.[22] PD-L1 is expressed by many tumors in order to evade the immune system. Chronic antigen exposure can upregulate PD-1 expression and lead to T-cell exhaustion, another mechanism that prevents detection of tumor cells by the immune system.[19] Blockade of the PD-1 pathway also enhances antitumor T-cell reactivity and prevents T-cell exhaustion. In 2014, the FDA approved nivolumab as the first PD-1 targeting therapy based on the results of the CheckMate-037 trial, which showed improved response rates to nivolumab versus investigator's choice chemotherapy among patients with unresectable or metastatic melanoma whose cancers had progressed despite treatment with ipilimumab and/or a BRAF inhibitor.[13] The number of indications for which CPIs have been approved has now increased to more than 20, with atezolizumab/anti–PD-L1 for triple-negative breast cancer as one of the latest indications.[23]

Table 1
Current Food and Drug Administration–approved immune checkpoint inhibitors

Checkpoint Inhibitor	Target	FDA-Approved Indications
Ipilimumab	CTLA-4	Metastatic melanoma
Nivolumab	PD-1	Metastatic melanoma, non–small cell lung cancer, renal cell carcinoma, Hodgkin lymphoma, head and neck cancer (squamous), mismatch repair deficient and microsatellite instability high colorectal cancer
Pembrolizumab	PD-1	Metastatic melanoma, non–small cell lung cancer, head and neck cancer (squamous), urothelial cell carcinoma, Hodgkin lymphoma, mismatch repair deficient and microsatellite instability high solid tumor
Atezolizumab	PD-L1	Urothelial cell carcinoma, non–small cell lung cancer, triple-negative breast cancer
Nivolumab + ipilimumab	PD-1, CTLA-4	Metastatic melanoma
Avelumab	PD-L1	Metastatic Merkel cell carcinoma, urothelial cell carcinoma
Durvalumab	PD-L1	Urothelial cell carcinoma

Adapted from National Cancer Institute. Annual plan & budget proposal for fiscal year 2019. Available at: https://www.cancer.gov/about-nci/budget/plan/2019-annual-plan-budget-proposal.pdf.

Tumor-Infiltrating Lymphocyte Therapy

ACT with TILs involves outgrowth of tumor-resident T cells followed by expansion ex vivo and transfer back into the same patient after the patient undergoes lymphodepletion.[24] Lymphodepletion involves the removal of regulatory T cells and cellular sinks such as natural killer cells that highly compete with the adoptively transferred T cells for the host homeostatic cytokines interleukin (IL)-7 and IL-15. IL-7 is important for the proliferation and survival of T cells and IL-15 is crucial for maintenance and function of the T cells.[25] Many studies have shown that infused T cells are supported by high-dose IL-2 to facilitate engraftment of the cells.[26] IL-2 is thought to enhance the antitumor response by providing continuous support of growth and activity of the TILs.[27]

The first demonstration of TIL clinical efficacy was among patients with metastatic melanoma in the 1990s and, since then, multiple clinical trials have shown objective responses varying between 40% and 70%.[27–30] The promising results of TIL therapy in melanoma have influenced numerous centers to replicate these studies.[14,29,31,32] Toxicities during TIL therapy are often caused by the effects of lymphodepleting regimens and subsequent IL-2 after TIL infusion, including hypotension, nausea, and anemia, although these tend to be transient.[33,34] TIL therapy has now been described for treatment of a variety of solid cancers other than melanoma, including ovarian, breast, colon, and cervical.[35–38]

Chimeric Antigen Receptor T Cells

Although the use of TILs has been promising in the treatment of metastatic melanoma, the success of TILs has been limited against other cancer types, possibly because melanoma is particularly immunogenic and has a higher affinity for immune clearance.[37,39] These limitations have led to the development of new methods by which peripheral mononuclear cells are genetically engineered to express exogenous T-cell receptor or CAR, rendering the cell tumor specific. The initial investigations of CAR T-cell therapies have largely focused on treatment of relapsed acute lymphocytic leukemia (ALL). In a trial of 75 patients with refractory ALL treated with a CD19-targeted CAR T-cell therapy, called tisagenlecleucel, remission with long-term persistence was observed, albeit with transient high-grade toxic effects.[40] Most patients experienced an adverse effect called cytokine release syndrome (CRS), which is a systemic inflammatory response caused by cytokines released by infused CAR T cells.[41] CRS may lead to widespread reversible organ dysfunction. Also evident among patients undergoing CAR T-cell therapy were neurologic toxicities, which may occur in the absence of CRS toxicities, suggesting the neurologic effects have a different mechanism.[40] Reported neurologic toxicities range from headaches and confusion to necessitation of mechanical ventilation for airway protection in the absence of respiratory failure.[42–45]

Since the use of CAR T cells to treat ALL, this therapy has shown unprecedented success in the treatment of relapsed or chemotherapy-refractory chronic lymphocytic leukemia[46–48] and non-Hodgkin lymphoma,[49–52] and clinical trials are currently underway to focus on translating this treatment to solid tumors, including brain tumors. The brain microenvironment, previously thought to be an immune-privileged site, does present unique challenges to the application of CAR T-cell therapy because the immune system access to the brain is tightly controlled to protect against immunologic attack.[53] Despite this challenge, CAR T cells have shown the ability to penetrate the BBB and infiltrate the brain diffusely, suggesting that the ability to mount a T-cell response against a brain tumor may overcome the challenges associated with poor drug delivery to the brain.[54]

BRAIN METASTASIS MICROENVIRONMENT

Several features make the TME of the brain distinctive from other tissues, and these include the composition of the extracellular matrix and unique tissue-resident cells such as microglia, astrocytes, and neurons. In addition, the brain environment is protected from systemic inflammation by the BBB. There are several proposed reasons for protection of the brain from an inflammatory reaction given the risk of cytotoxicity to neurons and resulting edema, which would lead to increased intracranial pressure.[2]

Although the TME of primary brain tumors has been described extensively,[55,56] there has been little literature describing the TME of metastatic brain tumors. Most research on the TME of metastatic brain tumors has focused on the role of reactive astrocytes. Only a small fraction of micrometastases reach a clinically significant size, and this is thought to be because of the protective actions of astrocytes.[57–59] Astrocytes are extremely abundant within the brain microenvironment and are not found in any other tissues. Therefore, metastatic cells must develop new mechanisms to interact with astrocytes and survive.[2,60] From an immunologic perspective, astrocytes and metastatic tumor cells may directly communicate with each other to support growth through gap junctions and release of cytokines and inflammatory mediators. Human and mouse breast and lung tumor cells express protocadherin 7, which causes astrocytes to construct gap junctions composed of connexin 43.[58] Brain metastatic cancer cells then use these channels to

transfer cyclic GAMP to astrocytes, which causes production of inflammatory cytokines interferon (IFN)-α and tumor necrosis factor (TNF)-α. These cytokines then activate Signal transducer and activator of transcription 1 (STAT1) and nuclear factor κB pathways in metastatic cells supporting tumor growth and resistance to chemotherapies. Also, IL-8 released by metastatic lung cancer cells may activate astrocytes leading to production of growth factors such as IL-6, IL-1β, and TNF-α.[61] Furthermore, in vitro studies showed that neurotrophic factors secreted by astrocytes such as IL-6, transforming growth factor-β, insulinlike growth factor-1, and chemokine ligand (CXCL) 12a may all play a role in breast cancer metastasis to the brain.[62,63]

The functions of microglia, the resident antigen-presenting cells within the central nervous system, are also used by metastatic cells for proliferation. Microglia densely infiltrate the peritumoral area of brain metastases,[64] and model systems using metastatic breast cancer cells show extensive reactive gliosis surrounding metastases followed by a 5-fold increase in metastatic cell proliferation caused by promitotic factors secreted by microglia.[65] However, cytotoxic activation of microglia seems to be minor, suggesting that brain metastatic cells may have protective mechanisms against NO-induced lysis.[64] Microglia may also enhance invasion of brain parenchyma through activation of WNT signaling–dependent pathways.[66]

In addition to resident astrocytes and microglia, TILs,[67] cells of the macrophage lineage,[68] myeloid-derived suppressor cells, and cancer-associated fibroblasts all assist in tumor growth and have been observed in the brain recruited by metastatic melanoma, breast, and colon cancer cells.[69] The number of TILs correlates positively with patient survival and peritumoral edema within the brain.[67] However, recruited immune cells enable tumor evasion by reducing expression of costimulatory molecules of T cells, including CD80, CD86, and CD40, which impairs antigen presentation.[55,70] As previously discussed, another effect of brain metastasis cell interaction with T cells is T-cell exhaustion, with CTLA-4 and PD-1 ligand binding both serving to downregulate T-cell proliferation.[71] Other mechanisms of T-cell exhaustion in brain metastasis remain an active area of investigation.

IMMUNOTHERAPY FOR DIRECT TREATMENT OF BRAIN METASTASIS
Melanoma

The first immunotherapy to be used in the treatment of metastatic melanoma was IL-2, a cytokine that plays a key role in activation and proliferation of T cells.[72] High-dose IL-2 led to a complete response among 5% of 270 patients with metastatic melanoma without intracranial metastases, although toxicities were severe, with 2% of patients dying from sepsis.[73] There is evidence of IL-2 efficacy intracranially, although patients with brain metastasis were generally excluded from trials to protect patients against vascular leak syndrome worsening intracranial edema and thrombocytopenia.[74,75]

Among patients with melanoma brain metastases, there have been several trials investigating the efficacy of CPI (**Table 2**). The first phase 2 prospective study (NCT00623766) investigated the efficacy of ipilimumab.[5] Intracranial efficacy of ipilimumab had previously been observed in a post hoc analysis of a phase 3 study showing improved overall survival (OS) among patients with metastatic melanoma treated with ipilimumab.[4] In the phase 2 study of patients with melanoma brain metastasis, unexpected toxic side effects were not observed. However, 2 years after the start of treatment, the OS for patients treated with ipilimumab alone was 26%, whereas symptomatic patients requiring steroid therapy had an OS of only 10%. These results may suggest that steroid treatment at the initiation of ipilimumab could downregulate the immune response expected with immune blockade therapy.[76] This effect of steroid therapy is a particularly important confounder given that high doses of steroids are often used among patients undergoing radiation, particularly whole-brain radiation therapy to mitigate intracranial edema. Since the publication of this study, many institutions use lower doses of steroids and for a shorter duration during stereotactic radiation, and some have even ceased the previous practice of using steroids for all patients with intracranial metastases.[77] Another study using ipilimumab to treat 146 patients with asymptomatic melanoma brain metastases showed a disease control rate of 27% with median progression-free survival (PFS) and OS of 2.8 and 4.3 months, respectively.[78]

Nivolumab and pembrolizumab, both monoclonal antibodies against PD-1, have both been approved for treating patients with metastatic melanoma, and randomized phase II and III trials have shown the superiority of this combination therapy among patients with untreated metastatic melanoma compared with ipilimumab alone, although in both trials patients with brain metastases were excluded.[79–81] One recent phase II trial of pembrolizumab for 23 patients with untreated brain metastases from NSCLC or melanoma showed median PFS and OS times of 2 and 17 months, respectively.[82]

Three combination therapy trials have been published and 1 is ongoing. Tawbi and colleagues[83] described a phase 2 study of 94 patients with previously untreated metastatic melanoma undergoing therapy with combined nivolumab plus ipilimumab. Intracranial responses were observed among 57% of patients and were concordant with extracranial activity, as previously shown with treatment using ipilimumab alone.[5] Another phase 2 trial showing outcomes of treatment with ipilimumab and fotemustine in patients with asymptomatic melanoma brain metastases showed control of brain metastases in 50% of patients and a median OS of 13.4 months.[84] Also, among patients who had undergone resection of melanoma brain metastases, subsequent ipilimumab was associated with prolonged survival.[85] In addition, there is an ongoing triple-arm phase III trial comparing the OS at 2 years of fotemustine monotherapy, combination ipilimumab and fotemustine, or combination ipilimumab and nivolumab among patients with brain metastatic melanoma. The study is expected to reach completion by the end of 2020 (NCT02460068).

Melanoma-targeted CD19 CAR T cells delivered systemically have been shown to successfully traffic to the brain and achieve complete and durable regression of melanoma brain metastases. Hong and colleagues[86] described a subset of patients who were retrospectively identified to have untreated melanoma brain metastasis and extracranial disease. Seventeen of these patients were treated with T cells that were either autologous tumor-infiltrating cells or cells transduced to express a receptor targeting a melanoma-specific antigen. Seven of these patients (41%) achieved a complete response in the brain and 6 (35.3%) achieved a partial response. One patient developed a subarachnoid hemorrhage caused by treatment-related thrombocytopenia. The bleed was thought to be caused by tumor necrosis from therapy because of the extensive lymphocytic infiltration within the tumor. These results suggest that brain metastases are as responsive to T-cell therapies as extracranial tumors.

Renal Cell Cancer

Immunotherapies have dramatically changed the treatment paradigm of metastatic renal cell carcinoma (RCC), with long-term studies showing a 3-year and 5-year OS of 35% to 41% and 34% among patients treated with nivolumab.[87] Currently there are only small prospective and retrospective series including patients with RCC with brain metastases treated with immunotherapy, and few of these trials have reported the

Table 2
Immunotherapy clinical studies for treatment of brain metastases

Study	Design	Phase	Drug	Results
Melanoma				
Di Giacomo et al,[84] 2012	RCT	II	Ipilimumab + fomustine	DCR 50%
Margolin et al,[5] 2012	RCT	II	Ipilimumab	RR 24% for asymptomatic patients, RR 10% for symptomatic patients
Goldberg et al,[82] 2016	RCT	II	Pembrolizumab	RR 22% all responses ongoing at 24 mo
Long et al,[85] 2018	RCT	II	Ipilimumab + nivolumab or nivolumab alone	RR 46%, 17% complete responses; 54% grade 3–4 adverse events
Tawbi et al,[83] 2018	RCT	II	Ipilimumab + nivolumab followed by nivolumab alone	RR 57%, 26% complete responses; 55% grade 3–4 adverse events
Kluger et al,[82] 2019	RCT	II	Pembrolizumab	RR 26%
Renal Cell Carcinoma				
Escudier et al,[91] 2017	Case series	NA	Nivolumab	RR 23%; neurologic deterioration requiring steroids 32%
Bracarda et al,[93] 2018	EAP	NA	Nivolumab	DCR 53%, 3% complete response, 16% partial response, 34% stable disease
Flippot et al,[94] 2019	RCT	II	Nivolumab	RR 12% among previously untreated brain metastases
Non–small Cell Lung Cancer				
Goldberg et al,[99] 2016	RCT	II	Pembrolizumab	RR 33%
Goldman et al,[98] 2016	RCT	II	Nivolumab	DCR 33%
Gadgeel et al,[99] 2019	RCT	III	Atezolizumab vs docetaxel	Among asymptomatic, untreated patients: OS 16.9 vs 11.9 mo, respectively. Among asymptomatic, previously treated patients: OS 13.2 vs 9.3 mo, respectively

Abbreviations: DCR, disease control rate; EAP, expanded access program; NA, not available; OS, overall survival; RCT, randomized controlled trial; RR, response rate.

Data from Aquilanti E, Brastianos PK. Immune checkpoint inhibitors for brain metastases: a primer for neurosurgeons. Neurosurgery. 2020.

outcomes of this subgroup (see **Table 2**).[88] One case report of a patient with clear cell RCC with metastasis to the brain had been treated with pembrolizumab as a fourth line and showed regression of all brain metastases despite continued steroid treatment of 4 mg of dexamethasone per day after 7 months of treatment.[89] A second case report of a patient with clear cell RCC with brain metastasis describes treatment with second-line nivolumab and progression following 9 months of stereotactic radiation.[90] This patient underwent surgery for resection of the presumed progression, but pathologic analysis showed radiation necrosis without viable metastatic tumor. Nivolumab was continued for 3.5 years without any disease progression.

There have been several case series describing outcomes of patients with clear cell RCC with brain metastasis treated with nivolumab. One of these studies described the outcomes of 69 patients with brain metastases not taking steroids.[91] Preliminary data of 55 of these 69 patients were reported after 2.4 months (range, 0–9 months) of nivolumab and showed a 3-month PFS of 60%. Forty-four patients were assessed for intracranial response, of which 23% had an objective response and 48% had local progressive disease. Neurologic deterioration requiring steroids was evident among 32%. Another evaluation of 8 asymptomatic patients with RCC metastatic to the brain as part of the Nivolumab in Patients With Metastatic Renal Cell Carcinoma Who Have Progresses During or After Prior Systemic Antiangiogenic Regimen (NIVOREN) trial (EudraCT [European Union Drug Regulating Authorities Clinical Trials Database] 2015-004117) showed, at a median follow-up time of 8.1 months, that all patients were still alive.[92] Six patients were treatment naive for their brain metastases and all required focal therapy for treatment of early disease progression. Seven of the 8 patients experienced disease progression of brain metastasis requiring steroid use and nivolumab discontinuation. A report from the Italian Expanded Access Program described a series of 32 patients with RCC with brain metastases who relapsed after at least 1 prior systemic treatment and were then treated with nivolumab.[93] These patients achieved a disease control rate of 53%, comparable with the overall study population, including 1 complete response (3.1%), 5 partial responses (15.6%), and 11 stable diseases (34.4%).[94] Overall, many questions remain unanswered with regard to the role of immunotherapies for brain metastases arising from renal cell cancers. For instance, the role of nivolumab in non–clear cell RCC was evaluated in 2 retrospective series but the outcomes of the brain metastasis subgroup of patients was not reported.[95,96] There are 4 ongoing clinical trials of immunotherapies for treatment of brain metastasis in RCC (NCT02886585, NCT02978404, NCT02982954, NCT02669914).

Lung Cancer

Classically, inhibitors of PD-1 and PD-L1 have shown promising clinical activity against primary lung cancers leading to the FDA approval of nivolumab, pembrolizumab, and atezolizumab in lung cancer treatment (see **Table 2**). The currently available clinical data studying the effect of these immunotherapies among these patients with brain metastases have been comparable. As briefly discussed previously, patients with NSCLC with asymptomatic brain metastases have been treated with pembrolizumab in a prospective phase 2 study.[97] Out of the 34 patients with PD-L1–positive NSCLC brain metastasis treated with pembrolizumab, 10 (29.4%) had an intracranial response to therapy. Five patients who were PD-L1 negative had no objective response. Nearly a third of all patients remained alive at 2 years.

Nivolumab has been also been studied in patients harboring NSCLC with untreated brain metastases.[98] Among a pool of 46 patients with NSCLC who were treated with nivolumab, 33% had no signs of intracranial progression and 52% had progressive disease. When comparing the group of patients treated with nivolumab versus docetaxel, the median OS was 8.4 months versus 6.2 months, respectively.

The phase 3 OAK trial compared patients with NSCLC with asymptomatic, treated brain metastases treated with atezolizumab versus docetaxel.[99] The median OS was longer with atezolizumab than with docetaxel (16 vs 11.9 months). Furthermore, there were fewer treatment-related adverse events reported in the atezolizumab group than with docetaxel. Atezolizumab may also have a preventive benefit because landmark analysis showed that patients in the atezolizumab group had a lower probability of developing new symptomatic brain lesions at 6 to 24 months.

Although these initial clinical data are promising, the efficacy of PD-L1 and PD-1 inhibitors against lung cancer with metastasis to the brain has been an area of research given the significant differences between the tumor microenvironment of primary lung cancers versus brain metastases. Many brain metastases from lung cancer lose PD-L1 expression or lack lymphocytic infiltration despite their findings in the primary lung cancer.[100] In a series of 146 paired lesions of primary lung cancer and brain metastases, 39% of primary lesions expressed PD-L1 and, of those, there was a 14% rate of discordance between primary lung cancer and paired brain metastasis. This tumor heterogeneity may be one of the factors responsible for the relative hindrance in response to anti–PD-1 therapy in brain metastasis versus primary lung cancer.[101]

IMMUNOTHERAPY AND RADIATION

Combining immunotherapy with radiation has gained significant attention given both the emerging success of immunotherapy as well as the fact that patients often experience a delayed response to immunotherapies, requiring about 3 to 5 months, and many patients cannot tolerate this delay if they are symptomatic.[96,102] An emerging body of literature is showing significant promise for combination therapy, especially for patients with melanoma metastatic to the brain.[103] Radiation therapy may synergistically work with immunotherapies because radiation induces an immune response through multiple pathways initiated by tissue injury induced by radiation, including inflammatory cytokines such as IFN-γ, TNFα, and CXCL16, which cause lymphocytic recruitment[104] and CD8+ T-cell activation.[105] Also, radiation causes upregulation of PD-L1 expression on cancer cells, hindering their ability to cause T-cell exhaustion.[106,107] The mechanism of this immune response may be related to the abscopal, or distant bystander, effect, in which radiation therapy reprograms the tumor microenvironment exposing previously unpresented tumor antigens, leading to recognition and destruction by immune cells even outside the field of radiation, a form of in situ vaccination.[108]

Clinically, there is emerging evidence that shows the abscopal effect of combining radiation therapy with immunotherapy.[109] One case report described a patient with metastatic melanoma treated with both ipilimumab maintenance therapy and extracranial stereotactic radiation surgery (SRS).[110] The SRS showed significant tumor shrinkage among lesions outside the radiation target field. Also, antigenic targets showed enhanced antibody responses after radiotherapy. Further evidence that the abscopal effect may be applicable to patients with brain metastases was shown in a cohort of 77 patients undergoing radiosurgery for melanoma brain metastasis who had an increased median OS of 21.3 months with both radiosurgery and ipilimumab therapy compared with 4.9 months with radiosurgery alone.[111] One review of 8 studies quantifying the abscopal response combining radiotherapy and ipilimumab in patients with metastatic melanoma concluded that radiotherapy plus ipilimumab significantly increases abscopal responses and OS without increasing toxicity.[112] Seven of the 8 studies analyzed included patients with brain metastases.

There are currently numerous ongoing clinical trials studying combination radiotherapy with immunotherapy for patients with brain metastasis. Choosing the best fractionation schedule for radiation therapy when used in combination with immunotherapy is currently being studied in preclinical models. Timing of radiation seems to be an important factor because 1 study showed increased rates of progression among patients treated with SRS before or during ipilimumab versus those who underwent SRS after ipilimumab.[113] There is 1 ongoing clinical trial (NCT02097732) studying the effect of SRS before or during ipilimumab induction.

ADVERSE EFFECTS OF IMMUNOTHERAPY

The progress of immunotherapy continues to be challenged by complications such as autoimmune reactions, neurologic toxicities, and tumor necrosis. Autoimmune reactions with CPIs are seen more frequently among patients with underlying autoimmune diseases.[114] These reactions tend to affect the skin, gastrointestinal tract, endocrine system, and lungs.[115] More common skin manifestations are eczemalike rashes or vitiligo that tend to occur within the first week of therapy initiation; however, severe reactions, although less likely, may occur, including blistering disorder, Stevens-Johnson syndrome, and toxic epidermal necrolysis. Gastrointestinal autoimmune disorders include colitis and hepatitis, and endocrine autoimmune disorders such as thyroid dysfunction, hypophysitis, and adrenal insufficiency can occur. Both gastrointestinal and endocrine manifestations are more common with anti–CTLA-4 agents. Pneumonitis may occur more frequently with anti–PD-1 agents and can be a severe event with immunosuppression using corticosteroids.[116]

Neurologic symptoms during immunotherapy for brain metastases may be caused by multiple factors, including perilesional edema, intralesional hemorrhage, necrosis, and tumor growth.[117] Radiation necrosis may occur with greater frequency among patients with immunotherapy than other systemic therapies,[117,118] which is particularly challenging because differentiation between radiation necrosis and tumor recurrence based on imaging can be difficult, and sometimes impossible.[117,118] Patients developing radiation necrosis may be treated with steroids to reduce edema. Bevacizumab, a vascular endothelial growth factor inhibitor, may be required among patients who cannot undergo immunosuppression with steroids in order to maintain a functional immune response for treatment.[119]

FUTURE DIRECTIONS

Given the new data supporting efficacy of immunotherapies in treating intracranial tumors, a new era in immunotherapy has been reached in which patients with brain metastases are no longer excluded from these new therapies and clinical trials. Gaining an understanding of the molecular determination for response to immunotherapies remains a major challenge. A focus on the specific microenvironment of the brain, a relatively immunosuppressed environment, is a crucial component of the emerging evidence that has the potential to address this challenge. Nevertheless, the positive clinical results of immunotherapy among patients with brain metastases may lead to dramatic changes in comprehensive management of these patients. Possible benefits of combining immunotherapy with other systemic chemotherapies, targeted therapies, or radiation and surgery are an active area of research.

DISCLOSURE

The authors have nothing to disclose.

REFERENCES

1. Peters S, Camidge DR, Shaw AT, et al. Alectinib versus crizotinib in untreated ALK-positive non-small-cell lung cancer. N Engl J Med 2017;377(9): 829–38.
2. Quail DF, Joyce JA. Microenvironmental regulation of tumor progression and metastasis. Nat Med 2013;19(11):1423–37.
3. Gong J, Chehrazi-Raffle A, Reddi S, et al. Development of PD-1 and PD-L1 inhibitors as a form of cancer immunotherapy: a comprehensive review of registration trials and future considerations. J Immunother Cancer 2018;6(1):8.
4. Hodi FS, O'Day SJ, McDermott DF, et al. Improved survival with ipilimumab in patients with metastatic melanoma. N Engl J Med 2010;363(8):711–23.
5. Margolin K, Ernstoff MS, Hamid O, et al. Ipilimumab in patients with melanoma and brain metastases: an open-label, phase 2 trial. Lancet Oncol 2012;13(5):459–65.
6. Osswald M, Blaes J, Liao Y, et al. Impact of blood-brain barrier integrity on tumor growth and therapy response in brain metastases. Clin Cancer Res 2016;22(24):6078–87.
7. Bai H, Han B. The effectiveness of erlotinib against brain metastases in non-small cell lung cancer patients. Am J Clin Oncol 2013;36(2):110–5.
8. Hata A, Katakami N. Afatinib for erlotinib refractory brain metastases in a patient with EGFR-mutant non-small-cell lung cancer: can high-affinity TKI substitute for high-dose TKI? J Thorac Oncol 2015;10(7):e65–6.
9. Prins RM, Vo DD, Khan-Farooqi H, et al. NK and CD4 cells collaborate to protect against melanoma tumor formation in the brain. J Immunol 2006; 177(12):8448–55.
10. Wilson EH, Weninger W, Hunter CA. Trafficking of immune cells in the central nervous system. J Clin Invest 2010;120(5):1368–79.
11. Shankaran V, Ikeda H, Bruce AT, et al. IFNgamma and lymphocytes prevent primary tumour development and shape tumour immunogenicity. Nature 2001;410(6832):1107–11.
12. Peggs KS, Quezada SA, Allison JP. Cancer immunotherapy: co-stimulatory agonists and co-inhibitory antagonists. Clin Exp Immunol 2009; 157(1):9–19.
13. Weber JS, D'Angelo SP, Minor D, et al. Nivolumab versus chemotherapy in patients with advanced melanoma who progressed after anti-CTLA-4 treatment (CheckMate 037): a randomised, controlled, open-label, phase 3 trial. Lancet Oncol 2015; 16(4):375–84.
14. Besser MJ, Shapira-Frommer R, Itzhaki O, et al. Adoptive transfer of tumor-infiltrating lymphocytes in patients with metastatic melanoma: intent-to-treat analysis and efficacy after failure to prior immunotherapies. Clin Cancer Res 2013;19(17): 4792–800.
15. Radvanyi LG, Bernatchez C, Zhang M, et al. Specific lymphocyte subsets predict response to adoptive cell therapy using expanded autologous tumor-infiltrating lymphocytes in metastatic melanoma patients. Clin Cancer Res 2012;18(24): 6758–70.
16. Pilon-Thomas S, Kuhn L, Ellwanger S, et al. Efficacy of adoptive cell transfer of tumor-infiltrating lymphocytes after lymphopenia induction for metastatic melanoma. J Immunother 2012;35(8): 615–20.
17. Garrido F, Ruiz-Cabello F, Aptsiauri N. Rejection versus escape: the tumor MHC dilemma. Cancer Immunol Immunother 2017;66(2):259–71.
18. Topalian SL, Hodi FS, Brahmer JR, et al. Safety, activity, and immune correlates of anti-PD-1 antibody in cancer. N Engl J Med 2012;366(26):2443–54.
19. Pardoll DM. The blockade of immune checkpoints in cancer immunotherapy. Nat Rev Cancer 2012; 12(4):252–64.
20. Peggs KS, Quezada SA, Chambers CA, et al. Blockade of CTLA-4 on both effector and regulatory T cell compartments contributes to the antitumor activity of anti-CTLA-4 antibodies. J Exp Med 2009; 206(8):1717–25.
21. Wei SC, Levine JH, Cogdill AP, et al. Distinct Cellular Mechanisms Underlie Anti-CTLA-4 and Anti-PD-1 Checkpoint Blockade. Cell 2017;170(6): 1120–1133,e7.
22. Buchbinder EI, Desai A. CTLA-4 and PD-1 pathways: similarities, differences, and implications of their inhibition. Am J Clin Oncol 2016;39(1):98–106.
23. Narayan P, Wahby S, Gao JJ, et al. FDA approval summary: atezolizumab plus paclitaxel protein-

bound for the treatment of patients with advanced or metastatic TNBC whose tumors express PD-L1. Clin Cancer Res 2020;26(10):2284–9.

24. June CH, Riddell SR, Schumacher TN. Adoptive cellular therapy: a race to the finish line. Sci Transl Med 2015;7(280):280ps287.

25. Gattinoni L, Finkelstein SE, Klebanoff CA, et al. Removal of homeostatic cytokine sinks by lympho-depletion enhances the efficacy of adoptively transferred tumor-specific CD8+ T cells. J Exp Med 2005;202(7):907–12.

26. Rohaan MW, van den Berg JH, Kvistborg P, et al. Adoptive transfer of tumor-infiltrating lymphocytes in melanoma: a viable treatment option. J Immunother Cancer 2018;6(1):102.

27. Dudley ME, Wunderlich JR, Robbins PF, et al. Cancer regression and autoimmunity in patients after clonal repopulation with antitumor lymphocytes. Science 2002;298(5594):850–4.

28. Rosenberg SA, Yannelli JR, Yang JC, et al. Treatment of patients with metastatic melanoma with autologous tumor-infiltrating lymphocytes and interleukin 2. J Natl Cancer Inst 1994;86(15): 1159–66.

29. Rosenberg SA, Yang JC, Sherry RM, et al. Durable complete responses in heavily pretreated patients with metastatic melanoma using T-cell transfer immunotherapy. Clin Cancer Res 2011;17(13): 4550–7.

30. Wu R, Forget MA, Chacon J, et al. Adoptive T-cell therapy using autologous tumor-infiltrating lympho-cytes for metastatic melanoma: current status and future outlook. Cancer J 2012;18(2):160–75.

31. Rosenberg SA. Raising the bar: the curative potential of human cancer immunotherapy. Sci Transl Med 2012;4(127):127ps128.

32. Besser MJ, Itzhaki O, Ben-Betzalel G, et al. Comprehensive single institute experience with melanoma TIL: Long term clinical results, toxicity profile, and prognostic factors of response. Mol Carcinog 2020;59(7):736–44.

33. Yang JC. Toxicities associated with adoptive T-cell transfer for cancer. Cancer J 2015;21(6):506–9.

34. Rosenberg SA, Packard BS, Aebersold PM, et al. Use of tumor-infiltrating lymphocytes and interleukin-2 in the immunotherapy of patients with metastatic melanoma. A preliminary report. N Engl J Med 1988;319(25):1676–80.

35. Webb JR, Milne K, Watson P, et al. Tumor-infiltrating lymphocytes expressing the tissue resident mem-ory marker CD103 are associated with increased survival in high-grade serous ovarian cancer. Clin Cancer Res 2014;20(2):434–44.

36. Hilders CG, Ras L, van Eendenburg JD, et al. Isola-tion and characterization of tumor-infiltrating lym-phocytes from cervical carcinoma. Int J Cancer 1994;57(6):805–13.

37. Yannelli JR, Hyatt C, McConnell S, et al. Growth of tumor-infiltrating lymphocytes from human solid cancers: summary of a 5-year experience. Int J Cancer 1996;65(4):413–21.

38. Turcotte S, Gros A, Hogan K, et al. Phenotype and function of T cells infiltrating visceral metastases from gastrointestinal cancers and melanoma: impli-cations for adoptive cell transfer therapy. J Immunol 2013;191(5):2217–25.

39. Christofi T, Baritaki S, Falzone L, et al. Current per-spectives in cancer immunotherapy. Cancers (Basel) 2019;11(10):3–10.

40. Maude SL, Laetsch TW, Buechner J, et al. Tisagen-lecleucel in Children and Young Adults with B-Cell Lymphoblastic Leukemia. N Engl J Med 2018; 378(5):439–48.

41. Brudno JN, Kochenderfer JN. Toxicities of chimeric antigen receptor T cells: recognition and manage-ment. Blood 2016;127(26):3321–30.

42. Brentjens RJ, Davila ML, Riviere I, et al. CD19-tar-geted T cells rapidly induce molecular remissions in adults with chemotherapy-refractory acute lymphoblastic leukemia. Sci Transl Med 2013; 5(177):177ra138.

43. Lee DW, Kochenderfer JN, Stetler-Stevenson M, et al. T cells expressing CD19 chimeric antigen re-ceptors for acute lymphoblastic leukaemia in chil-dren and young adults: a phase 1 dose-escalation trial. Lancet 2015;385(9967):517–28.

44. Davila ML, Riviere I, Wang X, et al. Efficacy and toxicity management of 19-28z CAR T cell therapy in B cell acute lymphoblastic leukemia. Sci Transl Med 2014;6(224):224ra225.

45. Grupp SA, Kalos M, Barrett D, et al. Chimeric anti-gen receptor-modified T cells for acute lymphoid leukemia. N Engl J Med 2013;368(16):1509–18.

46. Porter DL, Levine BL, Kalos M, et al. Chimeric anti-gen receptor-modified T cells in chronic lymphoid leukemia. N Engl J Med 2011;365(8):725–33.

47. Porter DL, Hwang WT, Frey NV, et al. Chimeric an-tigen receptor T cells persist and induce sustained remissions in relapsed refractory chronic lympho-cytic leukemia. Sci Transl Med 2015;7(303): 303ra139.

48. Brentjens RJ, Riviere I, Park JH, et al. Safety and persistence of adoptively transferred autologous CD19-targeted T cells in patients with relapsed or chemotherapy refractory B-cell leukemias. Blood 2011;118(18):4817–28.

49. Kochenderfer JN, Dudley ME, Carpenter RO, et al. Donor-derived CD19-targeted T cells cause regres-sion of malignancy persisting after allogeneic he-matopoietic stem cell transplantation. Blood 2013; 122(25):4129–39.

50. Kochenderfer JN, Dudley ME, Feldman SA, et al. B-cell depletion and remissions of malignancy along with cytokine-associated toxicity in a clinical

trial of anti-CD19 chimeric-antigen-receptor-transduced T cells. Blood 2012;119(12):2709–20.

51. Jensen MC, Popplewell L, Cooper LJ, et al. Antitransgene rejection responses contribute to attenuated persistence of adoptively transferred CD20/CD19-specific chimeric antigen receptor redirected T cells in humans. Biol Blood Marrow Transplant 2010;16(9):1245–56.

52. Savoldo B, Ramos CA, Liu E, et al. CD28 costimulation improves expansion and persistence of chimeric antigen receptor-modified T cells in lymphoma patients. J Clin Invest 2011;121(5):1822–6.

53. Kipnis J. Multifaceted interactions between adaptive immunity and the central nervous system. Science 2016;353(6301):766–71.

54. Sims JS, Grinshpun B, Feng Y, et al. Diversity and divergence of the glioma-infiltrating T-cell receptor repertoire. Proc Natl Acad Sci U S A 2016;113(25):E3529–37.

55. Quail DF, Joyce JA. The microenvironmental landscape of brain tumors. Cancer Cell 2017;31(3):326–41.

56. Charles NA, Holland EC, Gilbertson R, et al. The brain tumor microenvironment. Glia 2011;59(8):1169–80.

57. Garcia MA, Lazar A, Duriseti S, et al. Discovery of additional brain metastases on the day of stereotactic radiosurgery: risk factors and outcomes. J Neurosurg 2017;126(6):1756–63.

58. Chen Q, Boire A, Jin X, et al. Carcinoma-astrocyte gap junctions promote brain metastasis by cGAMP transfer. Nature 2016;533(7604):493–8.

59. Xing F, Kobayashi A, Okuda H, et al. Reactive astrocytes promote the metastatic growth of breast cancer stem-like cells by activating Notch signalling in brain. EMBO Mol Med 2013;5(3):384–96.

60. Massague J, Obenauf AC. Metastatic colonization by circulating tumour cells. Nature 2016;529(7586):298–306.

61. Farber SH, Tsvankin V, Narloch JL, et al. Embracing rejection: Immunologic trends in brain metastasis. Oncoimmunology 2016;5(7):e1172153.

62. Sierra A, Price JE, Garcia-Ramirez M, et al. Astrocyte-derived cytokines contribute to the metastatic brain specificity of breast cancer cells. Lab Invest 1997;77(4):357–68.

63. Hoelzinger DB, Demuth T, Berens ME. Autocrine factors that sustain glioma invasion and paracrine biology in the brain microenvironment. J Natl Cancer Inst 2007;99(21):1583–93.

64. Berghoff AS, Lassmann H, Preusser M, et al. Characterization of the inflammatory response to solid cancer metastases in the human brain. Clin Exp Metastasis 2013;30(1):69–81.

65. Fitzgerald DP, Palmieri D, Hua E, et al. Reactive glia are recruited by highly proliferative brain metastases of breast cancer and promote tumor cell colonization. Clin Exp Metastasis 2008;25(7):799–810.

66. Pukrop T, Dehghani F, Chuang HN, et al. Microglia promote colonization of brain tissue by breast cancer cells in a Wnt-dependent way. Glia 2010;58(12):1477–89.

67. Berghoff AS, Fuchs E, Ricken G, et al. Density of tumor-infiltrating lymphocytes correlates with extent of brain edema and overall survival time in patients with brain metastases. Oncoimmunology 2016;5(1):e1057388.

68. Hambardzumyan D, Gutmann DH, Kettenmann H. The role of microglia and macrophages in glioma maintenance and progression. Nat Neurosci 2016;19(1):20–7.

69. Jacobs JF, Idema AJ, Bol KF, et al. Regulatory T cells and the PD-L1/PD-1 pathway mediate immune suppression in malignant human brain tumors. Neuro Oncol 2009;11(4):394–402.

70. Liu Y, Komohara Y, Domenick N, et al. Expression of antigen processing and presenting molecules in brain metastasis of breast cancer. Cancer Immunol Immunother 2012;61(6):789–801.

71. Sharma P, Allison JP. The future of immune checkpoint therapy. Science 2015;348(6230):56–61.

72. Rosenberg SA. IL-2: the first effective immunotherapy for human cancer. J Immunol 2014;192(12):5451–8.

73. Atkins MB, Lotze MT, Dutcher JP, et al. High-dose recombinant interleukin 2 therapy for patients with metastatic melanoma: analysis of 270 patients treated between 1985 and 1993. J Clin Oncol 1999;17(7):2105–16.

74. Guirguis LM, Yang JC, White DE, et al. Safety and efficacy of high-dose interleukin-2 therapy in patients with brain metastases. J Immunother 2002;25(1):82–7.

75. Powell S, Dudek AZ. Single-institution outcome of high-dose interleukin-2 (HD IL-2) therapy for metastatic melanoma and analysis of favorable response in brain metastases. Anticancer Res 2009;29(10):4189–93.

76. Min L, Hodi FS, Kaiser UB. Corticosteroids and immune checkpoint blockade. Aging (Albany NY) 2015;7(8):521–2.

77. Schoenfeld JD, Mahadevan A, Floyd SR, et al. Ipilimumab and cranial radiation in metastatic melanoma patients: a case series and review. J Immunother Cancer 2015;3:50.

78. Queirolo P, Spagnolo F, Ascierto PA, et al. Efficacy and safety of ipilimumab in patients with advanced melanoma and brain metastases. J Neurooncol 2014;118(1):109–16.

79. Sunshine J, Taube JM. PD-1/PD-L1 inhibitors. Curr Opin Pharmacol 2015;23:32–8.

80. Postow MA, Chesney J, Pavlick AC, et al. Nivolumab and ipilimumab versus ipilimumab in

untreated melanoma. N Engl J Med 2015;372(21): 2006–17.

81. Larkin J, Chiarion-Sileni V, Gonzalez R, et al. Combined nivolumab and ipilimumab or monotherapy in untreated melanoma. N Engl J Med 2015; 373(1):23–34.

82. Goldberg SB, Gettinger SN, Mahajan A, et al. Pembrolizumab for patients with melanoma or non-small-cell lung cancer and untreated brain metastases: early analysis of a non-randomised, open-label, phase 2 trial. Lancet Oncol 2016;17(7):976–83.

83. Tawbi HA, Forsyth PA, Algazi A, et al. Combined nivolumab and ipilimumab in melanoma metastatic to the brain. N Engl J Med 2018;379(8):722–30.

84. Di Giacomo AM, Ascierto PA, Pilla L, et al. Ipilimumab and fotemustine in patients with advanced melanoma (NIBIT-M1): an open-label, single-arm phase 2 trial. Lancet Oncol 2012;13(9):879–86.

85. Long GV, Atkinson V, Lo S, et al. Combination nivolumab and ipilimumab or nivolumab alone in melanoma brain metastases: a multicentre randomised phase 2 study. Lancet Oncol 2018;19(5):672–81.

86. Hong JJ, Rosenberg SA, Dudley ME, et al. Successful treatment of melanoma brain metastases with adoptive cell therapy. Clin Cancer Res 2010; 16(19):4892–8.

87. McDermott DF, Lee J-L, Szczylik C, et al. Pembrolizumab monotherapy as first-line therapy in advanced clear cell renal cell carcinoma (accRCC): Results from cohort A of KEYNOTE-427. J Clin Oncol 2018;36(15_suppl):4500.

88. Kattan J, Rassy EE, Assi T, et al. A comprehensive review of the role of immune checkpoint inhibitors in brain metastasis of renal cell carcinoma origin. Crit Rev Oncol Hematol 2018;130:60–9.

89. Rothermundt C, Hader C, Gillessen S. Successful treatment with an anti-PD-1 antibody for progressing brain metastases in renal cell cancer. Ann Oncol 2016;27(3):544–5.

90. Lewis GD, Jonasch E, Shah AY, et al. Renal cell carcinoma brain metastasis with pseudoprogression and radiation necrosis on nivolumab after previous treatment with stereotactic radiosurgery: An illustrative case report and review of the literature. Pract Radiat Oncol 2018;8(5):e262–5.

91. Escudier BJ, Chabaud S, Borchiellini D, et al. Efficacy and safety of nivolumab in patients with metastatic renal cell carcinoma (mRCC) and brain metastases: Preliminary results from the GETUG-AFU 26 (Nivoren) study. J Clin Oncol 2017;35(15_suppl):4563.

92. Albiges L, Flippot R, Arfi-Rouche J, et al. Brain metastases (BM) from renal cell carcinoma treated with nivolumab: Evidence of early brain flare? J Clin Oncol 2017;35(6_suppl):520.

93. Bracarda S, Galli L, Maruzzo M, et al. Negative prognostic factors and resulting clinical outcome in patients with metastatic renal cell carcinoma included in the Italian nivolumab-expanded access program. Future Oncol 2018;14(14): 1347–54.

94. Flippot R, Dalban C, Laguerre B, et al. Safety and Efficacy of Nivolumab in Brain Metastases From Renal Cell Carcinoma: Results of the GETUG-AFU 26 NIVOREN Multicenter Phase II Study. J Clin Oncol 2019;37(23):2008–16. https://doi.org/10.1200/JCO.18.02218.

95. McKay RR, Bosse D, Xie W, et al. The clinical activity of PD-1/PD-L1 inhibitors in metastatic non-clear cell renal cell carcinoma. Cancer Immunol Res 2018;6(7):758–65.

96. Koshkin VS, Barata PC, Zhang T, et al. Clinical activity of nivolumab in patients with non-clear cell renal cell carcinoma. J Immunother Cancer 2018; 6(1):9.

97. Goldberg SB, Gettinger SN, Mahajan A, et al. Durability of brain metastasis response and overall survival in patients with non-small cell lung cancer (NSCLC) treated with pembrolizumab. J Clin Oncol 2018;36(15_suppl):2009.

98. Goldman JW, Crino L, Vokes EE, et al. Nivolumab (nivo) in patients (pts) with advanced (adv) NSCLC and central nervous system (CNS) metastases (mets). J Clin Oncol 2016;34(15_suppl): 9038.

99. Gadgeel SM, Lukas RV, Goldschmidt J, et al. Atezolizumab in patients with advanced non-small cell lung cancer and history of asymptomatic, treated brain metastases: Exploratory analyses of the phase III OAK study. Lung Cancer 2019;128: 105–12.

100. Mansfield AS, Aubry MC, Moser JC, et al. Temporal and spatial discordance of programmed cell death-ligand 1 expression and lymphocyte tumor infiltration between paired primary lesions and brain metastases in lung cancer. Ann Oncol 2016; 27(10):1953–8.

101. Kim R, Keam B, Kim S, et al. Differences in tumor microenvironments between primary lung tumors and brain metastases in lung cancer patients: therapeutic implications for immune checkpoint inhibitors. BMC Cancer 2019;19(1):19.

102. Motzer RJ, Tannir NM, McDermott DF, et al. Nivolumab plus ipilimumab versus sunitinib in advanced renal-cell carcinoma. N Engl J Med 2018;378(14): 1277–90.

103. Patel KR, Lawson DH, Kudchadkar RR, et al. Two heads better than one? Ipilimumab immunotherapy and radiation therapy for melanoma brain metastases. Neuro Oncol 2015;17(10):1312–21.

104. Frey B, Rubner Y, Kulzer L, et al. Antitumor immune responses induced by ionizing irradiation and further immune stimulation. Cancer Immunol Immunother 2014;63(1):29–36.

105. Lee Y, Auh SL, Wang Y, et al. Therapeutic effects of ablative radiation on local tumor require CD8+ T cells: changing strategies for cancer treatment. Blood 2009;114(3):589–95.

106. Dovedi SJ, Adlard AL, Lipowska-Bhalla G, et al. Acquired resistance to fractionated radiotherapy can be overcome by concurrent PD-L1 blockade. Cancer Res 2014;74(19):5458–68.

107. Deng L, Liang H, Burnette B, et al. Irradiation and anti-PD-L1 treatment synergistically promote anti-tumor immunity in mice. J Clin Invest 2014;124(2):687–95.

108. Vanpouille-Box C, Pilones KA, Wennerberg E, et al. In situ vaccination by radiotherapy to improve responses to anti-CTLA-4 treatment. Vaccine 2015;33(51):7415–22.

109. Ngwa W, Irabor OC, Schoenfeld JD, et al. Using immunotherapy to boost the abscopal effect. Nat Rev Cancer 2018;18(5):313–22.

110. Postow MA, Callahan MK, Barker CA, et al. Immunologic correlates of the abscopal effect in a patient with melanoma. N Engl J Med 2012;366(10):925–31.

111. Knisely JP, Yu JB, Flanigan J, et al. Radiosurgery for melanoma brain metastases in the ipilimumab era and the possibility of longer survival. J Neurosurg 2012;117(2):227–33.

112. Chicas-Sett R, Morales-Orue I, Rodriguez-Abreu D, et al. Combining radiotherapy and ipilimumab induces clinically relevant radiation-induced abscopal effects in metastatic melanoma patients: A systematic review. Clin Transl Radiat Oncol 2018;9:5–11.

113. Kiess AP, Wolchok JD, Barker CA, et al. Stereotactic radiosurgery for melanoma brain metastases in patients receiving ipilimumab: safety profile and efficacy of combined treatment. Int J Radiat Oncol Biol Phys 2015;92(2):368–75.

114. Johnson DB, Chandra S, Sosman JA. Immune Checkpoint Inhibitor Toxicity in 2018. JAMA 2018;320(16):1702–3.

115. Aquilanti E, Brastianos PK. Immune checkpoint inhibitors for brain metastases: a primer for neurosurgeons. Neurosurgery 2020. https://doi.org/10.1093/neuros/nyaa095.

116. Marin-Acevedo JA, Chirila RM, Dronca RS. Immune checkpoint inhibitor toxicities. Mayo Clin Proc 2019;94(7):1321–9.

117. Cohen JV, Kluger HM. Systemic immunotherapy for the treatment of brain metastases. Front Oncol 2016;6:49.

118. Martin AM, Cagney DN, Catalano PJ, et al. Immunotherapy and Symptomatic radiation necrosis in patients with brain metastases treated with stereotactic radiation. JAMA Oncol 2018;4(8):1123–4.

119. Weingarten N, Kruser TJ, Bloch O. Symptomatic radiation necrosis in brain metastasis patients treated with stereotactic radiosurgery and immunotherapy. Clin Neurol Neurosurg 2019;179:14–8.

Targeting the Tumor Microenvironment in Brain Metastasis

Nisha Giridharan, MD[a], Isabella C. Glitza Oliva, MD, PhD[b],
Barbara J. O'Brien, MD[c], Brittany C. Parker Kerrigan, PhD[a],
Amy B. Heimberger, MD[a], Sherise D. Ferguson, MD[a,*]

KEYWORDS

- Brain metastasis • Tumor microenvironment • Astrocytes • Targeted therapy • Immunotherapy

KEY POINTS

- Brain metastases are a growing issue in the field of oncology and are associated with a notable morbidity and mortality.
- A detailed understanding of the interplay between brain metastatic cells and the tumor microenvironment (TME) is critical for the development of new therapies.
- Aspects of the brain TME have emerged as key mediators of metastatic colonization, and targeting the TME is a potential therapeutic avenue for brain metastasis.

INTRODUCTION

Brain metastases are the most common brain tumors and represent a major challenge in multidisciplinary oncological care. Moreover, because of progress in systemic therapies lengthening the survival of patients with cancer and advances in imaging techniques, the incidence of brain metastases is increasing.[1,2] Brain metastases represent a major source of morbidity and mortality among patients with advanced cancer; hence, there is a need for a wider range of effective treatment options.

The components of the tumor microenvironment (TME) are emerging as crucial mediators of metastatic colonization and tumor progression. Tumor cells that metastasize to the brain possess characteristics that permit them to traverse the blood-brain barrier (BBB), evade the immune system, and survive within the unique brain microenvironment. Metastatic colonization is accomplished through complex and dynamic communication between metastatic cells and the surrounding TME, leading to a tumor-permissive milieu. In the era of immune-based and targeted therapies, interest in targeting the molecular and immune components of the brain TME has emerged. Accumulating preclinical data have demonstrated the clear impact of the TME in brain metastasis progression, and these new insights offer a potential for TME-directed therapies. In this review, the authors summarize the current data regarding the mechanisms within the TME contributing to brain metastasis. They also highlight specific TME targets and therapies that have shown potential for the treatment of brain metastases.

BLOOD-BRAIN BARRIER

The BBB is a specialized structural barrier and represents a significant challenge in the treatment of brain metastasis. It is composed of a network of endothelial cells, astrocytic foot processes, basement membrane proteins, and pericytes; microglia

[a] Department of Neurosurgery, The University of Texas MD Anderson Cancer Center, 1515 Holcombe Boulevard, Unit 422, Houston, TX 77030, USA; [b] Department of Melanoma Medical Oncology, The University of Texas MD Anderson Cancer Center, 1515 Holcombe Boulevard, Unit 430, Houston, TX 77030, USA; [c] Department of Neuro-Oncology, The University of Texas MD Anderson Cancer Center, 1515 Holcombe Boulevard, Unit 431, Houston, TX 77030-4009, USA
* Corresponding author.
E-mail address: sdferguson@mdanderson.org

Neurosurg Clin N Am 31 (2020) 641–649
https://doi.org/10.1016/j.nec.2020.06.011
1042-3680/20/© 2020 Elsevier Inc. All rights reserved.

additionally add to the BBB integrity.[3,4] Metastatic cancer uses a variety of mechanisms to compromise the integrity of the BBB to achieve metastatic colonization, including release of proinflammatory cytokines and proteolysis of tight junctions.[5,6] Two-photon imaging studies have allowed for the identification of the steps metastatic cells take following BBB disruption to promote colonization.[7] These steps include tumor cell arrest at vascular branch points, active extravasation of tumor cells into perivascular space, maintenance of physical contact to microvessels, and vascular cooption/angiogenesis.

Preclinical studies have identified multiple molecules implicated in BBB transmigration by metastatic cells, some of which have successfully been targeted in animal models. Metastatic cells express L1-cell adhesion molecule (L1CAM), an axon path-finding molecule, to facilitate cancer cell adhesion to endothelial cells and vascular cooption. If depleted of L1CAM, cancer cells fail to coopt the surface of brain capillaries, and metastatic outgrowth is hindered.[8] Transmembrane proteins in the disintegrin and metalloprotease family (ADAM) also facilitate tumor migration across the BBB. In breast cancer, ADAM8 is highly expressed and predictive of poor patient outcome. ADAM8 stimulates transendothelial cell migration via β1-integrin activation and angiogenesis through release of VEGF-A and upregulation of MMP-9.[9,10] Similarly, in lung cancer, upregulation of ADAM9 is associated with the development of brain metastasis.[11] In the setting of breast cancer, microvascular endothelial cells have been reported to secrete angiopoietin-2 (Ang-2), which increases BBB permeability via disruption of tight junctions, aiding tumor cell migration across the BBB. Ang-2 was shown to be targetable in a mouse model of triple-negative breast cancer, because inhibition with trebananib (Ang-2 peptibody) resulted in inhibition of brain metastatic

colonization.[12] The stromal cell-derived factor 1 (SDF-1)/CXCR4 signaling transduction has been considered essential in metastasis.[13,14] AMD3100 is a synthetic CXCR4-specific antagonist that targets CXCR4/SDF-1 signaling. In a lung cancer model, treatment with AMD300 hindered the development of brain metastasis by inhibiting this signaling axis, leading to increased tight-junction protein levels and decreased permeability of the BBB.[15]

In summary, penetration of the BBB and tumor extravasation are critical steps early in the metastatic cascade. Multiple studies have identified potentially targetable aspects of this process, but additional work is needed for clinical translation.

ASTROCYTES

Astrocytes are glial cell subtypes that normally function to prevent neuronal damage and represent the most abundant cell type in the central nervous system (CNS).[16] Successful metastatic brain colonization requires a favorable intercellular interaction between astrocytes and metastatic cells. As such, astrocytes have become accepted as a key player in the brain TME, mediating metastatic seeding and growth[17] (**Fig. 1**).

In response to injury or disease-related stimuli, astrocytes undergo a spectrum of functional and phenotypic changes referred to as reactive astrogliosis.[16] These reactive astrocytes are characterized by upregulation of the cytoskeletal intermediate filament protein, glial fibrillary acidic protein.[16,18] Reactive astrocytes are also are known to be a heterogeneous subpopulation, influencing the progression of multiple brain pathologic conditions, including metastasis.[8,19] In the setting of metastatic cancer, the role of reactive astrocytes is complex and multidimensional. Their influence on metastasis is accomplished by several methods, including the release of

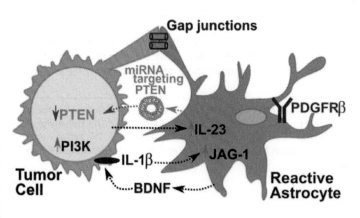

Fig. 1. The interaction between astrocytes and metastatic tumor. miRNA, microRNA. JAG1, Jagged1.

secretory products, direct interaction, formation of gap junctions, and modulation of the immune response.

In the early stages of the metastatic process, reactive astrocytes perform an antitumor function, initially limiting metastatic colonization. Specifically, in response to initial interaction with metastatic cells, reactive astrocytes produce plasminogen activators (ie, tPA and uPA), which transform plasminogen into the protease plasmin. Plasmin induces Fas ligand (FasL), a proapoptotic cytokine. Plasmin releases membrane-bound FasL from astrocytes, which binds to Fas and activates proapoptotic caspases, causing cancer cell death. Plasmin also inactivates L1CAM, which facilitates vascular cooption by metastatic cells in the brain.[8] To avert these killing mechanisms, metastatic cells express anti-PA serpins (eg, neuroserpin and serpin B2) to counteract the antitumor program derived from reactive astrocytes and promote metastatic colonization.[8]

Metastatic cells that successfully avert upfront destruction will continue to grow in the CNS. Multiple preclinical studies have demonstrated that reactive astrocytes cultivate a tumor-supportive, metastatic niche via the secretion of various molecules. In breast cancer, COX2 is upregulated in brain metastatic cells, and subsequent COX2-induced prostaglandins have been shown to support metastasis by promoting the expression of matrix metalloproteinase 1 (MMP1).[20] In response to stimulation, astrocytes also release neurotropins, such as brain-derived neurotrophic factor (BDNF). BDNF is a ligand for tropomyosin-related kinase B (TrkB), and binding activates the phosphoinositide-3 kinase (PI3K) pathway. BDNF-TrkB signaling has been suggested to promote tumorigenesis and treatment resistance,[21,22] and astrocyte-derived BDNF has specifically been linked to proliferation of breast-brain metastasis. Moreover, inhibition of this signaling pathway abrogated brain metastasis in a breast cancer animal model.[23] Klein and colleagues[24] reported bidirectional signaling between melanoma cells and astrocytes to promote tumor colonization. Specifically, they reported that melanoma cells induced the production of interleukin-23 (IL-23) in reactive astrocytes. This proinflammatory cytokine in turn promoted increased melanoma cell invasion/migration. Astrocytes also contribute to the invasive and migratory capabilities of brain-colonizing cells through secretion of MMPs (MMP-2 and -9) and heparanase, which degrades components of the extracellular matrix, altering cell adhesion and tumor migratory capacity.[25-27] Platelet-derived growth factor-β (PDGF-β) expression is a known mediator of angiogenesis,

promoting the integrity and function of vessels.[28,29] In a breast cancer metastasis model, Gril and colleagues[30] reported a subpopulation of metastasis-activated astrocytes that expressed an active (phosphorylated) form of PDGFRβ (p-PDGFRβ) in response to tumor-derived soluble factors. The presence of PDGFRβ-expressing astrocytes was confirmed in resected brain metastasis specimens of multiple cancer lineages. In this same study, pazopanib, an orally bioavailable multiple tyrosine kinase inhibitor, was demonstrated to decrease p-PDGFRβ expression in astrocytes in vitro and in an in vivo model and reduce metastasis.

Direct contact between astrocytes and tumor cells can also induce signaling cascades that facilitate brain metastases. Breast cancer brain metastases have been reported to express IL-1β, which activates astrocytes. This activation subsequently results in astrocyte expression of JAG1 and the interaction of astrocytes with cancer stemlike cells. This interaction stimulates Notch signaling in cancer stemlike cells, promoting self-renewal.[31] In addition to classic methods of cellular communication, exosomes, small vesicles of endocytic origin that carry a diverse range of bioactive molecules, have emerged as potential mediators of cancer progression. In a landmark study, Zhang and colleagues[32] demonstrated that PTEN (a known tumor suppressor) downregulation in brain metastatic cells was mediated by astrocytes. Specifically, astrocyte-derived exosomes facilitated intracellular transfer of PTEN-targeting microRNA to metastatic tumor cells. Furthermore, astrocyte-specific depletion of PTEN-targeting microRNAs or blockade of astrocyte exosome secretion rescues the PTEN loss and suppresses brain metastasis in vivo.

Gap Junctions

Gap junctions are formed by connexins and allow for passage of cytoplasmic molecules between cells and signal transduction.[33] Astrocytes couple with adjacent astrocytes into networks required for normal functions, including synaptic transmission and supporting neuronal activity.[34] When astrocytes become reactive, their activity and connectivity may be modified; hence, gap junctions can play a role in both normal and pathologic conditions.[35] Metastatic cells are able to communicate with astrocytes via gap junctions,[36,37] promoting tumor progression and chemoresistance. Chen and colleagues[38] demonstrated that cancer cells expressing protocadherin 7 (PCDH7) promote tumor-astrocyte gap junction formation by recruiting connexin 43 (CX43). These channels allow passage of cGAMP from cancer cells to astrocytes, triggering the secretion of inflammatory cytokines via STING pathway activation. This cascade activates signal transducer and activator of transcription 1 (STAT1) and nuclear factor κB pathways in cancer cells, promoting chemoresistance and tumor growth. Analysis of patient cohorts showed that the presence of PCDH7 and CX43 in primary tumors correlated with increased brain metastases in breast cancer and decreased metastasis-free survival in patients with lung cancer. These molecules could serve as potential biomarkers to assess the risk of developing brain metastases in patients and serve as prospective future molecular targets in the clinical setting.

Bidirectional signaling between astrocytes and cancer cells has also been shown to contribute to chemotherapy resistance. Reactive astrocytes can sequester intracellular calcium of metastatic cells via gap junctions. As cytoplasmic calcium levels are a hallmark of apoptosis, this presents a key mechanism by which astrocytes confer chemoresistance.[37] Moreover, pharmacologic inhibition or genetic knockdown of gap junctions in astrocytes reverses this process and renders cancer cells sensitive to chemotherapy. Preclinical data also indicate that reactive astrocytes can shield tumor cells from chemotherapy by upregulation of antiapoptotic genes. In an experimental breast cancer model, tumor-astrocyte gap junction signaling stimulated increased expression of IL-6 and IL-8 in cancer cells, which, in turn, increased endothelin peptide (ET-1) production in astrocytes and ET receptor expression in tumor cells. The endothelin axis results in activation of the AKT/MAPK signaling pathway and upregulation of survival proteins that mediate chemoprotection.[39] Lee and colleagues[40] evaluated the efficacy of a dual endothelin receptor antagonist (macitentan) in the treatment of experimental breast and lung cancer animal models. The investigators reported that combination chemotherapy (paclitaxel) and macitentan produced an increase in the number of apoptotic cells in both breast and lung cancer brain metastases compared with control animals and animals treated with monotherapy. Overall, these data imply that gap junctions are a key mechanism by which astrocytes protect malignant cells from chemotherapy and are a novel potential therapeutic target.

Immune Modulation

Astrocytes are also emerging as mediators of immune responses in brain metastasis. A recent study reported a subpopulation of reactive astrocytes with a high STAT3 modulated immune response in the presence of brain metastasis. The investigators demonstrated that reactive astrocytes expressing STAT3 have a negative effect on T-cell function, establishing an immunosuppressive microenvironment promoting tumor outgrowth.[41] This study also assessed therapeutic targeting of STAT3+ reactive astrocytes by treating tumor-bearing mice with Silibinin (a known STAT3 inhibitor that penetrates the BBB) that showed a decrease in brain metastasis growth.

Targeting Astrocytes—Clinical Perspectives

Preclinical studies provide critical insight into potential astrocyte-targeted therapies. A subset of preclinical studies targeting astrocytes has moved forward into the clinical setting. After demonstrating the effectiveness of STAT3 inhibition in reduction of brain metastases in preclinical models, Priego and colleagues[41] conducted a small clinical trial of 18 patients with metastatic lung cancer to the brain treated with Legasil (STAT3 inhibitor). Legasil was administered as a single agent in 3 patients and in combination concurrently with another therapy in the remainder. The study reported an overall response rate in the brain of 75%, including 3 complete responses (20%) and 10 partial responses (55%). In addition, the investigators compared their Legasil-treated group with a matched group of patients with brain metastases from lung cancer (n = 38) treated at the same institution who received whole-brain radiation therapy and standard-of-care chemotherapy. Survival after the diagnosis of brain metastasis was significantly longer in the Legasil-treated group than in the control cohort. These data support using STAT3 inhibition as a viable potential therapeutic in the setting of brain metastatic disease. Currently, another STAT3 inhibitor, WP1066 with BBB penetration, is being evaluated in a phase 1 clinical trial for patients with melanoma brain metastasis (NCT02429570). This trial is unique in that it includes a dose-expansion cohort in which patients are treated before surgical resection to ascertain blockade of STAT3 in the TME, including in the peritumoral reactive astrocytes, and antitumor immune modulation.

In preclinical studies of breast and lung brain metastasis, Chen and colleagues[38] pharmacologically blocked gap junctions using the anti-inflammatory compound meclofenamate, which inhibits gap junction gating,[42] and tonabersat, which has specific activity for binding to astrocytes and inhibiting gap-junction-mediated processes. Treatment with meclofenamate or tonabersat inhibited brain metastases in these animal models. In addition, administration of meclofenamate or tonabersat increased tumor chemosensitivity.[38] Based on these promising results, a clinical trial using meclofenamate in the treatment of recurrent/progressing brain metastasis has been completed (NCT02429570), and results are pending.

IMMUNE CELLS

The immune component of the TME plays a vital role in the progression of brain metastases. It is now well established that an in-depth understanding of the tumor-immune cell interaction is required for the development of rational and effective therapeutic strategies.

Lymphoid Cells

The lymphoid compartment of the immune system is composed of B cells, T cells, and natural killer cells. T lymphocytes are central in immunosurveillance; mature T cells are primed by engaging with antigen-presenting cells, leading to T-cell activation, clonal expansion, and ultimately, T-cell cytotoxicity.[43] Tumor cells can evade being immunologically destroyed by various mechanisms, and T cells are subject to profound dysfunction within the brain TME.

Because immunotherapy has become a topic of increasing interest, the interaction of brain metastasis with T cells has become a key issue. Several studies have confirmed the presence of infiltrating T cells in brain metastases across different cancers.[44] The prognostic value of T-cell infiltration in brain metastases has also been studied with mixed results. Berghoff and colleagues[45] reported that a high density of infiltrating T cells was associated with longer median overall survival regardless of primary tumor site, relative to a low CD3+ T-cell density. Similarly, in their analysis of 26 resected brain metastases, Zakaria and colleagues[46] reported that increased peritumoral CD3+ T-cell density was associated with a significantly prolonged survival time; specifically that patients whose metastases had the highest T-cell infiltration survived twice as long as those having metastases with low infiltration. Conversely, Harter and colleagues[47] found no significant association between patient survival and brain metastasis T-cell infiltration in their analysis of 204 patients. T-cell frequency does not necessarily associate with functional activity, and none of these studies directly addressed the confounding issues of T-cell-mediated immune suppression. Overall, the lack of consensus among these reports indicates that further investigation is warranted.

One of the well-known methods by which metastatic cells evade immune destruction is through expression of ligands that engage immune checkpoints, such as programmed cell death protein 1 (PD-1) and cytotoxic T-lymphocyte-associated protein 4 (CTLA-4) that suppress effector T-cell function and proliferation. PD-L1 is expressed on the surface of tumor cells and its interaction with PD-1 on T cells triggers apoptosis of cytotoxic T cells but inhibits apoptosis of regulatory T cells. CTLA-4 is a costimulatory pathway protein that interacts with HLA-B7-1 and HLA-B7-2 on T cells and delivers an inhibitory signal to effector T cells while promoting inhibitory function of regulatory T cells.[48,49] Together these pathways promote tumor cell survival and proliferation through immune evasion. In many instances, T-cell exhaustion is a key feature of CNS tumors that results from chronic, suboptimal antigen exposure and is characterized by expression of multiple immune checkpoints on the T-cell surface.[50] This profound form of T-cell dysfunction has now been described for both gliomas and intracranial metastases.[51]

T-cell dysfunction contributes to tumor immune escape in patients with cancer, including brain metastatic disease. A recent study revealed bone marrow sequestration as a novel mode of T-cell dysfunction in intracranial tumors, mediated by the S1P-S1P1 axis. This signaling axis is known for its role in lymphocyte trafficking, and decreased S1P1 expression on naïve T cells fosters their sequestration in bone marrow. Although the focus of this study was primary glioma, intracranial implantation of melanoma, breast, and lung cancer in mice also resulted in T-cell sequestration, indicating this is a potential mechanism of immune evasion in brain metastasis.[52] Notably, reversing T-cell sequestration by inhibiting S1P1 internalization was shown to increase the efficacy of immune checkpoint inhibitors.

Myeloid Cells

Cells of the myeloid compartment represent the most abundant nonmalignant cell types in the TME. In brain metastasis, myeloid cells (tumor-associated macrophages [TAMs] and microglia) can constitute up to 30% of the tumor mass.[5] TAMs have been shown to support tumor proliferation, invasion, and metastasis.[53] Microglia are the resident macrophages of the CNS[54] and are a major representative of the innate immune system constituting the first line of defense and response to multiple stimuli in the brain. The role of microglia in the progression of gliomas has been well described, specifically their role in promoting glioma immune system evasion.[55] In light of this, the role of microglia in the progression of brain metastasis has become an area of robust investigation. Imaging studies have shown a direct interaction between microglia and brain metastatic cells in experimental animal models and human specimens.[56,57] In addition, microglia have been shown to precede invading tumor cells, suggesting that they serve as guiding rails that assist in invasion and prepare the niche for colonization.[58]

Microglia and TAMs contribute to metastatic colonization through multiple mechanisms. Macrophages/microglia have been implicated in BBB disruption because of expression of high levels of MMP3, which is gradually upregulated during the development of the metastasis. Chuang and colleagues[59] demonstrated that tumor cells block proapoptotic functions of microglia and exploit tissue damage responses to increase their invasive capacity. The PI3K signaling cascade has also been linked to the progression of metastasis, and recent data indicate that PI3K is a mediator of metastasis-promoting macrophages/microglia during CNS colonization.[60] Wnt signaling is linked to various inflammatory pathways and has been identified as a key regulator of microglia-induced invasion in brain metastasis.[58,59,61] Coculture of breast cancer cells (murine and human) with microglia significantly enhanced the invasive ability of these cell lines. This invasive capacity was significantly diminished by treatment with Wnt inhibitors (DKK-1 and -2),[58] thus highlighting the impact of Wnt signaling for microglial-induced invasion. Another study investigated the role of tumor-derived exosomes during metastatic colonization and the contribution of microglia.[62] Cell migration-inducing and hyaluronan-binding protein (CEMIP) is a Wnt-related protein enriched in tumor-derived exosomes. Rodrigues and colleagues[62] reported that uptake of CEMIP+ exosomes occurs in endothelial and microglia, resulting in upregulation of proinflammatory cytokines in the metastatic niche, promoting vascularization and metastatic colonization. Notably, CEMIP was found in the brain metastatic samples of patients with breast and lung cancer. Analysis of brain metastases showed that tumor CEMIP expression was increased relative to surrounding brain stroma, and brain metastases from breast and lung showed significantly higher CEMIP expression than metastases from other organs. Furthermore, patients whose brain metastases had high CEMIP levels had significantly poorer survival relative to patients with low-CEIMP brain metastases. These data support exosomal CEMIP as a potentially powerful predictor of brain metastasis and a potential therapeutic target.

Targeting the Immune Compartment

The role of immunotherapy is discussed greater detail in a subsequent review ("Immune Therapy for CNS Metastases"), so it is only briefly addressed here. Thus far, most immune modulatory strategies have focused on reactivating T cells via immune checkpoint inhibition. Multiple clinical studies have proven this strategy to be very promising.[63,64] Although these data are very encouraging, a significant number of patients still succumb to the disease. One strategic approach is to combine with radiation therapy/radiosurgery, because this approach is thought to be synergistic.[65,66] Radiation can trigger cell death, thereby releasing antigens for presentation, and facilitating surface expression of major histocompatibility complex class I molecules, resulting in increased T-cell trafficking to the metastatic lesion.[67,68] This combination therapy has been evaluated clinically with favorable results,[69,70] and multiple ongoing clinical trials are evaluating this strategy (eg, NCT02886585, NCT02858869, NCT02696993).

Strategies have also been used to target the myeloid compartment in brain metastases. The colony-stimulating factor 1 (CSF1)/colony-stimulating factor 1 receptor (CSF1R) axis is central in the differentiation and survival of the mononuclear phagocyte system, particularly macrophages.[71] CSF1R+ macrophages have been correlated with poor survival in various tumor types[72,73]; hence, targeting CSF1R signaling in tumor-promoting myeloid cells represents a promising therapy. In their study of experimental melanoma brain metastasis, the investigators demonstrated that macrophages and microglia were significantly recruited in the presence of tumor. In a separate experiment, animals were pretreated with PLX3397 (a small-molecule inhibitor of CSF-1R) to deplete macrophages/microglia before melanoma cell inoculation (via carotid injection). Mice depleted of macrophages/microglia had an 83% reduction in number of metastases and a 65% reduction in tumor size,[57] suggesting the potential therapeutic utility of this therapy. STING is a widely expressed sensor of cellular stress, specifically the presence of DNA in the cytoplasm that bridges the innate and adaptive immune systems, both by triggering interferon release and through tumor recognition by innate immune cells.[74] Distinct from most other innate immune agonists, STING activation can reeducate tumor-supportive M2 macrophages toward a proinflammatory M1 phenotype and can reverse the suppressive phenotype of myeloid-derived suppressor cells. Furthermore, mouse tumors grow faster in STING knockout mice, demonstrating the critical role of this pathway in limiting tumor progression. Several injectable STING formulations have been devised and are now being developed for brain metastasis.[75,76]

SUMMARY

Brain metastases remain a challenge confronting multiple disciplines. The importance of the TME in the initiation and progression of cancer is increasingly being recognized. The development of more effective therapies will require a detailed understanding of how metastatic cells adapt to the brain microenvironment. Data are accumulating that are uncovering the molecular pathways facilitating brain metastatic colonization, opening a new opportunity for the development of unique TME-directed therapies to expand the potential therapeutic repertoire for this difficult patient population.

CONFLICTS OF INTEREST

The authors declare no conflicts of interest.

DISCLOSURE

N. Giridharan: nothing to disclose. I.C. Glitza: Research Support: BMS, Merck; Consultant: BMS, Novartis, ARRAY. B.J. O'Brien: Seattle Genetics: honorarium for educational talk; A.B. Heimberger: Advisory board: Caris Life Science, Western IRB; Stock: Caris; Licensed intellectual property/milestone payments: Celldex Therapeutics, DNAtrix; Other support: Moleculin; S.D. Ferguson: nothing to disclose.

REFERENCES

1. Eichler AF, Chung E, Kodack DP, et al. The biology of brain metastases-translation to new therapies. Nat Rev Clin Oncol 2011;8(6):344–56.
2. Rostami R, Mittal S, Rostami P, et al. Brain metastasis in breast cancer: a comprehensive literature review. J Neurooncol 2016;127(3):407–14.
3. Abbott NJ. Blood-brain barrier structure and function and the challenges for CNS drug delivery. J Inherit Metab Dis 2013;36(3):437–49.
4. da Fonseca AC, Matias D, Garcia C, et al. The impact of microglial activation on blood-brain barrier in brain diseases. Front Cell Neurosci 2014;8:362.
5. Sevenich L, Bowman RL, Mason SD, et al. Analysis of tumour- and stroma-supplied proteolytic networks reveals a brain-metastasis-promoting role for cathepsin S. Nat Cell Biol 2014;16(9):876–88.
6. Stamatovic SM, Keep RF, Andjelkovic AV. Brain endothelial cell-cell junctions: how to "open" the blood brain barrier. Curr Neuropharmacol 2008; 6(3):179–92.
7. Kienast Y, von Baumgarten L, Fuhrmann M, et al. Real-time imaging reveals the single steps of brain metastasis formation. Nat Med 2010;16(1):116–22.
8. Valiente M, Obenauf AC, Jin X, et al. Serpins promote cancer cell survival and vascular co-option in brain metastasis. Cell 2014;156:1002–16.
9. Romagnoli M, Mineva ND, Polmear M, et al. ADAM8 expression in invasive breast cancer promotes tumor dissemination and metastasis. EMBO Mol Med 2014;6:278–94.
10. Conrad C, Götte M, Schlomann U, et al. ADAM8 expression in breast cancer derived brain metastases: functional implications on MMP-9 expression and transendothelial migration in breast cancer cells. Int J Cancer 2018;142(4):779–91.
11. Lin CY, Cho CF, Bai ST, et al. ADAM9 promotes lung cancer progression through vascular remodeling by VEGFA, ANGPT2, and PLAT. Sci Rep 2017;7:15108.
12. Avraham HK, Jiang S, Fu Y, et al. Angiopoietin-2 mediates blood-brain barrier impairment and colonization of triple-negative breast cancer cells in brain. J Pathol 2014;232:369–81.
13. Amara S, Chaar I, Khiari M, et al. Stromal cell derived factor-1 and CXCR4 expression in colorectal cancer promote liver metastasis. Cancer Biomark 2015;15(6):869–79.
14. Tang CH, Tan TW, Fu WM, et al. Involvement of matrix metalloproteinase-9 in stromal cell-derived factor-1/CXCR4 pathway of lung cancer metastasis. Carcinogenesis 2008;29(1):35–43.
15. Li H, Chen Y, Xu N, et al. AMD3100 inhibits brain-specific metastasis in lung cancer via suppressing the SDF-1/CXCR4 axis and protecting blood-brain barrier. Am J Transl Res 2017;9:5259–74.
16. Sofroniew MV. Molecular dissection of reactive astrogliosis and glial scar formation. Trends Neurosci 2009;32:638–47.
17. Wasilewski D, Priego N, Fustero-Torre C, et al. Reactive astrocytes in brain metastasis. Front Oncol 2017;7:298.
18. Liddelow SA, Barres BA. Reactive astrocytes: production, function, and therapeutic potential. Immunity 2017;46:957–67.
19. Seifert G, Schilling K, Steinhauser C. Astrocyte dysfunction in neurological disorders: a molecular perspective. Nat Rev Neurosci 2006;7:194–206.
20. Wu K, Fukuda K, Xing F, et al. Roles of the cyclooxygenase 2 matrix metalloproteinase 1 pathway in brain metastasis of breast cancer. J Biol Chem 2015;290:9842–54.
21. Ho R, Eggert A, Hishiki T, et al. Resistance to chemotherapy mediated by TrkB in neuroblastomas. Cancer Res 2002;62(22):6462–6.

22. Thiele CJ, Li Z, McKee AE. On Trk–the TrkB signal transduction pathway is an increasingly important target in cancer biology. Clin Cancer Res 2009; 15(19):5962–7.

23. Choy C, Ansari KI, Neman J, et al. Cooperation of neurotrophin receptor TrkB and Her2 in breast cancer cells facilitates brain metastases. Breast Cancer Res 2017;19:51.

24. Klein A, Schwartz H, Sagi-Assif O, et al. Astrocytes facilitate melanoma brain metastasis via secretion of IL-23. J Pathol 2015;236:116–27.

25. Marchetti D, Li J, Shen R. Astrocytes contribute to the brain-metastatic specificity of melanoma cells by producing heparanase. Cancer Res 2000; 60(17):4767–70.

26. Shumakovich MA, Mencio CP, Siglin JS, et al. Astrocytes from the brain microenvironment alter migration and morphology of metastatic breast cancer cells. FASEB J 2017;31(11):5049–67.

27. Wang L, Cossette SM, Rarick KR, et al. Astrocytes directly influence tumor cell invasion and metastasis in vivo. PLoS One 2013;8(12):e80933.

28. Primac I, Maquoi E, Blacher S, et al. Stromal integrin α11 regulates PDGFR-β signaling and promotes breast cancer progression. J Clin Invest 2019;130: 4609–28.

29. Tsioumpekou M, Cunha SI, Ma H, et al. Specific targeting of PDGFRβ in the stroma inhibits growth and angiogenesis in tumors with high PDGF-BB expression. Theranostics 2020;10(3):1122–35.

30. Gril B, Palmieri D, Qian Y, et al. Pazopanib inhibits the activation of PDGFRβ-expressing astrocytes in the brain metastatic microenvironment of breast cancer cells. Am J Pathol 2013;182:2368–79.

31. Xing F, Kobayashi A, Okuda H, et al. Reactive astrocytes promote the metastatic growth of breast cancer stem-like cells by activating Notch signalling in brain. EMBO Mol Med 2013;5:384–96.

32. Zhang L, Zhang S, Yao J, et al. Microenvironment-induced PTEN loss by exosomal microRNA primes brain metastasis outgrowth. Nature 2015; 527(7576):100–4.

33. Oshima A. Structure and closure of connexin gap junction channels. FEBS Lett 2014;588(8):1230–7.

34. Giaume C, Koulakoff A, Roux L, et al. Astroglial networks: a step further in neuroglial and gliovascular interactions. Nat Rev Neurosci 2010;11:87–99.

35. Oberheim NA, Tian G-F, Han X, et al. Loss of astrocytic domain organization in the epileptic brain. J Neurosci 2008;28:3264–76.

36. Kim S-J, Kim J-S, Park ES, et al. Astrocytes upregulate survival genes in tumor cells and induce protection from chemotherapy. Neoplasia 2011;13: 286–98.

37. Lin Q, Balasubramanian K, Fan D, et al. Reactive astrocytes protect melanoma cells from chemotherapy by sequestering intra- cellular calcium through gap junction communication channels. Neoplasia 2010; 12:748–54.

38. Chen Q, Boire A, Jin X, et al. Carcinoma-astrocyte gap junctions promote brain metastasis by cGAMP transfer. Nature 2016;533:493–8.

39. Kim SW, Choi HJ, Lee HJ, et al. Role of the endothelin axis in astrocyte- and endothelial cell-mediated chemoprotection of cancer cells. Neuro Oncol 2014;16(12):1585–98.

40. Lee HJ, Hanibuchi M, Kim SJ, et al. Treatment of experimental human breast cancer and lung cancer brain metastases in mice by macitentan, a dual antagonist of endothelin receptors, combined with paclitaxel. Neuro Oncol 2016;18(4):486–96.

41. Priego N, Zhu L, Monteiro C, et al. STAT3 labels a subpopulation of reactive astrocytes required for brain metastasis. Nat Med 2018;24(7):1024–35.

42. Harks EG, de Roos AD, Peters PH, et al. Fenamates: a novel class of reversible gap junction blockers. J Pharmacol Exp Ther 2001;298(3):1033–41.

43. Chen L, Flies DB. Molecular mechanisms of T cell co-stimulation and co-inhibition. Nat Rev Immunol 2013;13:227–42.

44. Berghoff AS, Lassmann H, Preusser M, et al. Characterization of the inflammatory response to solid cancer metastases in the human brain. Clin Exp Metastasis 2013;30:69–81.

45. Berghoff AS, Fuchs E, Ricken G, et al. Density of tumor-infiltrating lymphocytes correlates with extent of brain edema and overall survival time in patients with brain metastases. Oncoimmunology 2015;5(1): e1057388.

46. Zakaria R, Platt-Higgins A, Rathi N, et al. T-cell densities in brain metastases are associated with patient survival times and diffusion tensor MRI changes. Cancer Res 2018;78(3):610–6.

47. Harter PN, Bernatz S, Scholz A, et al. Distribution and prognostic relevance of tumor-infiltrating lymphocytes (TILs) and PD-1/PD-L1 immune checkpoints in human brain metastases. Oncotarget 2015;6:40836–49.

48. Haanen JB, Robert C. Immune checkpoint inhibitors. Prog Tumor Res 2015;42:55–66.

49. Li B, Chan HL, Chen P. Immune checkpoint inhibitors: basics and challenges. Curr Med Chem 2019; 26(17):3009–25.

50. Wherry EJ, Blattman JN, Murali-Krishna K, et al. Viral persistence alters CD8 T-cell immunodominance and tissue distribution and results in distinct stages of functional impairment. J Virol 2003;77(8): 4911–27.

51. Woroniecka K, Chongsathidkiet P, Rhodin K, et al. T-cell exhaustion signatures vary with tumor type and are severe in glioblastoma. Clin Cancer Res 2018; 24(17):4175–86.

52. Chongsathidkiet P, Jackson C, Koyama S, et al. Sequestration of T cells in bone marrow in the setting

of glioblastoma and other intracranial tumors. Nat Med 2018;24(9):1459–68.

53. Mantovani A, Marchesi F, Malesci A, et al. Tumour-associated macrophages as treatment targets in oncology. Nat Rev Clin Oncol 2017;14(7):399–416.

54. Hanisch UK, Kettenmann H. Microglia: active sensor and versatile effector cells in the normal and pathologic brain. Nat Neurosci 2007;10:1387–94.

55. Zhai H, Heppner FL, Tsirka SE. Microglia/macrophages promote glioma progression. Glia 2011; 59(3):472–85.

56. Amit M, Laider-Trejo L, Shalom V, et al. Characterization of the melanoma brain metastatic niche in mice and humans. Cancer Med 2013;2(2):155–63.

57. Qiao S, Qian Y, Xu G, et al. Long-term characterization of activated microglia/macrophages facilitating the development of experimental brain metastasis through intravital microscopic imaging. J Neuroinflammation 2019;16(1):4.

58. Pukrop T, Dehghani F, Chuang HN, et al. Microglia promote colonization of brain tissue by breast cancer cells in a Wnt-dependent way. Glia 2010; 58(12):1477–89.

59. Chuang HN, Rossum DV, Sieger D, et al. Carcinoma cells misuse the host tissue damage response to invade the brain. Glia 2013;61(8):1331–46.

60. Blazquez R, Wlochowitz D, Wolff A, et al. PI3K: a master regulator of brain metastasis-promoting macrophages/microglia. Glia 2018;66(11):2438–55.

61. Klemm F, Bleckmann A, Siam L, et al. β-catenin-independent WNT signaling in basal-like breast cancer and brain metastasis. Carcinogenesis 2011; 32(3):434–42.

62. Rodrigues G, Hoshino A, Kenific CM, et al. Tumour exosomal CEMIP protein promotes cancer cell colonization in brain metastasis. Nat Cell Biol 2019; 21(11):1403–12.

63. Goldberg SB, Gettinger SN, Mahajan A, et al. Pembrolizumab for patients with melanoma or non-small-cell lung cancer and untreated brain metastases: early analysis of a non-randomised, open-label, phase 2 trial. Lancet Oncol 2016;17:976–83.

64. Tawbi HA, Forsyth PA, Algazi A, et al. Combined nivolumab and ipilimumab in melanoma metastatic to the brain. N Engl J Med 2018;379:722–30.

65. Lehrer EJ, McGee HM, Peterson JL, et al. Stereotactic radiosurgery and immune checkpoint inhibitors in the management of brain metastases. Int J Mol Sci 2018;19:3054.

66. Mouw KW, Goldberg MS, Konstantinopoulos PA, et al. DNA damage and repair biomarkers of immunotherapy response. Cancer Discov 2017;7:675–93.

67. Park B, Yee C, Lee KM. The effect of radiation on the immune response to cancers. Int J Mol Sci 2014;15: 927–43.

68. Sevenich L. Turning "cold" into "hot" tumors-opportunities and challenges for radio-immunotherapy against primary and metastatic brain cancers. Front Oncol 2019;9:163.

69. Chen L, Douglass J, Kleinberg L, et al. Concurrent immune checkpoint inhibitors and stereotactic radiosurgery for brain metastases in non-small cell lung cancer, melanoma, and renal cell carcinoma. Int J Radiat Oncol Biol Phys 2018;100(4):916–25.

70. Murphy B, Walker J, Bassale S, et al. Concurrent radiosurgery and immune checkpoint inhibition: improving regional intracranial control for patients with metastatic melanoma. Am J Clin Oncol 2019; 42(3):253–7.

71. Stanley ER, Chitu V. CSF-1 receptor signaling in myeloid cells. Cold Spring Harb Perspect Biol 2014;6(6):a021857.

72. Zhang QW, Liu L, Gong CY, et al. Prognostic significance of tumor-associated macrophages in solid tumor: a meta-analysis of the literature. PLoS One 2012;7(12):e50946.

73. Pyonteck SM, Akkari L, Schuhmacher AJ, et al. CSF-1R inhibition alters macrophage polarization and blocks glioma progression. Nat Med 2013;19(10): 1264–72.

74. Ager CR, Reilley MJ, Nicholas C, et al. Intratumoral STING activation with T-cell checkpoint modulation generates systemic antitumor immunity. Cancer Immunol Res 2017;5(8):676–84.

75. Ager CR, Zhang H, Wei Z, et al. Discovery of IACS-8803 and IACS-8779, potent agonists of stimulator of interferon genes (STING) with robust systemic antitumor efficacy. Bioorg Med Chem Lett 2019; 29(20):126640.

76. Woo SR, Fuertes MB, Corrales L, et al. STING-dependent cytosolic DNA sensing mediates innate immune recognition of immunogenic tumors. Immunity 2014;41(5):830–42.

Sellar Metastases
Diagnosis and Management

Mostafa Shahein, MD, MS[a,b], Thiago Albonette-Felicio, MD[a], Ricardo L. Carrau, MD[a,c],
Daniel M. Prevedello, MD[a,c],*

KEYWORDS

- Pituitary • Sella • Metastases • Skull base surgery

KEY POINTS

- Sellar metastases account for 1.8% of all surgically treated sellar masses.
- Breast and lung cancers are the most common sources.
- Mostly asymptomatic initially.
- They have a rapid progressive course with symptoms related to compression of surrounding neural structures or hormonal changes, mainly posterior pituitary gland.
- Treatment is usually palliative aiming at decompression and improving quality of life. Modalities include surgery, radiation, and to less extent chemotherapy.

EPIDEMIOLOGY

Sellar metastases (SM) include metastases to the pituitary gland, the stalk, or the surrounding structures (**Table 1**). One of the first reported cases in English literature was in 1913; this was preceded by a reported pituitary metastasis (PM) in German literature in the 1800s.[1] Sellar and PM are sometimes interchangeably used in the literature. Among all intracranial metastases, SM account for 0.87% in a recent meta-analysis.[2] They account for 1.8% of all surgically treated sellar masses.[3] Elderly patients within the seventh decade of life comprise the most affected age group; however, it may occur in younger patients.[4,5]

ORIGIN OF THE PRIMARY TUMOR

Breast and lung cancers account for 61.4% of all SM. Prostate, renal, thyroid, gastrointestinal, and other tumors are another possible origin. In some cases, the primary tumor maybe unknown. Breast cancer tends to metastasize to the pituitary gland more than other types of tumors due to the elevated hormonal levels, especially the prolactin in the pituitary gland,[6] or during treatment with anti-HER2 therapy.[2,7,8] SM, especially in bone-metastasizing primary tumors, maybe due to the close proximity of the posterior pituitary lobe to the sellar bone.[1]

ANATOMIC SITE OF METASTASES

The most common site of SM is the posterior pituitary lobe and pituitary stalk. An explanation maybe due to the pattern of blood supply that originates from the perforators of the internal carotid artery raising the chance of metastases directly from systemic circulation. However, the anterior pituitary receives blood supply from the hypothalamus through the portal venous circulation.[3] The metastases, however, can extend to suprasellar, sphenoorbital, or petroclival areas.[1]

MANIFESTATIONS OF THE DISEASE

SM maybe the first manifestation in some occult malignancies.[6] They can be symptomatic in only 7% of the cases.[1] These symptoms maybe

[a] Department of Neurological Surgery, The Ohio State University Wexner Medical Center, N-1049 Doan Hall, W. 10th Avenue, Columbus, OH 43210, USA; [b] Department of Neurological Surgery, Aswan University, Egypt; [c] Department of Otolaryngology–Head and Neck Surgery, The Ohio State University Wexner Medical Center, N-1049 Doan Hall, 410 West 10th Avenue, Columbus, OH 43210, USA
* Corresponding author.
E-mail address: dprevedello@gmail.com

Neurosurg Clin N Am 31 (2020) 651–658
https://doi.org/10.1016/j.nec.2020.06.012
1042-3680/20/© 2020 Elsevier Inc. All rights reserved.

Table 1	
Nutshells in suspecting pituitary metastases	
Age	Old patient in 60s or 70s age group
History	Known primary tumor, breast in woman or lung in men, or presented with nonspecific symptoms
Presentation	Diabetes insipidus, cranial nerve palsy, or nonspecific symptoms
Radiological examination	• MRI: sellar/suprasellar mass isointense on T1 and T2. Homogenously enhancing on T1W sequences. Loss of bright posterior gland or enhancing and/or thickening of the pituitary stalk or hypothalamus • CT: invasion rather than expansion of the sellar bone • Other radiological modalities showing primary tumor elsewhere, for example, PET/CT scan
Management	Main aim of treatment is palliative • Surgical in cases of neurologic deficit or to get a final pathologic diagnosis if primary is unknown • One of the radiation modalities for local control after surgery. Radiation with or without chemotherapy if wide spread metastases or surgery is contraindicated
Prognosis	Independent of the modality of the treatment. Local control maybe achieved; however, the burden of the primary tumor is the main factor

The most common findings are listed in each of the table component subheadings but variations are present in the literature.

nonspecific such as fatigue, headache, and general malaise. Manifestations maybe vision-related symptoms or endocrinological symptoms such as diabetes insipidus, selective anterior pituitary hormonal disturbance, or panhypopituitarism.[2]

Ophthalmologic Symptoms

The visual manifestations of these lesions are due to compression or direct invasion of the surrounding structures including the optic pathway and other cranial nerves mainly in the cavernous sinus. The optic pathway involvement presents, most commonly, with bitemporal hemianopsia.[1] When the parasellar region is involved, other cranial nerves can be affected manifesting with trigeminal nerve symptoms (facial pain or impaired sensation) or double vision with third, fourth, and sixth cranial nerve palsies.[1] The course of the cranial neuropathy is rapid due to the aggressive behavior of this disease and raises the suspicion of SM rather than pituitary adenoma if a sellar mass is visualized.[9] Retroorbital pain may also be encountered especially in cavernous sinus affection.[10]

Endocrine Symptoms

These patients may present with panhypopituitarism or selective anterior or posterior gland dysfunction.

Posterior pituitary: diabetes insipidus (DI): Commonly present in SM[6,11,12]; however, in recent studies, the incidence decreased due to the innovation in imaging techniques allowing early identification. It is a rare presentation in pituitary adenoma. DI with a sellar mass raises the suspicion of SM and warrants MRI evaluation even before scanning for the primary tumor.[6] Different theories have been described to explain the tendency of the metastases to the posterior pituitary lobe and thus causing DI.[13] This includes the pattern of blood supply explained earlier or by the close proximity of the dura to the posterior lobe.

Anterior pituitary: overproduction or underproduction of certain pituitary hormones maybe found in these patients.[1] *Hyperprolactinemia* is one of the probable findings, however, mostly not exceeding 200 ng/mL, indicating a stalk effect.[1] Cases of metastases to a pituitary prolactinoma, in which the prolactin level may exceed this level, have been reported.[14,15] Metastases to other pituitary adenoma tumors including nonfunctioning[16] or adrenocorticotropic hormone (ACTH)- and growth hormone (GH)-secreting tumors were described in the literature.[1] It is important to note that these metastases to tumors are rare findings and documented as case reports. SM may also be originating from ectopic secreting tumors such as ACTH-secreting tumors.[17]

Others

Gait instability, Horner syndrome and hearing loss are rare findings that are mostly related to the extension outside the sellar region.[1]

IMAGING

SM are rare tumors. It is usually difficult to distinguish the SM from other common sellar lesions, mainly the pituitary adenoma. Clinical and laboratory evaluation besides the radiological evaluation might be useful.

On MRI they usually have iso- or hypointense signal on T1-weighted image (T1WI) and hyperintense signal on T2WI. They are homogeneously enhancing on postgadolinium sequences.[1] Certain features may help in putting the SM higher in the differential. This includes invasion of the sellar bone or increased vascularity.[18] They usually respect the *diaphragma sellae* and appear as a dumbbell-shaped mass in sagittal planes.[1,19] Loss of the high signal on T2WI, a characteristic feature of the posterior pituitary, suggests an invasive rather than a benign lesion.[20] Briefly, sellar, suprasellar, and stalk/infundibular enhancement are the most commonly encountered findings but the extension to surrounding structures such as hypothalamus, cavernous sinus, and sphenoid sinus can be seen on imaging.[1] Magnetic resonance spectroscopy can be helpful differentiating an SM from a pituitary adenoma.[2]

On computed tomographic (CT) scans, they are iso- to hyperdense lesions. CT has the advantage of detection of invasion of the surrounding bone yet the MRI is still superior.[21] It has been hypothesized that pituitary metastases tend to erode but not expand the sellar bone due to the rapid aggressive behavior of the disease in contrast to the more slowly progressive pituitary adenoma that usually causes expansion of the sellae. All of the previous MRI/CT findings are not exclusively characteristic. Other sellar masses might have the same appearance (**Figs. 1** and **2**).

PET/CT scans are now a powerful tool for the detection of tumors. It plays an important role in designing and planning the treatment of patients with cancer. It can detect hypermetabolic lesions through the body; however, it does not differentiate between metastatic lesions, inflammatory or benign lesions within the pituitary gland. Pituitary adenomas may also show increased metabolism. Also, not all metastatic lesions are hypermetabolic or positive in PET/CT scans.[1] Certain uptake criteria, such as standardized uptake value greater than 4.1 in pituitary lesions means a higher probability of pathologic lesions; however, this should be evaluated in the context of each patient clinical, laboratory, and radiological data.[1]

MANAGEMENT

Management of these lesions is mainly palliative.[11] Surgery, chemoradiation, whole brain radiation, radiosurgery, and hormonotherapy are the modalities available for management. The aim of surgery is mostly to debulk the tumor or gross total resection when deemed safe, improve neurologic deficits, and to get a final pathologic diagnosis if the primary tumor is unknown.[22] Intraoperatively, the nature of the tumor is usually firm, vascular, and diffuse that leads to difficult removal. The preferred surgical approach is transsphenoidal for sellar, suprasellar, and parasellar lesions. Different open approaches can be used depending on the extension of the tumor.[1,23]

Surgical treatment will often improve neurologic function when the deficit is caused by compression. Visual field defects, double vision, and trigeminal pain can improve after tumor debulking and decompression. However, in situations where there is cancer invasion into the nerves, improvement is not observed. Surgery generally fails to improve any endocrinological deficiency as well due to the invasiveness of these tumors into the pituitary gland. In some previous studies, surgery also led to an increase in the survival period.[6] However, others concluded that there is no such improvement in the survival rate.[24]

Radiosurgery or conventional radiation can be used in different medical scenarios: as an adjuvant after surgery or preceding the surgery for control of disseminated diseases or in cases where surgery carries high comorbidity. There has not been any difference between the 2 modalities as regards the survival rate.[25] These modalities carry the risk of injury to surrounding structures. Improved neurologic deficits and diabetes insipidus but failed anterior pituitary dysfunction improvement have been reported in previous case series.[13,26] Radiosurgery achieved 67% tumor control in a previous series.[27] The recommended dose is widely variable and differ according to the surrounding structures being targeted. Most importantly, the optic nerves are usually in close proximity, and safe dose for these structures usually ranges between 8000 and 10,000 cGy for radiosurgery[28,29] and a total of 5400 cGy for fractionated radiotherapy.[30] The dose of radiation to the SM also differs according to the primary tumor being reported with variable response to radiation treatment. The reported dose for SM ranged from 8 to 40 Gy.[1,31–33] Local or whole-brain radiation for possible meningeal carcinomatosis or subarachnoid spread is a debate.[34,35]

Chemotherapy can be combined with radiation and is recommended as the treatment of choice

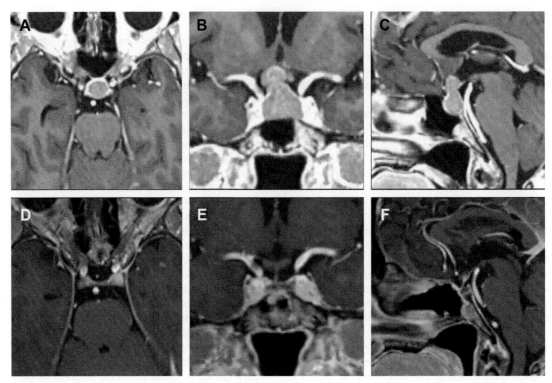

Fig. 1. Imaging of case #1. Preoperative (*A*) axial, (*B*) coronal, and (*C*) sagittal contrast-enhanced MRI, showing a lesion occupying the sellar and suprasellar spaces. Postoperative (*D*) axial, (*E*) coronal, and (*F*) sagittal contrast-enhanced MRI, showing gross total resection and preservation of the normal pituitary stalk and gland.

in widespread metastases cases.[1,6] It has been postulated that chemotherapy cannot penetrate blood brain barrier (BBB) and thus has no role in brain metastases; however, the BBB is disrupted in contrast-enhancing tumors and relatively larger metastases.[36] In addition, the pituitary gland, particularly, lacks a BBB. Chemotherapy agents used in SM mainly depend on the primary tumor. It has a role in chemosensitive tumors; however, the exact direct effect of these chemotherapeutic agents on these SM is not well defined.[37] Reported cases of sellar lesions in patients with breast cancer received a combination of fluorouracil, epirubicin, and cyclophosphamide followed by a taxotere a year later on lymph node involvement, then followed by vinorelbine and capecitabine. Despite all the previous chemotherapeutic agents the pituitary lesion continued to grow. During the course of the disease, DI and deterioration of vision occurred and the patient eventually died. In the same study, another case showed a stationary pituitary lesion although a craniopharyngioma was most likely.[37] A combination of stereotactic radiotherapy and chemotherapy with cisplastin and etoposide resulted in significant reduction of enhancing residual mass following a transsphenoidal resection of sellar mass proved to be

metastatic neuroendocrine carcinoma originating from the lung.[38]

In a recent systematic review of all cases reported for SM that included 657 cases, they concluded that chemotherapy and radiotherapy resulted in improving the survival rate in these cases. However, targeted radiotherapy and surgery did not improve the survival rate regardless of the degree of resection. Interestingly, chemotherapy was used in only quarter of these cases.[25] Hormone replacement therapy is also needed unless contraindicated.

PROGNOSIS

The aim of treatment in most of these patients is palliative. Choosing the appropriate modality should be focused on the quality of life. The mean survival rate ranges between 6 and 22 months irrespective of the modality of the treatment.[6,24] However, in a recent metanalysis, radiation and chemotherapy showed an improvement in the survival rate especially in the era after 2010 possibly due to improved diagnostic and treatment modalities.[25] The prognosis is related mainly to the number of metastases, the nature of the primary diseases, and the timing of the diagnosis.

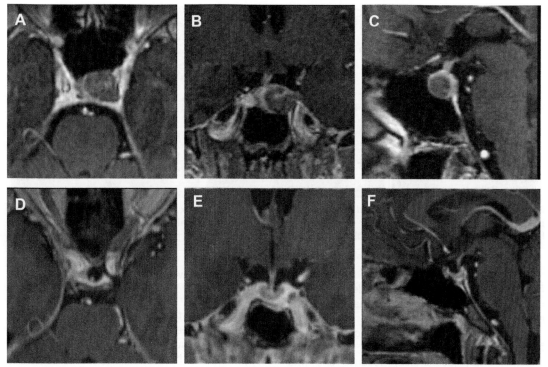

Fig. 2. Imaging of case #2. Preoperative (*A*) axial, (*B*) coronal, and (*C*) sagittal contrast-enhanced MRI, showing a sellar lesion pushing the pituitary gland to the right and invading the left cavernous sinus. Postoperative (*D*) axial, (*E*) coronal, and (*F*) sagittal contrast-enhanced MRI, showing complete resection and preservation of the normal pituitary stalk and gland.

Illustrative Cases

Case #1: metastatic lung cancer

History: a 71-year-old woman presented to the emergency department with severe acute left hip pain. She received a previous diagnosis of lung adenocarcinoma 5 months early.

Workup: the patient underwent a metastatic workup, which revealed a sellar and suprasellar lesion on MRI postcontrast (see **Fig. 1**A–C). It was homogeneously slightly enhancing to a lesser degree than the pituitary gland, and it compressed the optic chiasm. In addition, the brain MRI also showed multiple lesions in the falx and parafalcine locations, which enhanced avidly and homogeneously, had dural tail and no associated edema. Differential diagnosis for the sellar lesion included pituitary adenoma, meningioma, or SM especially with the known history of lung adenocarcinoma. For the remaining lesions, the differential diagnosis included meningioma and metastases. As part of her workup, a PET scan revealed the lesion in the sella as well as lesions in the mediastinum (bilaterally), left acetabulum, right humerus, and spleen to be hypermetabolic (**Fig. 3**). Hormonal workup showed no significant changes.

Presentation: the patient had a mild bitemporal hemianopsia on physical examination.

Management: because the lesion was symptomatic and in close contact to the optic chiasm, a decision to decompress the optic apparatus was made. Endoscopic endonasal transsellar transtubercular approach was planned to debulk the tumor in the sellar and suprasellar region.

Operative details (**Fig. 4**): the tumor was bloody and had a soft consistency. A total resection was achieved a combination of dissectors. We were able to obtain a gross total resection of the tumor from the sellar and suprasellar compartments. The tumor was followed superiorly avoiding a CSF exposure. After adequate hemostasis, focus was placed on reconstruction, which was undertaken using collagen matrix and, on top of the sellar opening, a mucosal graft from the middle turbinate, followed by pieces of gelatin sponges and bioresorbable nasal dressings, providing support to the construct.

Gross total resection of the tumor and adequate decompression of the optic apparatus were achieved. This was evidenced by a postoperative follow-up MRI (see **Fig. 1**D–F).

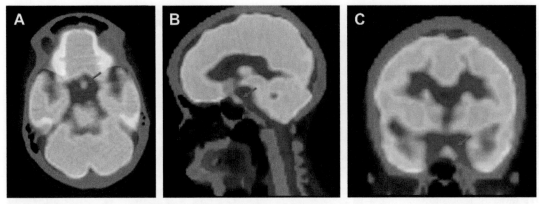

Fig. 3. Imaging for PET scan performed preoperatively with F18-fluorodeoxyglucose demonstrating hypermetabolic mass in the sellae and suprasellar space (*A*: axial; *B*: sagittal; *C*: coronal). The blue arrow is pointing to the hypermetabolic mass in the different planes.

Frozen pathology was equivocal; however, the final pathologic report showed the lesion to be a metastatic adenocarcinoma, originally from the lung.

Follow up: the patient had no complications from surgery. Then, she was initiated on immunotherapy (osimertinib) because she was positive for epidermal growth factor receptor exon 19 mutation, and radiation therapy was withheld. A brain MRI, after 14 months from the surgery, no sellar masses and no other enhancing brain lesions were present. On her last visit, 16 months after the surgery, she was doing well.

Case #2: metastatic neuroendocrine tumor

History: a 48-year-old man presented at our institution for a consultation after a discovery of a pituitary lesion on a brain MRI. The patient had already the diagnosis of stage IV lung cancer (neuroendocrine carcinoma with atypical carcinoid features) 16 months before this visit and also had a cerebellar metastasis, which was treated with radiation therapy.

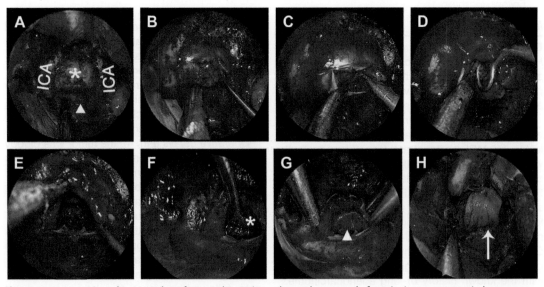

Fig. 4. Intraoperative photography of an endoscopic endonasal approach for pituitary metastatic lung cancer, showing tumor resection (case #1). (*A*). After the nasal phase and the wide opening of the sphenoid sinus, the bone forming the sellar floor is removed, exposing the dura (*asterisk*) between both internal carotid artery (ICA) and above the clivus (*arrowhead*). (*B*). Subsequently, the dura is opened in a booklet type fashion, and the tumor is debulked using a combination of (*C*) the 2-suction technique and (*D*) ringed curettes. (*E*). A 0-degree scope shows complete resection of the sellar component and (*F*) a 30-degree scope, the suprasellar component. It is possible to visualize the diaphragm sellae (*asterisk*) coming down. (*G*). Collagen matrix (*arrowhead*) is used for reconstruction, followed by (*H*) a mucosal graft (*arrow*) of the middle turbinate.

Workup: in addition to the already treated cerebellar metastasis, a brain MRI revealed a lesion isointense with the pituitary on T2WI, which did not enhance as much as the rest of the pituitary gland and was located on the left side of the sellae (see **Fig. 2**A–C). Endocrine workup was normal. PET scan showed hypermetabolic lesion in the sellae as well as lesions in the lung and lymphadenopathy in the supraclavicular, mediastinal, hilar, and gastrohepatic regions.

Presentation: the patient had no neurologic deficits on physical examination.

Management: a decision was made to operate his pituitary lesion in order to have specimen for definitive diagnosis. Endoscopic endonasal transsellar approach was planned. Gross total resection of the tumor was achieved, which was evidenced by a postoperative follow-up MRI (see **Fig. 2**D–F).

Operative details: the tumor was darker than a standard pituitary adenoma and much more fibrous and also bloodier. Despite that, we could carry out an extracapsular dissection. There was a portion of the tumor invading the left cavernous sinus, and, once this portion was removed, there was intense venous bleeding, which was controlled with thrombin foam. Once hemostasis was achieved, reconstruction was undertaken accordingly.

Frozen pathology and the final pathologic report showed the lesion was a metastatic neuroendocrine carcinoma, originally from the lung.

Follow up: the patient remained with no neurologic deficits. Then, the patient received radiation therapy and chemotherapy. At his last visit, 58 months after, he was doing well.

DISCLOSURE

D.M. Prevedello is a consultant for Stryker Corporation, Medtronic Corporation and Integra Life-Sciences Corporation. D.M. Prevedello has equity on 3 Rivers LLC, eLum Technologies LLC, and Soliton LLC. D.M. Prevedello receives royalties from KLS-Martin, Mizuho, and ACE-Medical. None is related wither directly or indirectly to the content of the article. The other authors have nothing to disclose.

REFERENCES

1. Javanbakht A, D'Apuzzo M, Badie B, et al. Pituitary metastasis: a rare condition. Endocr Connect 2018; 7(10):1049–57.

2. He W, Chen F, Dalm B, et al. Metastatic involvement of the pituitary gland: a systematic review with pooled individual patient data analysis. Pituitary 2015;18(1):159–68.

3. Fassett DR, Couldwell WT. Metastases to the pituitary gland. Neurosurg Focus 2004;16(4):1–4.

4. Javanbakht A, D'Apuzzo M, Badie B, et al. Pituitary metastasis: A rare condition. Endocr Connect 2018. https://doi.org/10.1530/EC-18-0338.

5. Freda PU, Post KD. Differential diagnosis of sellar masses. Endocrinol Metab Clin North Am 1999; 28(1):81–117.

6. Morita A, Meyer FB, Laws ER. Symptomatic pituitary metastases. J Neurosurg 1998;89(1):69–73.

7. Park Y, Kim H, Kim E-H, et al. Effective Treatment of Solitary Pituitary Metastasis with Panhypopituitarism in HER2-Positive Breast Cancer by Lapatinib. Cancer Res Treat 2016;48(1):403–8.

8. Peppa M, Papaxoinis G, Xiros N, et al. Panhypopituitarism due to Metastases to the Hypothalamus and the Pituitary Resulting From Primary Breast Cancer: A Case Report and Review of the Literature. Clin Breast Cancer 2009;9(4):E4–7.

9. Zager EL, Hedley-Whyte TE. Metastasis within a Pituitary Adenoma Presenting with Bilateral Abducens Palsies: Case Report and Review of the Literature. Neurosurgery 1987;21(3):383–6.

10. Supler ML, Friedman WA. Acute Bilateral Ophthalmoplegia Secondary to Cavernous Sinus Metastasis. Neurosurgery 1992;31(4):783–6.

11. McCormick PC, Post KD, Kandji AD, et al. Metastatic Carcinoma to the Pituitary Gland. Br J Neurosurg 1989;3(1):71–9.

12. Houck WA, Olson KB, Horton J. Clinical features of tumor metastasis to the pituitary. Cancer 1970; 26(3):656–9.

13. Chon H, Yoon K, Kwon DH, et al. Hypofractionated stereotactic radiosurgery for pituitary metastases. J Neurooncol 2017;132(1):127–33.

14. Abe T, Matsumoto K, Iida M, et al. Malignant carcinoid tumor of the anterior mediastinum metastasis to a prolactin-secreting pituitary adenoma: A case report. Surg Neurol 1997;48(4):389–94.

15. Hanna W, Davies D, Neal S. Pituitary apoplexy following metastasis of bronchogenic adenocarcinoma to a prolactinoma. Clin Endocrinol (Oxf) 1999;51(3):377–81.

16. Noga C, Prayson RA, Kowalski R, et al. Metastatic adenocarcinoma to a pituitary adenoma. Ann Diagn Pathol 2001;5(6):354–60.

17. Chandra V, McDonald LW, Anderson RJ. Metastatic small cell carcinoma of the lung presenting as pituitary apoplexy and Cushing's syndrome. J Neurooncol 1984;2(1):59–66.

18. Freda PU. Unusual causes of sellar/parasellar masses in a large transsphenoidal surgical series. J Clin Endocrinol Metab 1996;81(10): 3455–9.

19. Schubiger O, Haller D. Metastases to the pituitary-hypothalamic axis. Neuroradiology 1992;34(2): 131–4.

20. Chaudhuri R, Twelves C, Cox TCS, et al. MRI in diabetes insipidus due to metastatic breast carcinoma. Clin Radiol 1992;46(3):184–8.

21. Ginsberg LE. Neoplastic diseases affecting the central skull base: CT and MR imaging. Am J Roentgenol 1992;159(3):581–9.

22. Goulart CR, Upadhyay S, Ditzel Filho LFS, et al. Newly Diagnosed Sellar Tumors in Patients with Cancer: A Diagnostic Challenge and Management Dilemma. World Neurosurg 2017;106:254–65.

23. Dias ML, Abucham J. Pituitary and other sellar region metastases. Curr Opin Endocr Metab Res 2018;1:36–41.

24. Zoli M, Mazzatenta D, Faustini-Fustini M, et al. Pituitary Metastases: Role of Surgery. World Neurosurg 2013;79(2):327–30.

25. Ng S, Fomekong F, Delabar V, et al. Current status and treatment modalities in metastases to the pituitary: a systematic review. J Neurooncol 2020; 146(2):219–27.

26. Kano H, Niranjan A, Kondziolka D, et al. Stereotactic radiosurgery for pituitary metastasis. Surg Neurol 2009;72(3):248–55.

27. Iwai Y, Yamanaka K, Honda Y, et al. Radiosurgery for Pituitary Metastases. Neurol Med Chir (Tokyo) 2004; 44(3):112–7.

28. Carvounis PE, Katz B. Gamma knife radiosurgery in neuro-ophthalmology. Curr Opin Ophthalmol 2003; 14(6):317–24.

29. Leber KA, Berglöff J, Pendl G. Dose—response tolerance of the visual pathways and cranial nerves of the cavernous sinus to stereotactic radiosurgery. J Neurosurg 1998;88(1):43–50.

30. Indaram M, Ali FS, Levin MH. In search of a treatment for radiation-induced optic neuropathy. Curr Treat Options Neurol 2015;17(1):325.

31. Laigle-Donadey F, Taillibert S, Martin-Duverneuil N, et al. Skull-base metastases. J Neurooncol 2005. https://doi.org/10.1007/s11060-004-8099-0.

32. Iwai Y, Yamanaka K. Gamma Knife Radiosurgery for Skull Base Metastasis and Invasion. Stereotact Funct Neurosurg 1999;72(1):81–7.

33. Kocher M, Voges J, Staar S, et al. Linear Accelerator Radiosurgery for Recurrent Malignant Tumors of the Skull Base. Am J Clin Oncol 1998;21(1):18–22.

34. Max MB, Deck MDF, Rottenberg DA. Pituitary metastasis: Incidence in cancer patients and clinical differentiation from pituitary adenorna. Neurology 1981; 31(8):998.

35. Juneau P, Schoene WC, Black P. Malignant Tumors in the Pituitary Gland. Arch Neurol 1992;49(5): 555–8.

36. Schuette W. Treatment of brain metastases from lung cancer: chemotherapy. Lung Cancer 2004;45: S253–7.

37. Fortunati N, Felicetti F, Donadio M, et al. Pituitary lesions in breast cancer patients: A report of three cases. Oncol Lett 2015;9(6):2762–6.

38. Lin DS, Griffith B, Patel S, et al. Pituitary metastasis from lung carcinoma presenting as a pituitary adenoma. Appl Radiol 2018;47(7):34–6.

Management of Skull Base Metastases

Gautam U. Mehta, MD[a], Shaan M. Raza, MD[b],*

KEYWORDS

- Cancer • Metastasis • Skull-base • Surgery

KEY POINTS

- Skull base metastases are likely underrecognized in patients with cancer.
- Breast and lung cancers are the most frequent primary histologies among patients with skull base metastases.
- Presentation of skull base metastases often includes one or a combination of skull base clinical syndromes (orbital, sellar/parasellar, middle fossa, temporal bone, jugular foramen, occipital condyle).
- Optimal management of skull base metastases is histology dependent and should include a multidisciplinary approach.

INTRODUCTION

Although skeletal sites are a frequent location for cancer metastases, data on metastases to the skull base are scarce. Because of this infrequency, studies on skull base metastases typically have diverse criteria for inclusion, complicating our understanding of prevalence and management. For example, Berlinger and colleagues[1] described 5 patterns of involvement within the temporal bone by systemic malignancies: (1) distant metastasis, (2) direct regional spread of tumor, (3) meningeal carcinomatosis, (4) leptomeningeal spread of primary intracranial tumor, and (5) spread of a hematologic malignancy. Such varied criteria have been used to define inclusion among some studies of metastases to the skull base.[2] Lack of uniform data, in combination with the deep location and high concentration of neurovascular structures in the skull base pose challenges in the management of these metastatic lesions. Herein the authors review the existing literature on metastases to the skull base.

EPIDEMIOLOGY OF SKULL BASE METASTASES

Defining the prevalence of skull base metastases among patients with cancer remains challenging. First, patients with cancer typically do not undergo dedicated skull base imaging. Furthermore, imaging of the skull base is complex, with numerous vascular and soft-tissue structures potentially masking identification of small pathologic lesions. Regardless, information on the prevalence of skull base metastases can be extrapolated from autopsy study of temporal bones, which suggest that these lesions may be significantly underreported. Belal reported that among 357 patients with temporal bones available at the House Ear Institute, 13 demonstrated evidence of metastatic lesions,[3] and this suggests a prevalence of 4% in the general population at the time of death. Gloria-Cruz and colleagues[2] studied temporal bones of 212 patients with primary solid malignancies and found tumor involvement in 22% of patients (18% of temporal bones). This study included patients with temporal bone disease

[a] Division of Neurosurgery, House Clinic, 2100 West 3rd Street, Suite 111, Los Angeles, CA 90057, USA; [b] Department of Neurosurgery, The University of Texas M.D. Anderson Cancer Center, Room FC7.200, Unit 442, Houston, TX 77030-4009, USA
* Corresponding author.
E-mail address: smraza@mdanderson.org
Twitter: @GautamMehtaMD (G.U.M.); @DrShaanRaza (S.M.R.)

Neurosurg Clin N Am 31 (2020) 659–666
https://doi.org/10.1016/j.nec.2020.06.013
1042-3680/20/© 2020 Elsevier Inc. All rights reserved.

following any of Berlinger's 5 patterns of involvement; however, clinical data from 75% of involved temporal bones supported tumor seeding through hematogenous spread.[1]

Histology

Prior study has demonstrated that skull base metastases can cover a range of histologies (**Table 1**). It is important to recognize that treatment studies (surgery, radiation therapy, etc.) may be biased toward specific histologies that are amenable to that particular therapeutic modality. For example, Pan and colleagues[4] reported a series of 27 patients who were treated for skull base metastases with Gamma Knife stereotactic radiosurgery (SRS). The most common histologies in this cohort were breast cancer (27%) and nasopharyngeal cancer (19%), both of which are considered favorable candidates for radiation therapy. In 1981 Greenberg and colleagues[5] reported on 43 patients with skull base metastases who underwent conventional radiotherapy. They also reported the most common primary histology to be breast cancer (39%). Conversely, Chaichana and colleagues[6] reported 29 patients who underwent surgery for skull base metastases. In this cohort, the most common histologies were lung cancer (45%) and breast cancer (24%). Similarly, Chamoun and DeMonte reported on 27 patients with skull base metastases.[7] In their series, the most common histology was renal cell carcinoma (22%), which is considered relatively radioresistant. Most other large studies on skull base metastases have been location specific (sella, temporal bone), which may affect the likelihood of involvement by particular histologies.[2,8,9]

Only one study to date has included an unfiltered set of patients with skull base metastases. A systematic review by Laigle-Donadey and colleagues[10] in 2005 included a total of 279 patients with skull base metastases from all reports. They found prostate cancer to be the most common histology (39%), followed by breast cancer (21%), and lymphoma (8%). This study did include case studies and treatment series, which may have been subject to reporting bias.

The abovementioned study notwithstanding, breast cancer seems to be the most consistently reported histology (11%–47%), appearing as the first or second most common histology in all general studies (see **Table 1**). This is consistent with the high prevalence of breast cancer metastases among large studies of temporal bone (21%) and pituitary (22%) metastases.[2,8] Lung cancer skull base metastases were also consistently described (7%–45%). Not surprisingly, these histologies are the most highly represented among skeletal metastases in the general population (breast—36%, lung—16%).[11] Although the high prevalence of lung cancer in the general population likely accounts for its relatively high proportion among skull base metastases, breast cancer metastases seem to have a particular affinity for skeletal sites. Bone is the most common secondary site in breast cancer, and nearly 70% of patients with advanced disease develop skeletal metastases.[12] Mechanisms underlying this propensity are thought to be related to both tumor intrinsic factors and the bone microenvironment.[13,14]

CLINICAL PRESENTATION OF SKULL BASE METASTASES

Common locations of skull base metastases have been described by surgical series. Chaichana and colleauges[6] found the most common sites to be sellar/parasellar (24%) and orbital (21%). Similarly, Chamoun and DeMonte[7] described most lesions as involving the orbit (26%) and the sellar/parasellar region (19%). As these are surgical series, they are potentially biased toward lesions with histologies and locations that are amenable to surgery.

Because of the limitations in routine screening for skull base metastases in patients with cancer, these lesions are often identified based on location-specific clinical findings. Greenberg identified 5 clinical syndromes associated with location of skull base metastases: (1) orbital syndrome, (2) sellar/parasellar syndrome, (3) middle fossa (gasserian ganglion) syndrome, (4) jugular foramen syndrome, and (5) occipital condyle syndrome (**Table 2**).[5] Tumor involvement at these locations frequently causes cranial nerve dysfunction, leading to clinically relevant sequelae.[15] Chamoun and DeMonte also included temporal bone syndrome in a more recent description.[7] Finally, skull base metastases may also rarely present with hemorrhage.[16]

Orbital Syndrome

Orbital syndrome is present with approximately 7% to 13% of skull base metastases (see **Table 2**). In such cases, a lesion of the orbit can cause pain, difficulty with extraocular motility/diplopia, and/or proptosis. In some cases, patients may present with visual loss. Font and Ferry described a series of 28 patients with metastatic orbital tumors.[17] Breast cancer was the most common primary malignancy (29%). In this series, the most common clinical sign was proptosis (75%), followed by pain (29%) and decreased visual acuity (29%).

Table 1
Most common histologies reported by large series of skull base metastases

Author, Year	N	Population	Most Common Histologies
Greenberg et al,[5] 1981	43	Radiation therapy series	Breast—39% Lung—14% Prostate—12%
Laigle-Donadey et al,[10] 2005	279	Systematic review[a]	Prostate—39% Breast—21% Lymphoma—8%
Chamoun & DeMonte,[7] 2011; Chamoun et al,[26] 2012	27	Surgical series	Renal cell—22% Breast—11% Lung/Thyroid/Leiomyosarcoma—7%
Chaichana et al,[6] 2013	29	Surgical series	Lung—45% Breast—24% Primary bone—14%
Pan et al,[4] 2013	27	Radiosurgery series	Breast—27% Nasopharyngeal cancer—19% Lung—15%
Minniti et al,[22] 2014	34	Radiosurgery series	Breast—47% Lung—32% Colon—6%

[a] Includes series by Greenberg.

Sellar/Parasellar Syndrome

Tumor involvement of the sella or the parasellar region occurs with 16% to 29% of skull base metastases (see **Table 2**). Although involvement of the sella or pituitary may result in hypopituitarism, involvement of the parasellar region may result in a cavernous sinus syndrome (**Fig. 1**). The latter typically results in pain, ophthalmoplegia, and a decrease in visual acuity. Pituitary metastases have been summarized by several systematic reviews.[8,18] As with other skull base metastases, breast (26%–37%) and lung (24%–31%) cancers predominate.

Recent systematic review by Ng and colleagues[8] included 657 cases of pituitary metastases. Most common symptoms were anterior pituitary hormone dysfunction (54%), visual field defects (46%), and diplopia (35%). Mean diameter was 2.1 cm, with suprasellar extension in 63%. Cavernous sinus involvement was present in 22%. Approximately half of patients underwent some form of surgery, with 78% of patients undergoing biopsy or debulking and 22% with gross total resection. Recent study by Patel and colleagues[9] has suggested that surgical resection is associated with significantly improved survival, and this should be balanced against the concept

Table 2
Frequency of clinical syndromes associated with skull base metastases[a]

Clinical Syndrome	Common Findings	Greenberg et al,[5] 1981	Laigle-Donadey et al,[10] 2005[a]
Orbital	Proptosis, diplopia, pain	7%	13%
Parasellar	Diplopia, hypopituitarism	16%	29%
Middle fossa	Facial pain/numbness	35%	6%
Jugular foramen	Postauricular pain, hoarseness, dysphagia	21%	4%
Occipital condyle	Neck pain/stiffness, dysarthria, tongue weakness	21%	16%

[a] Includes series by Greenberg.

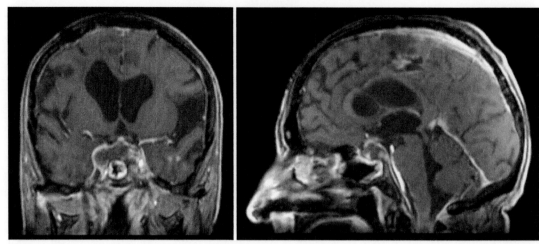

Fig. 1. T1 postcontrast MRI of a 72-year-old woman with multiple medical comorbidities who presented with 3 weeks of oculomotor palsy (*left*: coronal, *right*: sagittal). She was found to have a sellar mass involving her right cavernous sinus and abutting the optic chiasm. Computed tomography imaging of the body was negative for mass. Supraclavicular lymph nodes were noted; however, a biopsy of these was negative. Endoscopic endonasal biopsy revealed pathology consistent with colon adenocarcinoma. Colonoscopy confirmed a colonic mass. The patient refused oncologic treatment, and she died from septic shock related to central line–associated bacteremia 1 month later.

that patients selected for surgery may naturally have lesions more amenable to resection and/or a lower systemic burden of disease.

Middle Fossa Syndrome

Middle fossa syndrome has also been referred to as gasserian ganglion syndrome, as clinical presentation is largely related to compression of the trigeminal nerve in the middle skull base. Although this was relatively uncommon in the systematic review by Laigle-Donadey (6%), this was the most common skull base clinical syndrome in the series reported by Greenberg (35%).[5,10] In such cases, tumors involving the petrous apex or other regions of the middle cranial base may cause trigeminal symptoms including facial numbness, pain, or paresthesia. Autopsy study has revealed that the petrous apex is the most common site of involvement in patients with metastatic disease of the temporal bone.[2]

Temporal Bone Syndrome

Although temporal bone sequelae were not defined by Greenberg, this clinical syndrome was later described by Chamoun and DeMonte, given the high frequency of metastases to this location.[5,7] Tumors involving the temporal bone may affect the hearing and/or vestibular apparatus and the facial nerve. Hearing loss may be sensorineural, related to invasion of the optic capsule or cochlear nerve, or may be conductive in cases of

eustachian tube dysfunction. Retrospective chart review of 47 patients with temporal bone metastases identified at autopsy revealed hearing loss in 40%, vertigo in 15%, and facial asymmetry in 15%.[2]

Jugular Foramen Syndrome

In 4% to 21% of patients, the jugular foramen may be involved by metastasis (see **Table 2**). In such cases, the cranial nerves that exit through this foramen (glossopharyngeal, vagus, and accessory nerves) are at risk. This dysfunction of cranial nerves 9 through 11 is also termed Vernet syndrome. Clinical signs and symptoms at presentation may include asymmetry of the palate, vocal cord dysfunction, difficulty with shoulder shrug, hoarseness, and/or dysphagia (**Fig. 2**).

Occipital Condyle Syndrome

Sixteen to twenty-one percent of patients with skull base metastases present with occipital condyle syndrome (see **Table 2**). Lesions involving the occipital condyle typically present with unilateral pain (may be dynamic/worse with motion), dysarthria, and ipsilateral tongue weakness or fasciculations.[19] Patients often work hard to keep their neck straight to avoid pain. Capobianco and colleagues[19] reported 11 cases of skull base metastases resulting in occipital condyle syndrome. In 7 of 9 cases in which timing was recorded, occipital pain preceded hypoglossal weakness. All

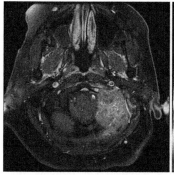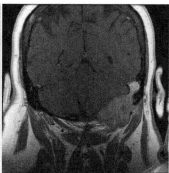

Fig. 2. T1 postcontrast MRI of a 64-year-old woman with a skull base renal cell carcinoma metastasis who presented with jugular foramen syndrome (hoarse voice) and occipital condyle syndrome (pain, tongue weakness).

patients had dysarthria on examination and 3 (of 11) patients had dysphagia.

MANAGEMENT OF SKULL BASE METASTASES
Diagnosis and (Re)staging

Histopathologic confirmation is critical to guide management of skull base metastases, as different treatment modalities are appropriate for specific histologies. Skull base metastases may present in the following 3 scenarios: (1) a skull base mass in a patient with known active malignancy, (2) a skull base mass identified concurrently with a noncranial mass and/or lymphadenopathy, and (3) a skull base mass identified in isolation. In the latter 2 cases histologic diagnosis should generally be determined before definitive treatment is directed at the skull base mass. In patients with both a skull base mass and another, more accessible lesion, biopsy of the systemic lesion is preferable. In cases where another lesion is not available for biopsy, and which seem suspicious for malignancy, biopsy of the skull base mass should be performed before definitive treatment if feasible.

For treatment planning, dedicated imaging should be performed to evaluate tumor involvement, which should include thin-slice computed tomography (CT) restricted to the area of involvement (orbits, sinus, temporal bone) as well as contrast-enhanced MRI. Fat-saturated MRI is particularly important for lesions that involve the orbit, as this will mitigate the T1 hyperintensity encountered with periorbital fat. With cranial nerve involvement, further diagnostic studies beyond the standard neurologic examination can be important to establish functional status. With suspected optic nerve or tract involvement, dedicated visual field examination (Humphrey automated perimetry) should be performed. Patients with involvement of the temporal bone should undergo otoscopy to evaluate for fluid in the middle ear

and undergo formal audiologic evaluation. In patients with involvement of the jugular foramen, or who present with swallowing difficulty, an evaluation of vocal cord and/or swallowing function can be useful before treatment planning.

Finally, in patients with metastatic cancer, an understanding of systemic disease burden is critical to determining optimal management. If not recently performed, body imaging including CT or PET can be useful for restaging.

Radiation Therapy

Because of their deep location and potential involvement of critical neurovascular structures, skull base metastases are attractive candidates for radiation-based treatment strategies. This is particularly relevant to patients with advanced stage cancer who may have multiple sites of disease. In addition, many of the common histologies among skull base metastases are typically considered radiosensitive (breast cancer, prostate cancer, and lymphoma) (see **Table 1**).[10] Greenberg and colleagues[5] reported 43 patients who underwent conventional radiation therapy for skull base metastases. Dosages were not reported; however, 86% of patients demonstrated symptomatic improvement. Prior study from Memorial Sloan Kettering has suggested that early treatment results in improved clinical outcome.[20] Based on early these findings, Greenberg dichotomized patients between those that underwent early initiation of treatment (<1 month after diagnosis) and late treatment (>1 month).[5] Symptomatic improvement was greater in the group who underwent early treatment (92% vs 78%). In addition, objective responses to radiation therapy were far more frequent in the group who underwent early treatment (72% vs 28%).

Focused, single-session radiation treatment using SRS has also been applied skull base metastases. Iwai and Yamanaka reported the results of Gamma Knife SRS for 11 patients with skull base metastases; however, these outcomes were mixed with the results of treatment of 7 patients with locoregional spread of nasopharyngeal carcinoma.[21] Mean margin dose was 16.2 Gy, and overall, 61% of patients demonstrated a symptomatic improvement. Complications included temporary nausea and vomiting (1 patient) and optic neuropathy (1 patient who previously underwent conventional radiation therapy). Pan and colleagues[4] reported a similar series in 27 patients with skull base metastases, also including a cohort of patients with locoregional spread of nasopharyngeal carcinoma. Median survival in this cohort was 15 months. In this series, nonsurvival outcomes were also mixed with the results of 16 patients with a primary skull base malignancy (hemangiopericytoma, olfactory neuroblastoma, etc.), further complicating interpretation of clinical outcomes and adverse radiation effects.

Finally, Minniti and colleagues[22] reviewed outcomes of a cohort of 34 patients with skull base metastases that involved the cavernous sinus or the optic apparatus who underwent hypofractionated SRS. Patients underwent 5 fractions of 5 Gy each. Local control at 2 years was 72%. Fifty-one percent of patients demonstrated a clinical improvement after therapy. One patient developed a new abducens nerve palsy 12 months after therapy, with full recovery after a course of oral corticosteroids.

Medical Management

Specific data on medical management of skull base metastases are not available. Regardless, chemotherapy, hormone therapy, and immunotherapy should be considered for skull base metastases based largely on histology and the burden of systemic disease. For patients with widespread disease, optimal management often prioritizes systemic therapy over local therapy. Furthermore, some histologies are uniquely sensitive to medical management, which includes, but is not limited to, hormone therapies for some breast and prostate cancers, targeted therapy for certain non–small cell lung cancers, and chemotherapy for some hematologic malignancies (ie, multiple myeloma). With expanding indications for targeted therapies and immunotherapies, the role of medical treatment of skull base metastases may increase over time (**Fig. 3**).

Medical management may also be used as part of a multidisciplinary approach to symptoms associated with skull base metastases.

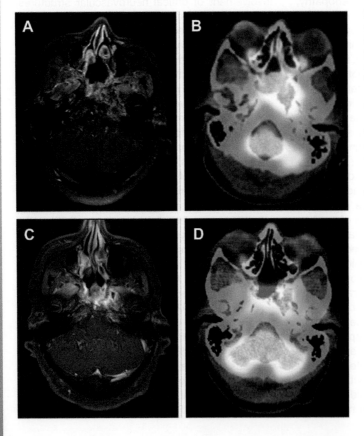

Fig. 3. Patient with known ovarian cancer presenting with conductive hearing loss. Before presentation, the patient had a previous endonasal biopsy and intensity-modulated radiotherapy. T1-weighted postcontrast MRI (*A*) and PET/CT (*B*) demonstrating mass involving the left nasopharynx, pterygoid plates, and middle cranial fossa demonstrating progression in comparison to initial postradiotherapy scans. Patient was initiated on anti-PD-1 therapy. Imaging (*C, D*) after 3 cycles of therapy demonstrates significant decrease in size. (Images are property of Department of Neurosurgery, The University of Texas M.D. Anderson Cancer Center.)

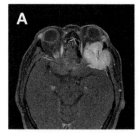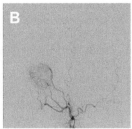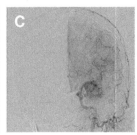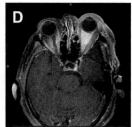

Fig. 4. Solitary renal cell carcinoma metastasis. Patient with known renal cell carcinoma presenting with proptosis, diplopia, and optic neuropathy. Postcontrast T1-weighted MRI (A) demonstrated an avidly enhancing mass centered in this sphenoid wing with extension into the middle cranial fossa and orbit. Systemic imaging demonstrated no other sites of disease. Cerebral digital subtraction angiography (B: lateral external carotid injection, C: AP common carotid injection) demonstrates vascular supply from the internal maxillary, middle meningeal, and ophthalmic arteries. Because of solitary site of disease and presenting symptoms, surgical resection was performed via orbitozygomatic craniotomy with anterior clinoidectomy, optic canal unroofing, wide dural, and periorbital resection. Gross total resection with resolution of symptoms was achieved (D). (Images are property of Department of Neurosurgery, The University of Texas M.D. Anderson Cancer Center.). AP, Anterior-posterior.

Corticosteroids may be useful in managing cranial neuropathies and brain edema. Furthermore, bone pain from skull base metastases can be managed using opioids, corticosteroids, and/or bisphosphonates.[23–25]

Surgical Management

Surgical resection of skull base metastases can be an effective strategy for local control but is appropriate in only a very specific patient population. Optimal candidates include patients with well-managed systemic disease with single or oligometastases (**Fig. 4**). Such patients indicated for surgery should have both high-performance status and long life expectancy and should be able to tolerate the physical recovery required after surgery.[15] Surgery may also be particularly beneficial in patients with intracranial extension, particularly in the posterior fossa, where resection may significantly affect life expectancy. Finally, patients with occipital condyle syndrome and pain from associated instability may benefit from instrumented fusion to reduce pathologic motion.

Among 27 patients who underwent resection for skull base metastases at M.D. Anderson Cancer Center, median overall survival was 11.4 months.[7,26] The most common histology was renal cell carcinoma (22%), as this cancer is relatively radioresistant. There were no mortalities and 2 patients had worsening of an existing cranial neuropathy. Greater survival was associated with lack of dural and/or brain invasion, higher performance status at the time of surgery, and favorable histologies (ie, follicular carcinoma of the thyroid). Gross total resection was achieved in 59% of cases but did not predict overall survival.[26] Most of the patients received postoperative radiation therapy. Chaichana and colleagues[6] reported

surgical outcomes of 29 patients with skull base metastases treated at Johns Hopkins Medical Institute. Gross total resection was achieved in 34% of cases. Median overall survival was 10 months, and the most common histology was lung cancer (45%). New postoperative motor deficits occurred in 10% of cases and new cranial neuropathies occurred in 10% as well.

SUMMARY

Autopsy studies suggest that skull base metastases are likely underrecognized in patients with cancer. Breast cancers have a particular predilection to skeletal sites and along with lung cancers are the most common histologies that metastasize to the skull base. Patients frequently present with one or a combination of skull base clinical syndromes that manifest as pain or cranial neuropathy. Once a skull base metastasis is suspected, establishing a histologic diagnosis, dedicated imaging, and restaging (if appropriate) are the first steps in management. A multidisciplinary approach should then be used to identify the optimal histology-based treatment strategy, taking into account the burden of systemic disease. Finally, definitive treatment may include one or a combination of surgical management, radiation therapy, or chemotherapy.

DISCLOSURE

The authors have nothing to disclose. The authors received no funding.

REFERENCES

1. Berlinger NT, Koutroupas S, Adams G, et al. Patterns of involvement of the temporal bone in

metastatic and systemic malignancy. Laryngoscope 1980;90(4):619–27.

2. Gloria-Cruz TI, Schachern PA, Paparella MM, et al. Metastases to temporal bones from primary nonsystemic malignant neoplasms. Arch Otolaryngol Head Neck Surg 2000;126(2):209–14.

3. Belal A. Metastatic tumours of the temporal bone A Histopathological Report. J Laryngol Otol 1985; 99(9):839–46.

4. Pan J, Liu AL, Wang ZC. Gamma knife radiosurgery for skull base malignancies. Clin Neurol Neurosurg 2013;115(1):44–8.

5. Greenberg HS, Deck MD, Vikram B, et al. Metastasis to the base of the skull: clinical findings in 43 patients. Neurology 1981;31(5):530–7.

6. Chaichana KL, Flores M, Acharya S, et al. Survival and recurrence for patients undergoing surgery of skull base intracranial metastases. J Neurol Surg B Skull Base 2013;74(4):228–35.

7. Chamoun RB, DeMonte F. Management of skull base metastases. Neurosurg Clin N Am 2011; 22(1):61–6.

8. Ng S, Fomekong F, Delabar V, et al. Current status and treatment modalities in metastases to the pituitary: a systematic review. J Neurooncol 2020; 146(2):219–27.

9. Patel KR, Zheng J, Tabar V, et al. Extended Survival After Surgical Resection for Pituitary Metastases: Clinical Features, Management, and Outcomes of Metastatic Disease to the Sella. Oncologist 2019. https://doi.org/10.1634/theoncologist.2019-0520.

10. Laigle-Donadey F, Taillibert S, Martin-Duverneuil N, et al. Skull-base metastases. J Neurooncol 2005; 75(1):63–9.

11. Hernandez RK, Wade SW, Reich A, et al. Incidence of bone metastases in patients with solid tumors: Analysis of oncology electronic medical records in the United States. BMC Cancer 2018;18(1):1–11.

12. Coleman RE, Rubens RD. The clinical course of bone metastases from breast cancer. Br J Cancer 1987;55(1):61–6.

13. Fornetti J, Welm AL, Stewart SA. Understanding the Bone in Cancer Metastasis. J Bone Miner Res 2018; 33(12):2099–113.

14. Roodman GD. Mechanisms of Bone Metastasis. N Engl J Med 2004;350(16):1655–64.

15. Harrison RA, Nam JY, Weathers SP, et al. 1st edition. Intracranial dural, calvarial, and skull base metastases, vol. 149. New York, NY: Elsevier B.V.; 2018. https://doi.org/10.1016/B978-0-12-811161-1.00014-1.

16. Woo KM, Kim BC, Cho KT, et al. Spontaneous epidural hematoma from skull base metastasis of hepatocellular carcinoma. J Korean Neurosurg Soc 2010;47(6):461–3.

17. Font RL, Ferry AP. Carcinoma metastatic to the eye and orbit III. A clinicopathologic study of 28 cases metastatic to the orbit. Cancer 1976;38(3):1326–35.

18. He W, Chen F, Dalm B, et al. Metastatic involvement of the pituitary gland: a systematic review with pooled individual patient data analysis. Pituitary 2015;18(1):159–68.

19. Capobianco DJ, Brazis PW, Rubino FA, et al. Occipital condyle syndrome. Headache 2002;42(2):142–6.

20. Vikram B, Chu FC. Radiation therapy for metastases to the base of the skull. Radiology 1979;130(2): 465–8.

21. Iwai Y, Yamanaka K. Gamma Knife radiosurgery for skull base metastasis and invasion. Stereotact Funct Neurosurg 1999;72 Suppl 1(2):81–7.

22. Minniti G, Esposito V, Clarke E, et al. Fractionated stereotactic radiosurgery for patients with skull base metastases from systemic cancer involving the anterior visual pathway. Radiat Oncol 2014; 9(1):1–8.

23. White P, Arnold R, Bull J, et al. The use of corticosteroids as adjuvant therapy for painful bone metastases: a large cross-sectional survey of palliative care providers. Am J Hosp Palliat Med 2018;35(1): 151–8.

24. Mercadante S, Villari P, Ferrera P, et al. Optimization of opioid therapy for preventing incident pain associated with bone metastases. J Pain Symptom Manage 2004;28(5):505–10.

25. Porta-Sales J, Garzón-Rodríguez C, Llorens-Torromé S, et al. Evidence on the analgesic role of bisphosphonates and denosumab in the treatment of pain due to bone metastases: A systematic review within the European Association for Palliative Care guidelines project. Palliat Med 2017;31(1):5–25.

26. Chamoun RB, Suki D, Demonte F. Surgical management of cranial base metastases. Neurosurgery 2012;70(4):802–9.

UNITED STATES POSTAL SERVICE®

Statement of Ownership, Management, and Circulation
(All Periodicals Publications Except Requester Publications)

1. Publication Title	2. Publication Number	3. Filing Date
NEUROSURGERY CLINICS OF NORTH AMERICA	010 – 548	9/18/2020

4. Issue Frequency	5. Number of Issues Published Annually	6. Annual Subscription Price
JAN, APR, JUL OCT	4	$434.00

7. Complete Mailing Address of Known Office of Publication *(Not printer) (Street, city, county, state, and ZIP+4®)*

ELSEVIER INC.
230 Park Avenue, Suite 800
New York, NY 10169

Contact Person
Malathi Samayan

Telephone *(Include area code)*
01-44-4299-4507

8. Complete Mailing Address of Headquarters or General Business Office of Publisher *(Not printer)*

ELSEVIER INC.
230 Park Avenue, Suite 800
New York, NY 10169

9. Full Names and Complete Mailing Addresses of Publisher, Editor, and Managing Editor *(Do not leave blank)*

Publisher *(Name and complete mailing address)*

DOLORES MELON, ELSEVIER INC.
1600 JOHN F KENNEDY BLVD. SUITE 1800
PHILADELPHIA, PA 19103-2899

Editor *(Name and complete mailing address)*

STACY EASTMAN, ELSEVIER INC.
1600 JOHN F KENNEDY BLVD. SUITE 1800
PHILADELPHIA, PA 19103-2899

Managing Editor *(Name and complete mailing address)*

PATRICK MANLEY, ELSEVIER INC.
1600 JOHN F KENNEDY BLVD. SUITE 1800
PHILADELPHIA, PA 19103-2899

10. Owner *(Do not leave blank. If the publication is owned by a corporation, give the name and address of the corporation immediately followed by the names and addresses of all stockholders owning or holding 1 percent or more of the total amount of stock. If not owned by a corporation, give the names and addresses of the individual owners. If owned by a partnership or other unincorporated firm, give its name and address as well as those of each individual owner. If the publication is published by a nonprofit organization, give its name and address.)*

Full Name	Complete Mailing Address
WHOLLY OWNED SUBSIDIARY OF REED/ELSEVIER, US HOLDINGS	1600 JOHN F KENNEDY BLVD. SUITE 1800 PHILADELPHIA, PA 19103-2899

11. Known Bondholders, Mortgagees, and Other Security Holders Owning or Holding 1 Percent or More of Total Amount of Bonds, Mortgages, or Other Securities. If none, check box ▶ ☐ None

Full Name	Complete Mailing Address
N/A	

12. Tax Status *(For completion by nonprofit organizations authorized to mail at nonprofit rates) (Check one)*
The purpose, function, and nonprofit status of this organization and the exempt status for federal income tax purposes:
☒ Has Not Changed During Preceding 12 Months
☐ Has Changed During Preceding 12 Months *(Publisher must submit explanation of change with this statement)*

PS Form **3526**, July 2014 *(Page 1 of 4 (see instructions page 4))* PSN: 7530-01-000-9931 PRIVACY NOTICE: See our privacy policy on www.usps.com.

---

13. Publication Title	14. Issue Date for Circulation Data Below
NEUROSURGERY CLINICS OF NORTH AMERICA	JULY 2020

15. Extent and Nature of Circulation			Average No. Copies Each Issue During Preceding 12 Months	No. Copies of Single Issue Published Nearest to Filing Date
a. Total Number of Copies *(Net press run)*			132	121
b. Paid Circulation *(By Mail and Outside the Mail)*	(1)	Mailed Outside-County Paid Subscriptions Stated on PS Form 3541 (Include paid distribution above nominal rate, advertiser's proof copies, and exchange copies)	52	44
	(2)	Mailed In-County Paid Subscriptions Stated on PS Form 3541 (Include paid distribution above nominal rate, advertiser's proof copies, and exchange copies)	0	0
	(3)	Paid Distribution Outside the Mails Including Sales Through Dealers and Carriers, Street Vendors, Counter Sales, and Other Paid Distribution Outside USPS®	47	45
	(4)	Paid Distribution by Other Classes of Mail Through the USPS (e.g., First-Class Mail®)	0	0
c. Total Paid Distribution *(Sum of 15b (1), (2), (3), and (4))* ▶			99	89
d. Free or Nominal Rate Distribution *(By Mail and Outside the Mail)*	(1)	Free or Nominal Rate Outside-County Copies Included on PS Form 3541	17	14
	(2)	Free or Nominal Rate In-County Copies Included on PS Form 3541	0	0
	(3)	Free or Nominal Rate Copies Mailed at Other Classes Through the USPS (e.g., First-Class Mail)	0	0
	(4)	Free or Nominal Rate Distribution Outside the Mail (Carriers or other means)	0	0
e. Total Free or Nominal Rate Distribution *(Sum of 15d (1), (2), (3) and (4))* ▶			17	14
f. Total Distribution *(Sum of 15c and 15e)* ▶			116	103
g. Copies not Distributed *(See Instructions to Publishers #4 (page #3))* ▶			16	18
h. Total *(Sum of 15f and g)* ▶			132	121
i. Percent Paid *(15c divided by 15f times 100)* ▶			85.34%	86.4%

* If you are claiming electronic copies, go to line 16 on page 3. If you are not claiming electronic copies, skip to line 17 on page 3.

16. Electronic Copy Circulation	Average No. Copies Each Issue During Preceding 12 Months	No. Copies of Single Issue Published Nearest to Filing Date
a. Paid Electronic Copies ▶		
b. Total Paid Print Copies (Line 15c) + Paid Electronic Copies (Line 16a) ▶		
c. Total Print Distribution (Line 15f) + Paid Electronic Copies (Line 16a) ▶		
d. Percent Paid (Both Print & Electronic Copies) (16b divided by 16c × 100) ▶		

☐ I certify that 50% of all my distributed copies (electronic and print) are paid above a nominal price.

17. Publication of Statement of Ownership
☒ If the publication is a general publication, publication of this statement is required. Will be printed in the OCTOBER 2020 issue of this publication. ☐ Publication not required.

18. Signature and Title of Editor, Publisher, Business Manager, or Owner

Malathi Samayan   Date 9/18/2020

Malathi Samayan - Distribution Controller

I certify that all information furnished on this form is true and complete. I understand that anyone who furnishes false or misleading information on this form or who omits material or information requested on the form may be subject to criminal sanctions (including fines and imprisonment) and/or civil sanctions (including civil penalties).

PS Form **3526**, July 2014 *(Page 3 of 4)* PRIVACY NOTICE: See our privacy policy on www.usps.com

Moving?

Make sure your subscription moves with you!

To notify us of your new address, find your **Clinics Account Number** (located on your mailing label above your name), and contact customer service at:

Email: journalscustomerservice-usa@elsevier.com

800-654-2452 (subscribers in the U.S. & Canada)
314-447-8871 (subscribers outside of the U.S. & Canada)

Fax number: 314-447-8029

Elsevier Health Sciences Division
Subscription Customer Service
3251 Riverport Lane
Maryland Heights, MO 63043

*To ensure uninterrupted delivery of your subscription, please notify us at least 4 weeks in advance of move.

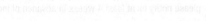